Debating Bioethics

This book studies the critical issues that dominate contemporary discourse on biomedical ethics. It brings together various debates highlighting the historical, philosophical, scientific and technological perspectives involved in modern medicine in different societies, with a focus on contemporary medicine in India. The volume provides a comprehensive look into the origin and evolution of bioethics with an examination of how complex bioethical issues are negotiated in different contexts. The author traces the transition from traditional to modern bioethics and examines important bioethical frameworks to deal with moral dilemmas and challenges. He also contemplates the future of bioethics with an emphasis on regulation in practice to prevent repression and exploitation in medicine.

A comprehensive study of contemporary approaches to bioethics, the book will be indispensable for students, professionals and researchers in public health, ethics, biomedical ethics, medicine, philosophy, sociology, public policy and anthropology.

Sreekumar Nellickappilly is Professor, Department of Humanities and Social Sciences, IIT Madras, India. He works in the areas of hermeneutics, phenomenology and bioethics. He completed his PhD in philosophy from the Central University of Hyderabad after obtaining an MPhil from the same institution. Prior to his appointment in IIT Madras in 2003, he worked as a lecturer in the Department of Humanities and Social Sciences, BITS Pilani, Rajasthan. A recipient of the Fulbright-Nehru Professional Excellence Fellowship (2017–2018), he has published articles in several peer-reviewed journals and has supervised students for PhD in different areas. He has coordinated national and international research projects and is a member of several academic boards and advisory committees. Besides IIT Madras, Nellickappilly has also taught in other institutes, such as NIT Calicut; IIT Palakkad; Syracuse University, USA; National Rail & Transportation Institute, Baroda; and Dr. B.R. Ambedkar School of Economics University, Bengaluru, as visiting faculty.

Debating Bioethics

Sreekumar Nellickappilly

Routledge
Taylor & Francis Group

LONDON AND NEW YORK

First published 2023
by Routledge
4 Park Square, Milton Park, Abingdon, Oxon OX14 4RN

and by Routledge
605 Third Avenue, New York, NY 10158

Routledge is an imprint of the Taylor & Francis Group, an informa business

© 2023 Sreekumar Nellickappilly

The right of Sreekumar Nellickappilly to be identified as author of this work has been asserted in accordance with sections 77 and 78 of the Copyright, Designs and Patents Act 1988.

Trademark notice: Product or corporate names may be trademarks or registered trademarks, and are used only for identification and explanation without intent to infringe.

British Library Cataloguing-in-Publication Data
A catalogue record for this book is available from the British Library

Library of Congress Cataloging-in-Publication Data
Names: Nellickappilly, Sreekumar, author.
Title: Debating bioethics / Sreekumar Nellickappilly.
Description: Abingdon, Oxon; New York: Routledge, 2023. |
Includes bibliographical references and index. |
Identifiers: LCCN 2022021445 | ISBN 9780367145675 (hbk) |
ISBN 9781032320625 (pbk) | ISBN 9781003312697 (ebk)
Subjects: LCSH: Medical ethics. | Bioethics.
Classification: LCC R724 .N437 2023 | DDC 174.2--dc23/eng/20220608
LC record available at https://lccn.loc.gov/2022021445

ISBN: 978-0-367-14567-5 (hbk)
ISBN: 978-1-032-32062-5 (pbk)
ISBN: 978-1-003-31269-7 (ebk)

DOI: 10.4324/9781003312697

Typeset in Sabon
by Deanta Global Publishing Services, Chennai, India

To
MY PARENTS

Contents

Preface

This book attempts to discuss some critical issues and problems that dominate contemporary debates on biomedical ethics. There are several accounts of the discipline of bioethics from various perspectives. This book does not provide a detailed account of the historical evolution of bioethics but highlights some critical milestones. More than tracing the history, it begins with examining the fundamental character of traditional indigenous bioethical concerns in different cultures. It tries to analyze how they fundamentally differ from how modern bioethics deals with various issues and dilemmas. We may find stark differences as well as continuities in this process.

The first chapter provides a broad outline of the discipline of ethics and also of medical ethics. I have discussed some important theoretical frameworks, both from the Western and the Indian perspectives, while introducing the idea of moral deliberations on the various practices that define the field of medicine in different civilizations. Different ethical theories are either directly or indirectly relevant while we deliberate upon the various ethical issues in medicine.

The second chapter problematizes the social context of ancient medicine by examining various indigenous traditions of medicine such as the Indian, Chinese, Hippocratic and Arabic. It also examines the nature and character of moral deliberations present in these ancient healing traditions. Historically, the influence of religious values is visible in many ancient healing traditions, as many healers were also spiritual heads of their community. Most of the ancient healing traditions hardly separated religious morality from medical morality. This chapter further discusses the common features shared by different ancient healing systems across cultures.

The third chapter traces the passage from ancient to modern bioethics, analyzing some significant historical incidents that fostered this passage more rapidly during the 20th century. The biotechnological innovations that changed the face of modern medicine have generated several new moral challenges to practitioners and the general public. Unethical clinical research, such as the Nazi inhuman experiments, the Tuskegee Study of Untreated Syphilis and the Willowbrook State School hepatitis experiments, has forced us to contemplate the place of values in medicine in the changing world. The global initiatives, like the formulation of the Nuremberg codes, become relevant and influenced the momentum of growth of the new orientation in bioethics. The new bioethics has to respond to many emerging challenges concerning clinical research, the domination of corporate interests, changes in family and social values, and the massive growth of technological application in medicine.

The fourth chapter begins with a close examination of the Nuremberg codes and other similar initiatives in formulating clinical research and practice guidelines, such as the Helsinki Declaration and the Belmont Report. All of them respond to some essential contemporary bioethics concerns like individual privacy, confidentiality, vulnerability, patient exploitation, trust, longevity, specific ethical issues related to end-of-life care, palliative care and the idea of death with dignity. Finally, it discusses the emergence of the principlist approach with an analysis of its scope and limits.

A critical feature of modern medicine is its extensive use of modern technology for diagnosis and cure. However, this trend has several serious consequences, as it makes treatment expensive and inaccessible to many people. The fifth chapter discusses such issues by analyzing the impact of technologization in healthcare and the various ethical issues generated in this context. It also focuses on the crucial role healthcare technologies play in controlling different phases of human life from conception, birth, well-being and death.

The next chapter primarily discusses the concepts of death, dying and end-of-life-related issues. Here too, technological interventions are crucial as all such phases associated with death are controlled by modern medical technologies. What often get neglected in such a mechanized medical environment are the interests of the dying patient. This chapter discusses the various ethical aspects related to the employment of modern technologies in addressing death and dying patients. The focus of modern medicine to extend the life of ailing patients, even at the cost of its quality, raises critical questions about what purpose medicine serves in the modern world.

The context of impressive technological growth in medicine poses several questions and anxieties concerning the very future of human societies. New-generation technologies like stem cell therapy, gene therapy and cloning offer remedies to many ailments, although their employment raises unprecedented ethical challenges. However, a closer look suggests that these ethical challenges are not entirely the products of the new technologies but are the inevitable consequences of the ways we have organized our societies. The last chapter addresses this issue, which elaborates on the moral crisis facing modern medicine and discusses its social organization. Some factors relevant here include the fundamental repressive nature of modern medicine, the tendency to prioritize artificial health over natural health, the emergence of individualism and the dominant market-oriented philosophy that treats market demands more important than genuine medical needs.

Modern bioethics owes a lot to the American oncologist Van Rensselaer Potter, who conceived it as a discipline that attempts to reunite ethical values with biological facts to know how to use knowledge for man's survival and good. However, the later developments in bioethics, particularly in the United States, centred around the development of the principlist approach, have oriented towards a more individualistic paradigm. The domination of this paradigm at the global level has generated many new puzzles and dilemmas. This book emphasizes the importance of a comprehensive approach in bioethics, different from the more individualistic approach adopted by the principlist framework. The need for understanding and appreciating the deeper environmental factors and evolutionary aspects related to diseases also points to the importance of a comprehensive approach in bioethics.

Acknowledgements

I wish to thank my institute, IIT Madras, for creating a flourishing environment for me ever since I joined in 2003. In 2017, it granted me a nine-month sabbatical to take up a Fulbright Professional Excellence Fellowship at Syracuse University, New York, during 2017–2018. It was during this time that I started writing this book. I thank the Fulbright Foundation for the support they extended so that I could spend time on this and a couple of other academic projects. I would also like to thank Falk College, Syracuse University, for hosting me and giving me a wonderful ambience for pursuing my work. I wish to thank Professor Sandra Lane and Professor Maureen Thompson, with whom I collaborated, for their valuable help and support.

I thank the Wellcome Trust, UK, for extending sponsorship for a project where I have examined the bioethics beliefs of Indian physicians. This project allowed me to understand some of the crucial historical and philosophical underpinnings in the perception and understanding of ethical principles and concepts, such as individual autonomy, agency, privacy, consent and justice, that bioethicists consider as vital in the contemporary world.

I am grateful to my sister, Dr Sreerekha N., and my students, Shyam Sundar Sridhar, Pritam Majumdar, Praveen Parasar and Ankur Ranjan. They read the early versions of this book carefully and gave their valuable suggestions. All of them took time off from their hectic schedule to fulfil the task I have bestowed upon them.

I would also like to remember my teachers, Professors K.S. Radhakrishnan, R.C. Pradhan, Suresh Chandra (late) and R. Balasubramanian (late) with gratitude. During my graduation days and after, their affection and encouragement gave me the courage to design my projects and believe that they make sense to others.

I thank my friend Professor David Bzdak of Onondaga Community College, Syracuse, with whom I discussed the idea of this book during my stay in Syracuse. Dr Nandini Kumar, former Deputy Director General (Senior Grade) of ICMR and Vice-President of Forum for Ethics Review Committees in India (FERCI), is another friend who owes my gratitude, as she has always been an inspiration and encouragement throughout these years. I wish to thank Professor Alastair Campbell, Visiting Professor in

Medical Ethics and Emeritus Director of Centre for Biomedical Ethics, Yong Loo Lin School of Medicine, National University of Singapore, for his support ever since I started working on issues related to bioethics. I am also grateful to Cecilia Coale Van Hollen, Professor and Head of Studies, Anthropology, Yale-NUS College, Singapore, for her friendship, encouragement and support in several of my academic pursuits.

I wish to acknowledge the friendship and support that my colleagues in the Department of Humanities and Social Sciences, IIT Madras, extended to me. I wish to mention my colleagues, Professor V.R. Muraleedharan and Dr John Bosco Lourdusamy, with whom I have discussed and shared some of the ideas illustrated in this book. Last but not least, I thank all my students with whom I had shared most of the ideas presented here before I started putting them down into one place with the idea of writing a book.

I thank my wife, Maya, and son, Harishankar, for allowing me the solitude to work on this project. My entire family stood with me and extended sincere support in carrying out my research, which culminated in writing this book and a few other articles.

I dedicate this book to my parents. They stood with me all along and taught me the value of family bonding in personal and professional lives.

1 Medical Morality and Medical Ethics

Ethics and Bioethics: An Overview

Bioethics studies questions of right and good concerning human behaviour that impacts different forms of life and the environment. In this sense, it is essential for bioethics to develop a proper understanding of the phenomenon of life by appreciating its diversity, complexity and, above all, essential interconnectedness.

Van Rensselaer Potter (1971), who popularised the term "bioethics" in academic circles during the 1960s, echoed such concerns when he commenced his project of developing the new discipline with an assumption that human ethics cannot be separated from a realistic understanding of ecology in the broadest sense and that ethical values cannot be separated from biological facts (vii). Potter's understanding of the term, as it is evident, relates to this original meaning in a broad sense. He conceives bioethics as a science of survival which embodies the essential wisdom that "provides the knowledge of how to use knowledge" for man's survival and good (1). This science of survival, according to him, is a very broad domain of human knowledge, as it is built on the science of biology and includes the essential elements of the humanities and social sciences, with an emphasis on philosophy conceived in its most original sense as the "love of wisdom." Bioethics, as envisaged by Potter, combined the two important ingredients of biological knowledge and human values that were needed in achieving the new wisdom he was talking about (2).

However, the term "bioethics" is widely used with a different connotation today. Bioethics, in principle, encompasses a wide range of concerns and can potentially address problems that emanate from several complex situations humans encounter individually as well as collectively. Phenomena like the climate crisis and ecological collapse have already begun to make drastic alterations in human life and humans cannot ignore their collective responsibility in such eventualities. It is clear that humanity is facing some momentous challenges in its long history of existence as a species as well as a member of the animate world. Our response to these challenges is further crippled by a profound moral crisis facing humankind accompanied

DOI: 10.4324/9781003312697-1

by the loss of purpose and reference points that make everyday life a painful persecution. Friedrich Nietzsche (2006) aptly captured the philosophical kernel of this moral crisis with his idea of the "death of god." Although the emergence of the industrialized modern world brought material progress, it ultimately compelled the forfeiture of the idea of a meaningful life as it expedited the fragmentation of society into different autonomous functional units, societal and individual fragmentation, which had severe repercussions on social life. The diminishing influence of religious and metaphysical ideals subverted the undifferentiated unity that characterized human societies. Societal modernization eventuated the ultimate fragmentation of society into different relatively autonomous units. This fragmentation was not confined to the separation of the state from the church. The age had witnessed the emergence of several relatively independent functional spheres in the society which distanced themselves from the demands of the moral community. The loss of a common purpose was evident and this promulgated moral nihilism. Of course, such developments have not remained exclusive to the Western world. The spread of industrialized modernity to other parts of the world due to historical and economic factors made the moral crisis a universal phenomenon.

In other words, the current moral crisis is caused by the fragmentation of human reality, and the solution to the crisis lies in reestablishing that unity. Fritz Jahr (2010), who initially coined the term "bioethics" in a paper published in 1927, attempted to develop a global bioethics that integrates ideas from different cultures. Potter, as we have seen above, envisioned it as a new discipline with a strong foundation in biological sciences that aims to bridge the gap between the two cultures of sciences and the humanities. Over time, the focus of the discipline was narrowed down in order to more directly address moral issues in the domain of life.

Ethics as a branch of philosophy has, from its very beginning, endeavoured to study morality in relation to both the ends of human life and the means to attain those ends (Skutch 2007, xiii). Hence, the primary concern of ethics is to critically study morality, a term which comes from the Latin word *mos*, meaning custom. Morality consists of specific rules, principles and practices that aim at establishing harmony between individuals in society and between humans and their environment as well (xiii). Different societies have adopted different measures and practices in order to ensure social harmony, which over a while has given shape to a set of moral ideals they consider as constituting the foundations. Morality is a product of the social, economic and cultural factors that shape society. Religious traditions, customs, conventions and several ritualistic practices reflect the spirit of these moral foundations. Of course, ethical deliberations need not necessarily reiterate the validity of those morals. Instead, by reformulating them in the light of contemporary realities and political sensibilities, they are critically appropriated by the current ethical environment. For example, most ancient moral frameworks assume a patriarchal social order that finds stern protestations from the modern democratic ecosystem, even as modern philosophers look back to ancient philosophy for answers to the problems of modernity.

It is important in this context to reiterate the essential differences between ethics and morality. Morals or morality stand for those assumptions and practices that guide or determine human behaviour in a society. Every society may have a set of such guiding moral principles. These principles are further subjected to change over time. Several factors influence such changes as all significant aspects of the social, political and cultural realities are intimately linked with the moral environment. On the other hand, ethics is a philosophical enterprise that addresses morality and moral judgements from a rational perspective. In other words, it involves reflection and is a rational endeavour. Hence, though every society indeed has morals, not every society has developed ethical reflections.

However, many civilizations have formulated very advanced theories of ethics and have deliberated upon significant moral challenges that human societies have encountered in their historical existence. In the ancient Greek world, Socrates constantly debated the question of justice in order to seek clarity on the concepts and principles people employ in moral debates. Similarly, the Indian epics of *Ramayana* and *Mahabharata* contain elaborate discussions of such ethical conundrums. Some such challenges are general and ask questions such as: Why is honesty important? Why should one be moral? What is the importance of integrity? Many others have to bear upon specific situations such as the conflicts of interest an administrator or a ruler faced in their respective career domain. They ask questions like: Whether tradesmen should spend a portion of their earnings for charity? What are the moral responsibilities of a soldier? We could broadly classify these concerns under two types of ethics: general ethics and applied or practical ethics. Bioethics is an example of the latter.

Different Paradigms and Diverse Moral Frameworks

While ethics, in general, deals with the question of right and wrong actions, there is significant disagreement between different ethicists on the criteria that distinguish right action from wrong, or good from evil. The German philosopher Immanuel Kant emphasized duty and universalizability, whereas the utilitarian philosopher J.S. Mill treated only those actions that brought forth maximum utility to a maximum number of people as ethically right. Meanwhile, Aristotle, whose writings laid the very foundations of ethics as a discipline, conceived cultivation of good character as forming the very crux of ethics. These differences are fundamental as they point to the criteria which each framework has upheld as determining the characteristic features that distinguish right from wrong.

Again, different periods in human history have shaped the moral sentiments of that age differently. Post-Vedic India's ethical debates have arguably surrounded the idea of *dharma*. We find mention of this concept in philosophical texts across traditions, social and political treatises such as the *Arthasastra* of Kautilya, the *Dharmasasthras*, the *Smritis* of Manu, Yajnavalkya, Parashara and Narada, and various literary and poetic works like the *puranas* and *ithihasas*. Ancient Indians encountered the question of *dharma* both as a paramount philosophical idea and a guiding moral ideal. The philosophical traditions in India, despite their differences on metaphysical and epistemological points of view, broadly agree upon the centrality of this moral notion. The only exception is the *Lokayata* school of thought which advocates materialism.

Such differences of moral sentiments in accordance with changing historical eras are more visible in Europe, which has undergone drastic social, cultural, economic and political upheavals in its eventful history during the past two millennia. While the idea of the good was determined through politics in the city-state (or *polis*) in ancient Greece, the historical developments of the Age of Enlightenment during the 17th and 18th centuries in Europe fundamentally altered social, political and economic relations in the continent and reconstituted the moral frameworks of modernity. Several other developments like the two world wars, the growing democratic predicament, the Cold War that continued till late 1980s, the peculiar features of the new world order that emerged after the dissolution of the Soviet Union, the emergence of the internet and the cyberworld, the increasing globalization facilitated by several international treaties, the emergences of new political alliances at the international level and many more such economic and political movements and initiatives at the international level have all in some way contributed in the formation and reformulation of several moral ideas and ideals.

Unlike ancient days where a single moral precept governed the conduct of everyone in a society—like the idea of virtue in ancient Greece and *dharma* in ancient India—the contemporary democratic environment permits individuals to hold on to different ideologies, value systems and paradigms. On the one hand, this may result in a constant modification and reformulation of values by everyone as we tend to learn from others. But more often, the value diversity creates confusion and conflicts, as there is no universal agreement on any criterion that distinguishes the right from the wrong. However, it is incontestable that there are some actions, which most people with democratic predicament may reasonably consider as wrong. Child abuse, sexual harassment and racial discrimination fall into this category. Here too, the meanings of the terms "abuse" and "harassment" may differ from culture to culture. Conversely, there are certain kinds of actions, which most people reasonably believe to be laudable.

However, despite such differences, people of different value environments can communicate and establish different types of relationships with each other with reasonable success. The world today is primarily shaped by some economic and political considerations, and they necessitate a world order that links people faster and closer. Such phenomena may stimulate and enthuse people from different value environments to learn from each other and slowly cultivate a moral order with more and more common considerations and interests. This scenario may eventually shrink the gap between different value environments and ultimately promote better mutual understanding and cooperation.

We may wonder whether it is the property of the action itself or our attitude towards it or our reasons for acting in a particular way that makes it morally objectionable or praiseworthy. Ethics, as a discipline, tries to primarily respond to such queries along with a set of other issues we may encounter in our social life. It discusses what we do when we identify actions as right or wrong. Often, we find people claiming that they "feel" a certain kind of action is right or wrong. Here it is unclear what makes the action right or wrong, as there is hardly anything other than the feeling that guides us in evaluating the moral quality of an action. The fact that feelings can be highly subjective prevents us from forming judgements based on them that have any social value. It is almost irrefutable that morality is beyond personal feelings and feelings themselves are the product of a conceptual horizon that emanates from the social interactions of a moral community. This moral community is a complex formation that integrates historically evolved ideas about what society treats as right and wrong. Such ideas nevertheless are highly fluid and contain within them diverse perspectives—religious, scientific, economic and political—and consequently, do not exhibit any homogeneity. Ethics as a discipline needs to be aware of this complexity and the fundamentally historical nature of moral ideas and their fluid character. Not only moral ideas but also the laws that regulate human behaviour in a society are the products of such complex social and cultural horizons. Hence, there is an intimate link between ethics and law, though there are also fundamental differences between their nature, import and function in the society.

The traditional definition of ethics as a "normative science of the conduct of human beings living in societies" (Lillie 1957, 2) is not entirely irrelevant today, though we prefer to have a broader understanding of the discipline emphasizing other aspects like its social function. Besides, it is also liberated from its Aristotelian conceptual environment, which keeps the habitual disposition of a virtuous character—the idea of conduct—at the centre of ethical explorations. Today we stress more on ideas such as "reasonableness" and fairness and realize them as part of our various endeavours in bringing about social harmony and peaceful coexistence. Ethics thus deals with reasonable and fair standards of human behaviour that instruct us about the kinds of human behaviour we need to refrain from and those that we need to adopt and emulate. For instance, ethics supplies us with reasons for why we must value compassion and honesty or why we must respect human rights and individual autonomy. We thus have to know the importance of those values we need to follow in order to make social life harmonious and meaningful and direct social progress in the right direction.

Understanding Moral Deliberations

Several factors prevent us from comprehending the nature of moral deliberations, both when we attempt to grasp it historically and when we analyze the contemporary moral judgements of people from different walks of life. Among the numerous factors that determine the fundamental nature of our moral judgements, the historical and cultural rootedness of moral concepts is an important one. Moral assumptions may also overlap with the sentiments that stem from religious, scientific and the other social institutions that shape human life. Finally, the philosophical deliberations that emerge historically reflecting the moral conventions and the nature of moral evaluations play a crucial role in determining the ways people make moral judgements. Since the meanings of the terms we employ in moral deliberations may vary according to time and place, it is crucial to situate these concepts in their historical contexts for arriving at a proper understanding of their conceptual import.

We can understand this better by examining any moral precept that was accorded paramount importance in some period of history. The term *dharma*, as used by ancient Indians as a fundamental moral dictum, is a classic example. We find the term in the *Upanishads* (1000–500 BCE), reflecting the Vedic notion of *rta*, which stands for a very general idea that encompasses the harmonious coexistence of the animate and the inanimate entities of the whole universe. For the Vedic people, *rta* stands for the cosmic and moral order and is considered to be the very principle that upholds life in the world. During the post-Vedic era, more specific interpretations of *dharma* became relevant. With the constitution of a more complex social order, it became associated with the different functional units in the society, each characterized by a set of obligations. Such obligations stem from the individuals' *varna*, which is understood in two different ways. On the one hand, it is defined in terms of a person's aptitudes and corresponding capabilities. Here the individual's social obligations are determined in terms of such capabilities he/she possesses by virtue of his/her inherent nature and inclinations. On the other hand, when the term *varna* is understood as a synonym for caste, it is determined hereditarily. This was largely the case in the post-Vedic society in India. Indian society is stratified in terms of several castes and sub-castes *for several centuries. Dharma then* became the caste duty of each individual, which not only determines the role each individual plays in the society but also decides the latter's social status. Kautilya's *Arthasasthra* (Kangle 2010), one of the prominent post-Vedic orthodox Hindu texts that belonged to the *Smriti* tradition, identifies specific *dharmas* (*vishesha dharmas*) for the four castes of *Brahmins, Kshatriyas, Vaisyas* and *Sudras*, along with ascribing a unique set of duties to the householder, the students of the *Vedas*, the forest-anchorite and the wandering ascetic, etc. (1.3.5 to 1.3.12). In addition to such specific obligations, Kautilya also refers to a set of ordinary duties, which are called the *samanya dharmas*, such as non-violence, truthfulness, uprightness, freedom from malice, compassion and forbearance (1.3.13).

What is characteristic of the post-Vedic concept of *dharma* is its identification with caste duties. Each person's obligations to others and to the society are determined by such caste duties. Any violation of this was ethically and legally wrong. During this period, we find a visible shift in emphasis from the moral and philosophical approaches to a more social and political outlook, both in elucidation and application of the concept of *dharma*. While the Vedic and the Upanishadic conceptions primarily treat *dharma* as a universal cosmic principle that harmonizes everything in the universe, the post-Vedic cosmology accentuates more on the social and political aspects and is preoccupied with the project of establishing harmony in the social world. Even when it was philosophically conceived as the most intricate and incomprehensible concept, social and political life was strictly ordered with its dictates, and the prevalence of *dharma* in the society was primarily ensured by austerely mandating the nature of the interrelationship between different castes and their mutual obligations.

Dharma thus remained as a residual notion within the Indian culture for a long time. Even those heterodox traditions like Buddhism and Jainism did not deviate from its broad framework while they deliberated upon morals. However, the meaning of the concept was different for them as they stressed more on the notion of non-violence. Almost all moral deliberations and discussions ultimately centred on the idea of *dharma*. It was only in the rebuttal by the nihilist *Charvakins* that we find an indictment of the concept of *dharma* in the Indian tradition. Nevertheless, here also *dharma* has not been uprooted from its moral pedestal; rather, the *Charvakins* deplored the entire discourse on morality as meaningless.

If *dharma* is a unique moral precept of the ancient Indians, virtue constituted a central ethical principle for the ancient Greeks. As indicated above, participation in the *polis* was central to shaping the Greek moral ideas. As Alasdair MacIntyre (1998) suggests, moral concepts are embodied in and are partially constitutive of forms of social life (1). MacIntyre further points out how the concept of justice is understood and analyzed differently by different philosophers like Plato, Hobbes and Bentham in different ages in the history of moral philosophy (1). This is in line with the differing interpretations of *dharma* by the different philosophical traditions and schools in India. Due to such differences, the understanding of moral concepts is difficult today. We need to understand each word in the context of the social life where it finds its historical origin and grasp the rules that governed the language used in that original context since different forms of social life will provide different roles for concepts to play (1).

All these suggest how heavily the moral sensibilities of people depend on their historical, political and economic conditions. This factor may seem to support the argument that favour moral or cultural relativism, which states that different cultures uphold different ethical frameworks that may or may not correlate with other frameworks, and there are no culture-neutral parameters with which we may decide among them. As MacIntyre himself points out, though moral practices and the content of moral judgements may vary from society to society and from person to person, and hence what is held to be right or good is not always the same, roughly the same concepts of right and good are universal (1). People across cultures and civilizations hold certain practices as good and right in contrast to certain other practices that are evil and wrong and form moral evaluations based on such assessments. They come to conclusions about the quality of being morally good or evil, employing a particular process of evaluation that is based on certain assumptions. Such assumptions are obviously determined by historical factors, and different cultures entertained moral rules with contents different from each other.

However, only the contents differ from each other; the very idea of some actions being right or wrong/good or evil does not. Hence, some like Jonathan Haidt and Craig Joseph (2007) have endeavoured to identify some common foundations of intuitive ethics that, according to them, may function as building blocks from which cultures create moralities. They identified five such foundations: harm/care, fairness/reciprocity, in-group/loyalty, authority/respect and purity/sanctity (16). The harm/care foundation responds to the fact that mammals, by definition, face the need to care for vulnerable offspring, which is central to evolutionary success. The fairness/reciprocity foundation reflects the emotions that have evolved that help social organisms reap the gains of reciprocal altruism with non-kin or distant kin. The in-group/loyalty foundation organizes phenomena related to the well-studied human tendency to aggregate into tribes, gangs and teams based on some similarities and competes with other tribes, gangs and teams. The authority/respect foundation responds to the patterns of dominance and submission across species and across cultures that suggest how such hierarchies are formed based on the principle of the subordinates showing respect to the authority of the superior in return to the protection they receive from them. The fifth foundation, purity/sanctity, responds to the adaptive challenge that is nutritive, which human beings encounter owing to their omnivorous food strategy combined with their relatively large group sizes. Humans have always been exposed to very high levels of threat from bacteria and parasites, which spread by physical contact, and this demanded a strict food evaluation and rejection system that has been adapted for social evaluation and rejection (17–18).

We may be able to add more to this list of foundations, and it is a fact that we continuously modify our moral rules and perspectives. As mentioned above, religious and philosophical influences may actively shape our moral rules. In some ancient traditions, moral texts appeared as law books that claimed divine authority, while in other texts, especially those from India,

China and Greece, the emphasis was on the idea of the habitual formation of virtues and the idealizing of exemplary characters employing the personification of such virtues. The depiction of Rama, the protagonist in the principal epic *Ramayana* (Rao 2004), as the embodiment of righteousness, where he is an equable person with truthfulness as his valour, announces the unique manner in which morality was understood in terms of virtues and their personification. Different characters in the epics personify the various virtues like valour, truthfulness, righteousness, integrity, compassion and respect. The ancient Greeks endorsed a similar approach to moral deliberations right from the Homeric days, and the eudaimonic and virtue ethics that followed became prominent in the thoughts of Socrates, Plato and Aristotle. It was only during the Enlightenment era that moral deliberations became a matter of rational reflections predominantly. John Locke (2010) in the 17th century contemplated the centrality of freedom, which became a defining feature of man. Locke imagines about a state of nature where all men are naturally in and contends that a state of perfect freedom to order their actions, and dispose of their possessions and persons, as they think fit, within the bounds of the law of nature, without asking leave or depending upon the will of any other man. He then argues that this state of nature has a law of nature to govern it, which is reason. This reason, according to Locke, teaches all mankind that no man ought to harm another in his life, health, liberty or possessions, as they are all equals (114).

The overlapping of religious sentiments with moral deliberations and the crucial features both endeavours share often make it difficult for us to delineate one from the other. The morals held by many societies often reflect religious feelings and ideas. Ethics is primarily concerned with the questions of good and right. There is also a strong feeling for the prosperity of others. These concerns intersect with the predominant religious interests that are preoccupied with the questions of good and evil. However, many religions in the world link such questions with certain metaphysical eventualities or with the divine will. Being good is to follow an order that has been established by the divine will, and quite often what is good itself is decided by the divine will. Even in those religions that do not explicitly endorse any divine will—like Buddhism—the idea of an esoteric moral order is predominantly present. In all such cases, the motivation for being good is ascribed to factors that are beyond human creation or control. Hence, the scope of human will is limited, though it is not absent. The moral will here is expected to deliver the divine will. Morality, on the other hand, may value freedom of will and presume humans to enjoy a great deal of control over what they do.

Historically, many factors have obscured the boundaries between faith-based value judgements and moral evaluations. The virtue-based moral evaluations of ancient societies were in harmony with the sentiments of religious morality that prevailed in those societies. For instance, in the ancient Greek and Indian societies, people valued some virtues and considered those people in which such virtues personify with high esteem. The wisdom and valour of various mythical characters find mention with high esteem in both Greek and Indian epics. However, with the development of modern ethical frameworks since the 17th century in Europe, the bifurcation became more pronounced. The modern and later the Enlightenment Age ethical systems developed a new set of vocabularies in order to articulate their ideas and perspectives concerning the right and the good, which radically separated them from the religious vocabularies. They brought to the forefront the moral significance of some ideas that was never recognized before. The Enlightenment era treated them as preeminent. For example, the concept of autonomy became a central notion in ethical deliberations since Immanuel Kant's and J.S. Mill's ethical theories. After that, the autonomous individual has become the epicentre of moral evaluations, and this has contributed heavily in shaping the nature of modern-day ethical deliberations and reflections in many parts of the world.

With more such ideas taking centre stage, the modern-day ethical systems gradually developed a set of distinct vocabularies employing which moral evaluations are carried out, while significantly minimizing the role of cultural and civilizational differences in the process. Though there exists hardly any universal moral frameworks, this broad set of vocabularies is capable of capturing several moral concerns that are raised by people across cultures in diverse situations. Despite differences in the moral acceptability of certain practices, everyone is fairly aware of the reasons for such disagreements and often can remain nonpartisan to other perspectives. The growing democratic sentiments and scientific temperament have induced momentous alterations to most of our conventional values. Such new scenarios generate serious clashes between the old and new paradigms. Notwithstanding such undesirable occurrences, modern democracies flourished with the installation and advocacy of constitutional ethics, which reiterated the Enlightenment values. Modern societies also recapitulate the importance of the rule of law. This scenario has contributed heavily to furthering egalitarian values and spreading a democratic culture in society.

With the spread of democracy and its values to many cultures that remained traditional until recently, the clashes between social morality and constitutional ethical codes have started to occur more frequently. Such clashes and the ongoing negotiations between incompatible moral frameworks are part of the increasing democratization process many cultures witness today. Often constitutional ethics is enforced as law, and this often obscures the nature of moral evaluation as it traverses with law. For the common man, ethical reasoning closely resembles legal reasoning. Laws may mainly reflect moral assumptions and convictions, which often function as their basis. For instance, the law against drug abuse is reinforced by strong moral sentiments. Both are to a great extent products of reflections that have been shaped by historical factors and both are deeply concerned with the questions of right and good. Different people endorse different moral norms as well as espouse different legal systems. Nevertheless, in reality, they are two different exercises. People internalize morals by virtue of their membership in a social or cultural organization either by birth or by choice. However, the legal system that regulates their conduct sometimes embraces them externally. For example, someone who changes his citizenship to a different state after that has to endorse the legitimacy of the legal system that prevails in his new domicile. Morals cease to change even after this new association, as people who change their citizenship may not substantially distance from the value system that shapes their lives. However, they may keep persuading each other and often may change following the impelling demands of the one over the other. The changing moral evaluations about the rights of the LGBT community in many societies are an example. Again, while the modern democratic values are implemented in many societies, they are reasonably appropriated to the cultural conditions of that community.

Morality, therefore, has some deeper concerns, as it is grounded on the fundamental values that not only define the significance of our lives but also determine our destiny. Our morals reflect some of our most fundamental worries concerning our lives; our ideas about the meaning, purpose and destiny of human life; our relationship with others; our understanding of our commitments and obligations, etc. However, these concerns can never be easily captured into any single theoretical framework and hence are often not rationally justifiable. Many laws reflect strong moral sentiments.

However, not all laws may find such strong moral foundations. Moreover, we keep evaluating and revising our laws. Modern democracies make amendments to their constitution following the changes that happen in society. Such revisions and amendments are to be primarily from a pedestal external to law and hence should be fundamentally from a moral perspective. As Edward Major points (2012) out, without an independent moral review, we lose much of our impetus to change law and correct imbalances (62). The *Medical Ethics Manual* (2005) brought out by the World Health Organization notes that quite often, ethics prescribes higher standards of behaviour than does the law, and occasionally ethics requires that physicians disobey laws that demand unethical behaviour. It further adds that, while laws differ significantly from one country to another, ethics is applicable across national boundaries.

Today the language of morals is often obscured by certain vital factors that shape our social relationships and political dynamics. In Europe, ever since societal modernization began during and after the Enlightenment, the role of moral values and the nature of their regulative power have begun to dwindle. Societal modernization happened with the emergence of different and relatively autonomous functional spheres, with no single all-encompassing moral fabric to establish their intimate links. Society fails to effectively communicate its fundamental moral anxieties directly to these autonomous and fragmented social units. It does it with the formulation of various laws, which vaguely reflect the moral concerns but nevertheless characteristically differ from the latter, as they scarcely presuppose any intimate link between the fragmented functional spheres (Pratley 1997, 30–33).

The Process of Moral Decision-Making and the Theories of Ethics

The process of moral decision-making is a complicated exercise, as individuals try to justify or provide reasons why do they think a particular course of action is the right or appropriate one instead of other available options. They often do it by taking resort to the various theoretical frameworks, such as deontologism, utilitarianism, virtue ethics, rights ethics and relativism. These theoretical frameworks supply them the necessarily required platform where they can ground their moral arguments. For instance, one may justify the need for mandatory vaccination from the perspective of an argument that supports the idea of the common good. However, one may oppose it emphasizing individual freedom and rights. It is often difficult to adjudicate between such opposing value frameworks. However, a multiplicity of value perspectives does exist in a democracy, and one needs to resolve such conflicts every time they occur with persistent negotiation and patient dialogue.

As it is clear from the above discussions, the process of moral decision-making was relatively a straightforward exercise in ancient societies, where the moral consciousness of people was not so diversified and complex. Many societies had a dominant religious outlook that determined their moral values. Mythology and literature influenced moral perspectives, conventions and ethical evaluations, and customs played essential roles. The Homeric epics in the Greek world and the *Ramayana* and *Mahabharata* in Indian cultures are examples. Although today the influence of religions is not to be denounced thoroughly, their all-encompassing authority is not as extensive and comprehensive as it was earlier. In the day-to-day affairs, ordinary morals in society foster usual ethical deliberations without much difficulty. A critical feature of modern societies is the presence of various professional institutions and organizations. They primarily comprise the economic system and also influence the social structure in crucial ways. People have to continually negotiate their lives with varied interests of these institutions and organizations. For instance, our modern healthcare establishment is a complex network of several institutions such as hospitals, laboratories, diagnostic centres, pharmaceutical firms, manufacturers of technological equipment and dealers. Individuals have to negotiate with each one of them when they fall sick.

Ethical issues surface more in such relationships where institutions and organizations are involved. As Dennis F. Thompson (2005) observes, the institutionalization of the professions in recent years is the result of a social trend commencing with a shift from "social trustee professionalism" to "expert professionalism." Here the focus is more on ethical issues salient in institutions than in relations among individuals or in structures or states. What is characteristic of this phenomenon is the

> traditional ideal in which professionals alone or in small groups serve their patients and clients in accord with a public-spirited goal has moved more toward practices in which professionals serve in organizations that value mainly their expertise and expect them to act in accord with the organization's goals.
>
> (267)

Thompson adds that the market often determines those goals, and economic pressures are an important part of the trend.

Negotiating ethical issues therefore requires serious attention, and any decision made should be justifiable. On many occasions, an ethical problem presents in the form of a dilemma, which will have more than one alternate choice. To choose the morally right alternative is a task that requires theoretical, technical and practical knowledge. However, this is not always part of the professional education curriculum, and the relative ignorance and indifference to many such issues may create difficulties in professional life. While the practical knowledge and skills can be acquired with experience and technical knowledge is gained as part of professional education, the theoretical knowledge about ethics is one aspect that is completely neglected. Four primary concerns become relevant in this context. The first concern, metaethics, is one needs to know what aspects would properly describe the nature of moral reasoning. The second concern, normative ethics, ventures to devise moral norms or standards that regulate the right conduct. The third concern, moral psychology, deals with the psychological aspects of ethical reasoning, and the fourth concern, applied ethics, deals with practical issues. The first two and the last one are even treated as the essential branches of ethics, as moral psychology is a different category of concern altogether. Ethics as a discipline is conventionally understood to be embracing these three branches.

Metaethics deals with the description of the nature of moral reasoning that distinguishes it from other modes of reasoning, such as logical, scientific, mathematical, aesthetic and even legal. It explores whether ethical judgements are true or false or whether they are just expressions of our emotions and desires. In continuation of this basic query, it examines whether moral truths are absolute or relative. Normative ethics analyzes the meaning of ethical terms such as good, right, fair, obligation, etc. It examines what makes an action morally acceptable and tries to devise rules and principles in determining it. The third branch of ethics is applied ethics, which deals with the application of moral ideas and theories in our day-to-day lives. This practical aspect of ethics has been gaining importance since the second half of the past century, and now we find several such approaches prevailing in the academic circles, each of them dealing with the practical application of ethics. Each functional sphere in society raises unique and serious ethical issues. For instance, general moral arguments are insufficient to address the unique moral dilemmas we confront in the domains of law, business, healthcare and so on. Again, within the sphere of the corporate world, professionals of different departments like manufacturing, software, robotics, automation, etc. encounter distinct moral issues. The typical ethical issues originating from each domain demand unique approaches in understanding their specific nature and character. So we may device appropriate strategies and policies to tackle them.

Theories of Ethics

Absolutism, Subjectivism and Relativism

Plato documented one of the oldest philosophical debates concerning the question of justice in his *Republic* (in Warmington and Rouse 1984), where the philosopher Socrates encountered the Sophists. The latter famously declared that the individual man was the measure of all things and affirmed that might could be equated with right. Socrates found these assumptions fundamentally problematic, and in a series of arguments, he established that these could not be the case. Through Socrates, Plato was trying to ascertain the fact that, despite the apparent differences in its application, moral ideas have absolute universal validity. Plato's theory of ideas facilitates this, as he considered moral ideas to be transcendental and transcultural. They are valid for all times for all people. Ethical absolutism demands that norms are valid absolutely; for all people, all times.

While Plato's theory provided the philosophical justification for moral absolutism, the Abrahamic tradition asserted its religious sanctity. The Ten Commandments prohibited all men from certain acts, which were proclaimed to be absolutely wrong. There are many others who can be classified as absolutists in ethics, such as Immanuel Kant. They all proposed ethical theories that identified a criterion of evaluation that was both ahistorical and objective. Consequently, they formulated ethical ideas that have universal validity. Thus, they proposed ethical precepts that would enable us to decide whether an act would be right or wrong under all circumstances. For example, moral absolutists would argue that acts like killing, promise-breaking and lying were morally wrong under all circumstances, even in cases where such acts may prevent extreme disasters. This complete disregard for the consequences and other circumstantial elements of the act makes moral absolutism problematic. Thus, it goes too far in one direction and seems to neglect the disaster cases (Shafer-Landau 2013, 437).

The idea of relativism is often projected as an alternate theory to absolutism. However, moral relativism is not an antithesis to moral absolutism. In a broad sense, ethical relativists are also cultural relativists, as they content that it is differences in culture that result in holding to different ethical principles.

The "Kishkindha Kanda" of the *Ramayana* narrates a conversation between Bali, the valiant Vanara king, and Rama, who shot him from a hide. The wounded Bali fell and accuses Rama of violating the moral law, *dharma*. Rama informs Bali that he has not done anything wrong, as being a Kshatriya and a member of the Ikshvaku clan and also a subject of Bharata, the king, it is his duty to protect *dharma* and ensure that this eternal moral law is not violated. By laying his hands on his younger brother's wife, Bali has violated the moral law, which insists that one should consider one's younger brother as his son and his wife as a daughter-in-law. However, the substance of Bali's accusation, which preceded this reply, was that a different set of laws ruled his clan (the Vanaras). Bali was alluding to a form of relativism, and hence what is *dharma* for Rama need not necessarily be so for Bali. Rama assumed that *dharma* is universally valid, and hence its violation, wherever it has happened, needed to be confronted. While Bali seems to be referring to a moral relativist outlook, Rama holds firmly to an absolutist moral standpoint.

The position of moral relativism can be brought out more accurately with an examination of the nihilistic and individualistic stance adopted by the Sophists of ancient Greece. The Sophists condemned the possibility of any rational moral ideas and advocated moral relativism and nihilism and opposed all forms of absolutism and foundationalism. In the absence of any universal position in morality, all positions become equally valid. The aim was to denounce the universal validity of any moral ideas. To substantiate this outlook, Protagoras advocated the idea of *dissoi logoi* or different words. This view proclaims that every issue has two opposite sides to it and could be seen from two different perspectives. Protagoras deplored the possibility of any transcendental reality that decided the values of human life and disapproved of the validity of any absolutely and universally correct moral positions or criterion independent of the individual who acts and takes decisions. The Sophists, in general, alluded to the general nature of moral values and laws and considered them to be the creation of the weak, who constitute the majority, in order to restrain the strong who are a minority. Hence, for them, moral values were non-natural, and what was naturally right was what was right to the stronger. It was against this relativism and nihilism, particularly the moral position that equated might with the right, that Socrates lashed out his attacks.

Etymologically, the Greek word *ethos* and the Latin word *mores* mean customs. The link between morality and customs is not confined to the word's etymological roots. Customs play a very crucial role in facilitating harmony in society by regulating human behaviour. Some customs are observed by society for an extended period, and they eventually become the standard of behaviour or even law that cannot be violated. For instance, uncle-niece marriages are prevalent among some communities in Asia,

Africa, the Middle East and some parts of Europe. Such consanguineous marriages are quite common in the states of Tamil Nadu and Andhra. Among some communities, the nieces marry only their maternal uncles, and in some other communities, they marry both maternal and paternal uncles. However, in some other parts of the world, such marriages are not customary, and in many places, they are legally and ethically forbidden. Is there anything fundamentally wrong with such marriages? What makes consanguineous marriages acceptable or forbidden are not any factual or scientific aspects or features, but customs. They become valid because they constitute the "acceptable ways of doing things" by people in a particular society, owing to historical reasons and conditions such as geographical, climatic, economic and political. In this sense, they are contingent and conditional and are sometimes subject to changes. Until more demanding historical factors challenge them, they remain valid and acquire the status of the moral law.

Many of our morals are indeed the products of our customs that are contingent upon historical factors. Customs are different for different people and societies, and hence morals too are different. This makes different people subscribe to and follow different values and viewpoints. Since people evaluate things and events in the light of their values and viewpoints, they may arrive at different judgements. Hence, one may conclude that peoples' evaluations are bound to be relative to their value systems that can ultimately be traced to their culture. Notwithstanding its binding nature, our relative value systems are not rigid. They are products of historical factors and may change in response to their interactions with other value systems. While living in a multicultural society, we engage with other people from different cultural backdrops, and the increasingly globalized world also brings people from different cultures together to work and live together. Despite such fusions that happen between value systems, the differences and incommensurability between them may generate serious problems. There is no final solution to them as it is impossible to situate moral judgements on any ahistorical pedestal that is neutral to any cultural influences. Hence, moral judgements are different. They lack any claim to truth; they are relative to people, culture and society. They also change from time to time as new factors keep influencing people.

Can we conclude from these contentions that ethical judgements lack any universal validity, and they are valid only locally? Since *ethos* and *mores* can claim only local validity, can we conclude that ethics and morality too can claim only local validity? Ethical relativism affirms so and denies the possibility of any moral value that has absolute validity. It confines their validity to the historical, social and cultural horizon of the individual. Consanguineous marriages are, therefore, neither right nor wrong in the absolute sense. They are right in certain societies where they form part of the social ethos of such places. The numerous cultural practices that prevail in different human societies have always been a matter of wonder and astonishment to others and often attract extensive critic.sm from them. For example, male circumcision is widely practised among Jews and Muslims all over the world, despite its opposition from human rights activists. While the believers find it as an essential religious prerequisite, such a practice is criticized for the violation of child rights it involves. Some studies have also stressed its therapeutic benefits. However, the fact that they are performed on individuals who are unable to make informed decisions make them objectionable from a secular ethical perspective. Even more controversial is the practice of female circumcision or female genital mutilation, which has no medical benefit and is also harmful, but is common among certain groups of people in some parts of Africa, Asia and the Middle East, and this is treated as a clear violation of human rights and is illegal in all democratic countries in the world. Again, among the Danis, who constitute one of the many ethnic groups in Papua, which is an Indonesian province, the death of a relative is considered to be a matter of great grief, which is expressed by the female members amputating their finger joints!

One important feature of all such controversial practices is their disapproval outside the community where they are performed either as a religious predicament or as a cultural practice. Their validity is local, and for the groups of people who practise them, they are "right," and any failure in practising them is viewed as "unholy" or "wrong." The conflicting perspectives on such practices may generate huge moral confusions and anxieties. The solution to this problem seems to be lying in finding out a universal value framework, which enables us to adjudicate between various conflicting perspectives. However, the relativists deny the availability of such a framework. For them, there are no ultimate moral truths and facts.

Opposing such a conclusion, those who argue for the universal validity of moral truths venture to situate them in some ahistorical and transcendental platform. There are various types of moral absolutism such as Platonic idealism, Aquinas's "natural law theory," Kant's deontologism and Bentham's utilitarianism. They all endeavour to identify some criterion that everyone could accept when they make moral evaluations. Plato is arguably the complete moral absolutist, as he placed the moral ideas in the transcendental world of abstract realities, where the ideas exist as essences, untouched and untainted by the objects of the physical, sensual world. The two Enlightenment moral frameworks of deontologism and utilitarianism, despite their fundamentally different perspectives on the question of the good, attempt to identify the ahistorical criterion that makes human actions good and right; for the former, it was the universal reason and for the latter, pleasure (Hayry 2005).

Strict moral absolutism has not many takers in the contemporary world, though many do not find it appropriate to argue for an absolute relativist and nihilist position of morality. On the other hand, the claims of relativism are not altogether discarded. One reason for this relative sympathy for a broad relativism is its openness and inclusiveness perspective towards different approaches and frameworks. A relativist would view all perspectives as equally valid and therefore does not treat any single framework as more valid. In this sense, it is more progressive. However, many ethicists hold that it is also essential to recognize some moral principles as valid for everyone. There seems to be an impasse, which needs to be overcome.

Historically, ethical relativism has been a product of cultural relativism, arguing that moral codes and customs are products of culture. With the disenchantment around post-Enlightenment scientism, there has been a corresponding rejection of the model of knowledge that became prominent during the Enlightenment, with its emphasis on empirical observation and laboratory investigations. Sociologists and anthropologists have proposed a broader approach to knowledge and truth with a greater emphasis on lived experiences, social constructivism and cultural diversity. These are the foundations of ethical relativism.

Many view an extreme version of cultural relativism as a danger to humanity, as it hinders us from criticizing certain practices, rituals and policies of governments. For instance, if cultural relativism were true, then we may not be able to critically evaluate practices like female genital mutilation, caste system, gender discrimination, etc. We may then have to adopt a morally neutral standpoint towards oppressive religious practices prevalent in some societies and allow all practices that claim the legitimacy of custom and tradition. This, however, is against the spirit of the egalitarian and emancipatory political ideologies that constitute the foundation of our democratic predicament.

James and Stuart Rachels (2012) bring out a number of things implied by cultural relativism (19–20). If we take this position seriously, they argue, then we may not be able to consider others' views as inferior to us, and subsequently, we may not be able to criticize their views. It also makes us blind to our pitfalls and casts doubt on the very idea of moral progress. We thus lose the weapon to oppose objectionable practices that happen in other societies, such as the political oppression in China. We may also fail to see the evils of our practices like the caste system, which then deprives us of the opportunity of learning from others and improving our presumptions and evaluations. Finally, cultural relativism forbids us from making moral progress, whereby we replace the old ways with new ones that are better than the former. However, if cultural relativism were true, then we may not arrive at such assumptions, as there is no transcultural criterion that enables us to judge that the present is better than the past, which is the case. James and Stuart Rachels affirm that we should not overestimate the extent to which cultures differ. They affirm that there exists no difference between the value systems of two different cultures. They differ only in their belief systems. They try to demonstrate that "there are some moral rules that all societies must embrace because those rules are necessary for society to exist," such as the rules against lying and murder, which exist in all cultures (21, 23–24).

Cultural relativism as an ethical principle opposes absolutism and objectivism, which argue that the moral criterion of evaluations lies outside all conceptual schemes and frames of references. They refuse to accept the ahistorical and transcendental status of moral criteria. However, when relativism itself becomes an absolute theoretical position, it becomes problematic. It is essential to acknowledge the existence of differences and diverse perspectives on moral issues. Once we privilege any one of the frameworks, we tend to ignore the plurality of cultural and customary outlooks that enable us to shape our moral perspectives. Cultural relativism helps us to perceive different viewpoints and approaches with tolerance and change our perspective to make it fit more appropriately to existing situations. To acknowledge the importance of relativism helps us to come out of our prejudices and belief that our perspective is right and true. We would slowly tend to accept that other viewpoints might also be authentic and valid. It brings us to the realization that many of our beliefs, which we treat as absolutely valid, are only valid relatively, as they are the products of our historically evolved customs and conventions.

The denial of objectivism of values may stem from either a sceptic or a subjectivist. Even nihilists too oppose an objective or absolutist moral framework. However, the nihilist's position is different from the other two as she treats all morality as hollow. While neither the sceptic nor the subjectivist conclusively denies the existence of moral truth, the nihilist denies it completely. The subjectivist denies its objective status and situates it in her subjective universe. The sceptic, on the other hand, does not raise any doubts about the possibility of having moral truths, but she merely says that to discern it is impossible. Moral nihilism throws the very idea of moral truth out of the window.

Moral nihilism has two prominent strands: first, the error theory of J.L. Mackie, which argues that all value judgements are systematically false as they do not refer to any objective values, since such values do not exist; and second, the expressivism of A.J. Ayer, which argues that value judgements are neither true nor false, since they do not refer to anything in the world. According to Ayer, actual ethical judgements do not belong to any branch of philosophy or science (Ayer 1971, 105).

The three important ethical theories that still find references in the evaluations of ethicists are virtue ethics, deontologism and ethical consequentialism, which is also known as ethical hedonism. However, none of these three theories constitute a single unified framework. The approach of virtue ethics is derived from the Aristotelian framework, which can more specifically be treated as a form of eudaimonism. Among eudaimonists, there are different philosophers like Socrates and Epicurus, who ultimately argued for fundamentally different things. Again, ethical hedonism is a broad school of thought, which has egoists like Ayn Rand and utilitarians like J.S. Mill. Then there is deontologism, which emphasizes duty. Here also the approaches vary among diverse practitioners. There are divine command theorists who emphasize God's commands as forming the basis of duties; contractarians consider the idea of contracts between human beings as the basis; libertarians underscore rights; and Immanuel Kant underlines the idea of good will.

Eudaimonic Ethics and Virtue Theory

Eudaimonia does not have a directly corresponding word in English, but its pretty near translation is "flourishing," "happiness," or "good life." It is the goal one has to pursue and achieve by realizing a happy life as this is equated with a good life. Hence, goodness's intrinsic relationship with happiness or flourishing is affirmed upfront. More precisely, it emphasizes the agent's happiness or good, and in this sense, it is a form of egoism. However, the proponents of eudaimonism in the Greek world were not egoistic hedonists in the ordinary sense of the term. Again, although different thinkers who are eudaimonists differ among themselves in their respective theoretical positions, they all share some common features such as the emphasis on the agent's well-being, raising the question what sort of life is best and what sort of life constitutes "happiness" (Sharples 2003, 83) and finally, placing the notion of virtue at the centre of their ethical theory.

Virtue in Greek is *aretê*, which means excellence, and it is understood as a settled disposition to act in a certain way. The Greeks considered wisdom, courage, temperance and justice as cardinal virtues, and all of them become virtues when they are found in people as settled dispositions. A courageous man is courageous on all occasions, and we do not find him contrary to that on any occasion. Hence, a virtuous character is essential for the realization of eudaimonia.

The spirit of eudaimonism was prevalent in the ancient Greek world much before and after the philosophers like Socrates, Plato and Aristotle. These three philosophers represent significant phases in the development of this perspective, with Aristotle's theory of ethics outlined in the *Nicomachean Ethics*, being the most elaborate one. The Greek world was familiar with moral debates through the works of Athenian tragic dramatists and historians who discussed moral and political questions in detail. Although earlier philosophers like Pythagoras have deliberated upon the notion of virtue as a moral concept, Socrates is hailed as the first moralist in the Western world (Irwin 2007, 13). Socrates's treatment of moral concepts and inquiry into the nature of moral knowledge was thoroughly unconventional. Instead of developing a scholarship on moral knowledge, he preferred to engage in conversations with fellow human beings, including both lay and learned men. Such collective endeavours hardly concluded with any final definition of the subject matter.

Socrates's encounters with the Sophists paved the way to the development of his moral theory. The Sophists largely held a relativist or subjectivist moral perspective, and considered moral claims as fundamentally hollow and lacking any substance. Sophists advocated the famous doctrine, "man is the measure of all things." This *homo-mensura* canon is originally attributed to Protagoras, a disciple of Democritus, who was arguably the most famous among the Sophists in ancient Greece. Protagoras's perspectivism ultimately saw morality as lacking any substance and truth, as all truth about it are reducible to mere conventions. Since the question of good is dissolved with the extreme perspectivism that made all knowledge a matter of perception and hence subjective and relative, morality too is relative, and the prevailing moral norms in a society are nothing more than conventions. Since such conventional moral norms cannot uphold any objective moral ideas, they have no claim to truth. Each individual, therefore, has to pursue her self-interest by negotiating with these conventions.

Socrates opposed this perspectivism and conventionalism, and demonstrated that morality was not merely conventional. He believed that there is an inherent connection between morality and truth. Ethical knowledge is knowledge about the ultimate good, and this can be known through the employment of the right method. Socrates alluded to the notion of virtues and affirmed that knowledge of virtues was also knowledge of the good and morally right. Such knowledge has inculcated in us what was good for us so that we could venture to realize it in our life. This is to realize our own good and well-being. This well-being of the individual is known as eudaimonia. We read in Plato's *Apology* the following passage, where Socrates summarized his philosophical and ethical positions.

> For I do nothing but go about persuading you all, old and young alike, not to take thought for your persons or your properties, but first and chiefly to care about the greatest improvement of the soul. I tell you that virtue is not given by money, but that from virtue comes money and every other good of man, public as well as private. This is my teaching, and if this is the doctrine which corrupts the youth, I am a mischievous person. But if any one says that this is not my teaching, he is speaking an untruth.
>
> (Plato 2018, 15)

Virtue is the only thing that is good, and everything becomes good when flowing from virtue. Courage is good only when it is present in a virtuous person. Similarly, wisdom and moderation are good only when they are found in a virtuous person. In such people, they become a learned disposition that defines their character. The life of a virtuous person realizes what is good and hence also happiness. The happiness of such a person is not merely sensual pleasures, which are conditional and momentary, but is unconditional and everlasting.

Aristotle's theory is very close to this Socratic-Platonic view but also differs from it in significant ways. Aristotle examines the nature of many ethical concepts like virtue and happiness in detail and develops a complete system of moral and political philosophy that supplements his metaphysical and epistemological endeavours. According to him, eudaimonia is the highest good for man, and it is with such an idea of the good he is interested in. Aristotle's ethical theory advocates a form of naturalism, as he considers the highest good for man is realized in the gratification of human nature, which, in turn, is defined in terms of the rational aspect of the soul. Human beings alone have the rational faculty, in addition to the nutritive, loco-motive and perceptual faculties that other animals too possess. He holds that virtues like wisdom, courage, etc. are displayed in action. However, they become virtues only when they emanate from someone habitually and consistently and are guided by right reason (Aristotle 1893, 79). Aristotle's ethics emphasizes a lot on the character of individuals. Aristotle affirms that a habit or trained faculty that is praiseworthy is what we call excellence or virtue (33).

Character refers to the totality of an individual's character traits. They become virtuous when they are admirable. A virtuous person consistently and without exception exhibits admirable character traits. Aristotle argues that emotions and appetites do not rule a virtuous person. On the other hand, he follows the dictates of reason. He is neither influenced by the emo-tional aspects of his soul nor is apprehensive of the consequences of his actions. Aristotle asserts that man's function is to exercise his vital faculties both in obedience to reason and with reason (16). Another important aspect of Aristotle's ethical theory is the avoidance of the extreme and the adoption of the mean. Every virtue is, therefore, a golden mean, which is rational. Virtue, he adds, is a kind of moderation inasmuch as it aims at the mean or moderate amount (46).

While other moral theories focus either on duty or on consequences, virtue ethics emphasizes character. One important aspect of Aristotle's moral theory is its identification of goodness not necessarily in good acts but also in the person's learned and habitual dispositions. Hence, we find goodness in the virtuous individual's character. As Joe Sachs (2019) puts it, an action counts as virtuous when and only when one holds oneself in a stable equilibrium of the soul, in order to choose the action knowingly and for its own sake. Sachs concludes that this stable equilibrium of the soul is what we mean by having character and character, in turn, gives a moral equilibrium to a life.

All eudaimonist thinkers have alluded to "happiness" as the goal of human life, though, for different thinkers, the nature of this happiness and the means to attain it were different. Hence, in a broad sense, all eudaimon-ist ethical theories aim to secure the agent's well-being. However, this self-referential aspect of eudaimonism does not make all eudaimonists egoistic hedonists. It is evident that Socrates, Plato and Aristotle are not oriented towards self-interest.

However, not all eudaimonists in the Greek tradition considered happi-ness or eudaimonia as these three great thinkers. Some of them like Epicurus have treated pleasure as the goal of life, where a happy life consists in hav-ing a surplus of pleasure over pain, both physical and psychological. Hence, for achieving this goal, Epicurus proposes to pursue pleasure and eliminate pains that hinder this undertaking. According to him, the fear of death and punishments for the deeds of this life after death is the primary cause of anxiety, which humans need to overcome with a clear knowledge about the real nature of the self. Being a disciple of Democritus, Epicurus held an atomist conception of reality and maintained that even the human soul is atomic and hence does not exist after death. Thus, Epicurus urges his followers to enjoy the pleasures in life by indulging in activities that keep the surplus of pleasure, although he was against pursuing pleasure without self-control and restraint. The possibility of pain resulting from such ventures should be avoided. Sharples (2003) makes the following observation about Epicurean approach towards pleasure.

> Bodily pleasures are fundamental for Epicurus, it seems, not in the sense that we should pursue them indiscriminately, but in that freedom from anxiety or ataraxia, itself a pleasure in the mind, is ultimately freedom from anxiety about physical pain—in the form of punishments in the afterlife, for example.
>
> (90)

Sharples adds that Epicureans will never shy off from enjoying life, as it is the only opportunity for enjoyment we have, although they do not pursue pleasure indiscriminately and do it cautiously (98).

Though examples for eudaimonist and virtue ethics approaches discussed here are chosen from the European tradition and particularly the Greek tradition, there are moral frameworks that are akin to them in other civilizations as well. For instance, the Chinese tradition and Indian tradition were largely eudaimonist in nature and spirit. Confucius in China raises questions similar to those that were raised by Socrates and even Aristotle. For Confucius, the question was, "where is the *dao* or way of being a human" and this query is similar to Aristotle's questions about the character and eudaimonia. As Jiyuan Yu (2005) observes, "[J]ust as Greek ethicists are all concerned with eudaimonia, Chinese philosophical schools in the classical period (which roughly corresponds to the flourishing period of Greek philosophy) offer competing accounts of what *dao* is" (179).

The traditional Indian philosophy in general was eudaimonist in nature, with very few exceptions like the *Lokayatha* school. Both the orthodox and heterodox systems of thought have propounded some idea of spiritual emancipation: *Nirvana* for *Buddhism*, *Moksha* for *Advaita*, *Kaivalya* for *Sankhya*, etc. They all conceive such a concept of emancipation as the ultimate goal and good, which consists in the realization of the human self. Parallel to the notion of virtue in the west, ancient Indian ethics projected the notion of *dharma*. Similar to Aristotle's ethics that had the virtuous individual at the centre, who possessed excellence in character, the

Bhagavad Gita had projected the *yogi*, who excels in his field of activity. Such excellence, according to the *Gita*, is the result of virtuous character traits of the *yogi*.

The eudaimonist framework and virtue ethics that stress more on the character of individuals become gradually less significant. With the emergence of Enlightenment philosophical and ethical theories, rational theories that underscore the rights of the individual became predominant. However, the strands of egoism and hedonism that had originated during the Greek era continued to exert influence even in the contemporary age.

Consequentialist Theories: Ethical Egoism and Utilitarianism

Unlike the eudaimonist ethical theories and approaches, egoism as an ethical theory focuses exclusively on the agent's well-being and maximizing her self-interest. Some varieties of this normative egoism presuppose a psychological theory that affirms that each individual has her welfare as the ultimate goal. Psychological egoism is, therefore, a descriptive theory about general human behaviour, which argues that each individual ultimately aims at her own welfare. On the other hand, normative egoism is an ethical theoretical position, which claims, "each person ought to seek her own welfare." Psychological egoism is a theory about all human beings and all human actions. It not only affirms the universal egoistic intention behind every human action but also asserts that altruistic actions are not possible. James and Stuart Rachels (2012) summarize this distinction by arguing that while psychological egoism makes a claim about human nature, or about the way things are, ethical egoism makes a claim about morality, or about the way things should be (66).

An event happened that in the life of Abraham Lincoln, the former president of the United States, is often cited to bring out some psychological aspects involved in the ethical decision-making process. Lincoln once stopped his carriage to save a sow and its piglets from drowning. Later he remarked that he should have had no peace of mind all day had he let them drown. Lincoln himself argued that saving the piglets was a selfish act as he did it for himself (for his peace of mind). The essence of the story suggests that all acts, including those which are altruistic, are in substance rooted in selfishness and self-interest. Lincoln's act is an egoistic act that aims at the agent's welfare (in this context, mental peace).

However, this psychological thesis sounds problematic. Though many of our actions endeavour to safeguard our own interests, not all actions are oriented towards selfish goals. It is not that we are exclusively concerned only about us, and as James and Stuart Rachels argue, common sense might tell us to balance our own interests against the interests of others (65). They further try to demonstrate some fundamental flaws in the theoretical position of psychological egoism, which affirms that all examples of altruistic actions could be seen as fundamentally stemming from self-centred motives.

They find two fundamental flaws in the argument, which asserts that when people indulge in altruistic actions, they are actually doing what they want to do, and hence they do not deserve any praise. The first flaw in this argument, according to them, is that there are things that we do, not because we want to, but because we feel that we ought to. We may want to do the contrary, but as a matter of conscience, we do the right course of action. The second flaw consists in confusing between what is the desire and the content of the desire. We may have a desire and act on it, but if our action aims at the happiness of others and not just of ourselves, then the acts are not based on self-interest (68).

Ethical egoism, as mentioned earlier, states that every man ought to seek his own pleasure. However, this need not necessarily stop an individual from helping other people. Nevertheless, the chief intention should be self-interest, and when this self-interest coincides with others' interests, it never stops from being altruistic. But genuine altruism is not ethically warranted (68). The basic rule of an ethical egoist is that each individual should care for her own welfare and if everyone does it, then that may result in the total improvement of the society. The Russian-born American novelist and philosopher Ayn Rand (1964), who proposed a radical form of rational self-interest, popularized this ethical position. The idea of rational selfishness, according to Rand, refers to the values required for man's survival qua man, i.e., values required for human survival. She says that she uses the word "selfishness" in its real sense, where it means "concern with one's own interests." She argues that nature does not provide man with an automatic form of survival, and man has to support his own life with his efforts, and hence, it is important to be oriented towards self-interest (6). She criticizes the ethics of altruism because it considers self-interest as evil. Rand's objectivist ethics maintains that the actor must always be the beneficiary of his action and that man must act for his own rational self-interest (7). Ethical egoism vehemently opposes altruism, which emphasizes that ethics must be essentially other-regarding, by reminding us that we need to value the individual and that altruism, which urges us to sacrifice the individual for the sake of others, fails to do so.

Contrary to ethical egoism, utilitarianism is an other-regarding theory that has numerous applications in the various efforts we take in making ethical decisions in our personal and professional lives. The famous statement, "maximum happiness to the maximum number of people," is associated with utilitarianism. Though the emphasis is on utility, the proponents of this stream of thought equate utility with happiness. Hence, utilitarianism, like ethical egoism, alludes to human happiness or pleasure in a significant way. The difference between them is that, while the latter is too narrowly agent-centric, the former affirms that the consequences in terms of the benefits of the utility should reach the maximum number of people. Unlike many other systems of ethics, notably eudaimonism and deontologism, utilitarianism emphasizes the consequences of an action. Hence, actions themselves do not have any moral worth. They become morally good or bad by their utility or usefulness as a means to some end.

As stated above, utilitarianism equates utility with pleasure and considers the latter as intrinsically valuable. Every other thing, which we consider as good, is so in terms of their contribution to producing pleasure. Jeremy Bentham (2000), the English utilitarian philosopher and social reformer, observes:

> Nature has placed mankind under the governance of two sovereign masters, pain, and pleasure. It is for them alone to point out what we ought to do, as well as to determine what we shall do.
>
> (14)

Therefore, utilitarianism suggests how men ought to act and what men ought to desire by presenting pleasantness as the only quality because of which an experience is good or valuable (Lillie 1957, 184). Since the stress is on maximum happiness, utilitarianism affirms that, among the various courses of action available, the morally right action produces the greatest net happiness for all concerned. Hence, as a moral theory, utilitarianism not only is explicitly other-regarding but it also envisages to produce a better world where a large number of people are happy by alluding to produce maximum happiness to a maximum number of people. The maximalist criterion of utilitarianism makes it an excellent social theory that can potentially influence policymaking in society.

By making pleasure intrinsically good, Bentham even constructs a pleasure calculus by suggesting the factors such as certainty, propinquity, fecundity, purity and extent, which have to be taken into account while considering the moral worth of actions. He thought this would make moral evaluations more objective. Bentham's theory is known as "act utilitarianism," as it focuses on the acts performed by individuals while making moral evaluations. However, Bentham's focus on acts became problematic since it never differentiated between different kinds of pleasures. Some kinds of pleasure are qualitatively superior to others. John Stuart Mill proposes his "rule utilitarianism" in order to overcome such issues with an emphasis on the consequences of rules on the basis of which they were performed instead of acts. His framework proposes to differentiate between different types of pleasure produced by focusing on whether they conform to justified moral rules or not. It examines whether a particular action is right or wrong in terms of certain rules the society would hold after reaching an agreement about whether adopting a rule would lead to good or evil consequences in society.

The utilitarian approach is widely adopted in many fields in framing policies and making decisions. It aims at the greater good of the society by promoting maximum utility of maximum number of people. It also offers an objective method in evaluating the moral worthiness of actions. However, while making moral decisions, in order to evaluate the utility/pleasure that results from the performance of actions, utilitarians make a cost-benefit analysis, which may often quantify the various factors. For example, a chemical factory has to make an important decision about whether to continue operations or to close down, as there are several complaints about pollution. In order to make a decision, the utilitarians may compare the cost required for treatment and death and medical insurances for the people who are affected by pollution with the investment required for the implementation of measures to prevent pollution. If the cost of the pollution control is higher than the other alternative, then the rational conclusion for the utilitarian is to maintain the status quo and meet the expenses for the health and death insurance of the people affected. This may invite criticism as the utilitarian may have to face the accusation of being insensitive to the life and health of human beings and their anxieties. Again, its extreme focus on consequences may have total disregard for the motives and intentions behind actions and may sometimes go against our common moral beliefs.

Deontologism

In a broad sense, deontological ethical theories emphasize on duty. The term *deon* in Greek means duty. The basic questions they address are "What is duty?" and "How do we ascertain our duty?" The answer to the first question is straightforward: "what is the right thing to do" is one's duty. To the second question, there are different answers possible, such as "what human reason warrants," "what is in accordance to the custom," "what is suggested by one's conscience," "what is prescribed in the scriptures or revealed by God" and so on. Immanuel Kant, to whom the deontological perspective is often attributed, subscribes to the first alternative.

Kant alludes to the universal moral law, to which any rational person has to be obedient. The idea of good is intrinsically related to this notion of the moral law. Every rational person has to oblige to this law, and she ought to do so while she makes choices and performs actions. The only moral consideration in making decisions is that her choice is what the moral law authorizes. The "good will," which occupies a central place in Kant's ethical theory, is the will to act in accordance with the moral law, which is one's duty. Good will, which is the only thing that is unconditionally good, is the constant motivation to do one's duty for its own sake, and its only motive is to do its duty for the sake of doing it. All other things which we consider as good, such as health, wealth and intellect, are good only insofar as they are used well. Kant (2018) asserts the unconditional nature of the good will to reiterate the non-consequential and non-teleological character of what is morally right. He observes:

> [I]f with its greatest effort the good will should still achieve nothing, and there should remain only the good will, then, like a jewel, it would still

shine by its own light, as a thing which has its whole value in itself. Its usefulness or fruitfulness can neither add nor take away anything from this value.

(Kant 2018, 8)

At the outset Kant announces that good will's only motive is to do its duty for the sake of doing duty. This implies four important things. First, Kant disapproved duty done with any interests other than the motive to do duty, which is a rational urge. Second, according to Kant, "to do the right" is important than realizing the desired consequence, even if it is the good of the entire humankind. Hence in one sense, what is "right" is more important than what is "good" (Alexander and Moore). Third, some people have a natural inclination to perform dutiful actions. However, Kant does not consider them as morally right, as they are not done "for the sake of duty." Fourth, Kant considers moral principles and laws as categorical imperatives and emphasizes their essential obligatory nature. The moral law, according to him, has an unconditional authority, and he disapproves of any external authority—even of God—as commanding it. On the other hand, it should be a command that comes from within, from one's reason, which is universal. It is enforced as a matter of rational compulsion.

Kant maintains that all human actions are based on some principle. However, not all our principles are rational and hence cannot be treated as a criterion to decide moral accuracy. "The Golden Rule," which is found in the New Testament, is a deontological principle and is often used as a criterion. It urges to "do unto others as you would have them do unto you." Kant's categorical imperative reflects this Golden Rule and he formulates it and proposes it also a test for the principle upon which one should base one's actions. He affirms that one must "act only in accordance with that maxim through which you can at the same time will that it become a universal law" (Kant 1997, 4.421). This according to him is the single categorical imperative.

As indicated above, the deontological theory has various other forms, and Kantian theory is arguably one that reflects the spirit of the Enlightenment thought the most. The ancient moral theories of many other societies are essentially deontological, as many of them emphasize the notion of duty. The question "what is duty" resembles the question "what is *dharma*," which we find was repeatedly raised in the ancient Indian scenario. *Dharma* is said to be the principle that supports life in the world, and its moral precursor is the Vedic concept of *rta*, which refers to the cosmic and moral order the universe exhibits. The reference is to the notion of "absolute order."

Other Theories

There are several other important theoretical approaches, particularly those that have originated during the modern period, which are still relevant in many fields. In the 16th and 17th centuries, many European countries witnessed several cultural, social, political and economic changes alongside the revolutionary changes in science. The unprecedented growth of trade and the emerging individualist spirit in the society due to the collapse of traditional social structures following the downfall of the feudal society had crucial moral implications.

The social contract theory, which is primarily a political theory that legitimizes the authority of the sovereign, proposes a moral outlook that announces that all morality is conventional. Hobbes proposes a primarily mechanistic theory of human nature, which argues that human actions can be explained in terms of universal laws of nature. The motives that are behind the choices we make are the products of internal bio-mechanical processes, and it is hard to find any room for anything that is absolutely and objectively good or evil. On the other hand, good and evil depend on the individual and her appetites and desires. Moreover, since the life of each man is fundamentally "solitary, poor, nasty, brutish and short," the idea of absolute goodness is impossible to find in human nature.

Hobbes refers to a "natural state" of man, which is a state of private judgement, as each man will search only for the satisfaction of his desires. Hence, in the natural state, there is no morality, no government, no social order and no civilization or culture. It will be a state of perpetual war, and continual fear, and people have strong reasons to avoid it. This reason will fundamentally legitimize an external public authority to which everyone will submit and ensure mutual cooperation. In the state of nature, everyone has absolute freedom. However, reason suggests that this idea of absolute freedom serves no one's interests, and for the best interest of all, it is good to renounce it. This is done with the enforcement of contracts, where everyone's rights are limited. Reason suggests that it is beneficial to collectively and reciprocally renounce these rights to establish a civil society. The contracts ensure that if we restrain our rights, others will also do so, and if others violate the contract, we are not obliged to pursue peace. The Hobbesian framework, therefore, asserts the purely conventional nature of all morality and law.

Jean-Jacques Rousseau proposes a social contract theory, which is significantly different from Hobbes's. According to him, the state of nature was not a state of disorder and war but a state where men were free. It is the civil state and the laws that people created eventually enslaved them. The state of nature was a state where people pursued peace and happiness without indulging in conflicts and competition for private possessions. In opposition to Hobbes, Rousseau argued that human natural impulses are not exclusively rooted in self-interest. In the state of natural and simple living, humans were endowed with moral purity, which was lost with the advancement of society. When human societies became complex, contracts became necessary for the establishment of order. Complex social organizations could function only with the establishment of private property, which replaced the state of nature where everyone was equal. The social contracts were created and governments were established in order to prevent the conflicts that may surface under such circumstances. They protect the right to private property, but they also proliferate inequalities and injustice.

Rousseau urges man to pursue the path of reason by applying it for the regulation of his conduct. He alludes to the notion of conscience, which obliges us to pursue the path of justice. Conscience is the voice of duty, which urges man to overcome his physical impulses that are self-indulging and rise to the level of a rational and intelligent human being from the state of a mere stupid and unimaginative animal.

Despite such crucial differences, the moral position of social contract theory ultimately states that morality is essential for enabling social organization. Fundamentally what constitutes moral rules is nothing but conventions, as nature is amoral. These moral rules are dictated by reason, as it is rationally clear that human beings benefit from following them. Morality benefits everyone. In other words, morality consists of a set of conventional rules that is obligatory to everyone since following them would benefit everyone.

Political ideologies like Marxism and Gandhian approaches propose strong moral positions. Marx addresses a moral problem concerning human alienation and realizes that the fundamental cause of this is the exploitative social structure. He problematizes it in the context of a capitalist economic system, which, according to him, alienates the working class from both their labour and each other. Production, according to him, is a distinctively human activity, and it is manifested through human labour. The end result of every labour process is an object which the labourer produces, which has already existed in the imagination, and in the process of production, she brings it out through her labour. By bringing this out, she realizes a purpose, and hence the product which she brings out from her imagination through her labour is her own essence. However, Marx complains that in the exploitative capitalist environment, the labourer has no right over it as it does not belong to her because she has already sold out her labour, which is responsible for its creation. The labourer does it for money, and hence money is the alienated essence of human labour and life. The more humans worship money, the more they lose their freedom and get alienated. Marx's solution for the abolition of alienation, therefore, consists in the abolition of money and also private property! The ultimate solution for the problem consists of the reconstitution of production relations in society and the establishment of a political and social order that propagate socialism. In general, Marxian scholars address the professional scenarios that involve social and ethical worries, which ultimately result in alienation.

The Gandhian ethical approach is rooted in the ideals of non-violence or *ahimsa*, and he considered the human journey as a voyage to be concluded in the realization of truth. Both Marxian and Gandhian approaches have rich insights in framing a non-capitalist moral outlook in the contemporary world, as they both fundamentally denounce free market system, private property and capitalist model of development. Gandhi particularly emphasizes on the idea of self-rule or *swaraj*, which for him was not merely a political idea but a very comprehensive ideal that touches upon all aspects of human life. They both can serve the ventures that attempt to develop a non-exploitative and non-market-oriented health policy in the contemporary world.

Ethical Theories and Decision-Making

Our day-to-day moral decision-making happens more or less unreflectively, and the lay public is hardly aware of the moral theories. Nevertheless, quite often, we do appreciate a good "character," take into account of "consequences" of our actions, and also may try to base our actions on what is rationally compelling for us to do. However, in the context of professional life, we need to be more careful and should take into account different aspects involved while we make a decision. The decisions made by a physician may have significant impacts on the life of her patients, and in this sense, she is "responsible" for what she does. She should be able to "justify" the choices she makes to the entire world, and on such occasions, she may refer either to consequence or to duty.

Though from the outset, it appears that these two ethical theories of utilitarianism and deontology adopt conflicting criteria for making ethical judgements—consequences and duty, respectively—in actual life situations, professionals may combine them as they may have to make decisions at various levels, with varied complexities. It is a matter of personal choice, whether an individual should give more importance to consequences or to duty. But when the individual has to make a professional decision, the matter has to go beyond her personal choices. She may have to examine both aspects, depending on the situation.

For example, when a doctor decides to administer a particular therapy to her patient, she has to take into account whether it is going to benefit the patients significantly and whether the risk taken is reasonable. Here the focus is on consequences. Although the final decision to be taken lies with the patients, it is crucial how the doctor presents the scenario to them. Here the doctor's personal moral preferences may play an important role. The ethical way out in such situations is to follow the basic principles, particularly the principle of nonmaleficence or the do–no-harm principle.

In day-to-day life, we recurrently come across ethical quandaries and negotiate with different scenarios and situations. The layman is hardly aware of the diverse theories, and they subsequently make their decisions sound and reasonable, citing various justifications. However, the professional needs to be more precise and avoid contradictions. They should possess better clarity about the moral position they adopt while attempting to negotiate the complex scenario constituting professional decision-making.

Such scenarios may involve several stakeholders and may give rise to severe disagreements and conflicts of interest. At least a broad awareness about the various theoretical approaches may help the professionals to arrive at a better decision.

The Science of Medicine and Ethics

Though Van Rensselaer Potter first used the word "bioethics" in 1970, physicians, philosophers and religious scholars debated the ethical aspects related to the practice of medicine since antiquity. The codes of Charaka and Susruta were popular among Indian physicians since the 3rd century BCE. These ancient physicians contemplated several other aspects of medical morality in their texts and even gave more importance to such aspects other than those of medicine. Similar debates could be found in Chinese and Arabic civilizations as well. The underlying paradigm of Chinese medical ethics of the ancient days was a Confucian ideology, and it also derived values from Taoism and Buddhism. The 7th-century text, *On the Absolute Sincerity of Great Physicians*, written by the Taoist physician and alchemist Sun Szu-miao (581–682 CE), reflects these insights. Besides "compassion" (*tz'u*) and "humaneness" (*len*), Sun Szu-miao highlighted values like care for the patients, self-discipline, nonmaleficence, abstaining from material goods, killing, desire for fame, etc. Sun Szu-miao also insists that physicians should exert equal treatment to all patients, rich and poor. The Arab physician Ishaq bin Ali al-Rohawi's book on biomedical ethics, composed in the 9th century AD is the first concise document on the subject in the Arabic language. The oath for physicians composed by the 3rd-century BCE Greek physician Hippocrates is another example of ancient medical ethics. The principles of beneficence and nonmaleficence are the two important values, besides many other values like compassion, care, integrity, etc., which Hippocrates had highlighted in his work.

Despite their diverse cultural affiliations, the moral values endorsed by all these ancient systems have certain things in common. They all highlight certain general and fundamental human values, which reflect the religious sentiments of their times. Along with abstinence from greed and lust, they all allude to the importance of altruism. For all of them, the physician was a moral exemplar. However, such an image of medical practice underwent drastic changes during the Middle Ages. Magner and Kim (2017) make the following observation.

> The transition from Greco-Roman culture to medieval Christianity transformed the status of the healing art. The Hippocratic tradition based on the love of the art, intellectual curiosity, glorification of the human body, and passionate pursuit of physical wellbeing were foreign to the spirit of medieval Christianity. ... as a branch of secular learning, medicine was considered inferior to and subordinate to theology. If it

were true that all sickness was the consequence of sin, or a test of faith, suffering through such trials and tribulations might well be the only appropriate response.

(89)

Herbal remedies were widely used during the Middle Ages, and medical schools were established, which helped in more systematic explorations. However, all medical exploration and activities were dominated by religious sentiments, and Christian beliefs were treated as fundamental and several superstitions prevailed during this period, which overshadowed some achievements medicine made during this time. Several monasteries functioned as hospitals and medical schools and they provided care to the public, though they failed to understand the causes of diseases and consequently made several mistakes in diagnosis and treatment. For instance, the bubonic plague that took away a large number of lives in the 14th century continued to be a major public health threat till the 17th century mainly because the actual cause of the disease remained unknown.

Around this time, the Arabic and Islamic medicines made some advancements and the Islamic civilization was at its peak during the 11th century AD. Alluding to the Quran, which urged people to take care of the needy and the responsibilities that the rich has towards the poor, Islamic civilization by and large patronized medicine and medical establishments. Under the Umayyad Caliphate and after that under the Abbasid Caliphate, the Arabs exhibited great enthusiasm to learn from the Hellenic civilization and important Greek works were translated into Arabic. The Arabs established several hospitals and developed techniques, such as distillation, crystallization and use of alcohol as an antiseptic, which are in use even today (Majeed 2011, e4). Despite all these developments, medical practice in the Islamic world was firmly rooted in a religious worldview. These Islamic physicians considered ethical conduct very important. Ishaq bin Ali al-Ruhawi, the author of *Adab al-Tabib*, which deals with ethics for physicians, considers medicine as a divine art. He brings together insights from the Abrahamic tradition of religion, Greek ethics and the ideals of Hippocratic ethics and presents a comprehensive view about ethical conduct in medicine (Padela 2007, 172).

The nature and scope of modern biomedical ethics are characteristically different from these ancient contemplations on medical morality. Modern medicine, in all sense, is the product of Western civilization or, more precisely, of modern science. With the emergence of modern science and its unique methods, the several healing practices prevalent among Western society were remodelled after its peculiar procedures and methods. The important characteristic features of modern science are its emphasis on empirical observation and the method of explaining natural phenomena in terms of their causes. Newtonian science has influenced physicians during the Enlightenment period. This new science has avowed the regularity and order of the world and tried to explain the functioning of the universe in terms of certain laws and principles. Enlightenment physicians emulated to do the same in understanding the human body and diseases. They have "elaborated a rational theory of medicine which could provide comprehensive explanations of disease causation and effect, while simultaneously supplying a firm foundation for medical practice" (Risse 1992, 155). After that, the medical practice gradually excluded all its metaphysical, religious assumptions and also replaced the old Hippocratic framework with the new theoretical model of modern science.

Along with such developments, the ethical aspects that were at the centre of the Hippocratic tradition failed to find an appropriate place and role in the practice of modern medicine. The focus of the new science of medicine was entirely directed towards scientific advancements in the development of medicine, new and novel therapies and technologies. The pace of such developments revolutionized medicine and made it a domain of practice of highly skilled professionals from different fields. Medicine as science was isolated from other social concerns, and with all such new developments, it raises certain pertinent conflicts of interests between the profit-oriented drives of the various professional communities and the healthcare requirements of the people. Again, the use of technologies has introduced several complex ethical issues.

The practice of medicine today raises several problems, which were unfamiliar to our predecessors. For example, the new technological advancements can assist people in reproduction and even at the level of making very fundamental and minute choices that may decide many features of the offspring such as bodily features and health. Such possibilities raise serious ethical concerns. We need to adopt different theoretical approaches to addressing such issues.

An important feature that distinguishes contemporary approaches to ethics from the ancient, and particularly the Greek conception, is the emphasis on individuality. Aristotle held an essentially social conception of individuality, as opposed to the "egoistic individualism" which the modern liberal political theory has at its centre (Blackledge 2012, 22). The virtues that are central to Aristotle's ethics aim at the improvement of the character of the individual so that she will be able to fulfil her own as well as society's well-being. On the contrary, many contemporary theories are keen to protect the individual from the coercion of others. The "rights" of the individual are at the centre of ethical deliberations.

Contemporary bioethics too shares this fundamental concern. Tom Beauchamp and James Childress developed the four principles approach, which many argue affords a good and widely acceptable basis for practising good medical ethics (Gillon 2015, 111). The four principles are respect for autonomy, beneficence, nonmaleficence and justice. Beauchamp and Childress (1997) maintain that "[T]hese principles initially derive from considered judgements in the common morality and medical tradition" and

"[B]oth these principles and the content ascribed to the principles are based on our attempts to put the common morality as a whole into a coherent package" (37). Therefore, the ethical approach of principlism is not to be treated as an ethical theory. On the other hand, it borrows from various available theories, and their legitimacy can be derived from the existing theories. They offer a broad framework from where actual problems can be discussed and negotiated. The principlist approach is discussed in detail in the fourth chapter.

The Important Concerns of Medical Ethics

While discussing the specialty of medical ethics, the World Health Organization's *Medical Ethics Manual* states that though compassion, competence and autonomy are not exclusive to medicine, physicians are expected to exemplify them to a higher degree than other people, including members of many other professions (Williams 2005, 17). The *Manual* adds that besides this, medical ethics differs from the general ethics by being publicly professed in an oath such as the World Medical Association Declaration of Geneva and/or a code. Though there are differences between the oaths of various countries, there are certain common features as well. The promises that physicians will consider the interests of their patients above their own, will not discriminate against patients on the basis of race, religion or other human rights grounds, will protect the confidentiality of patient information and will provide emergency care to anyone in need are some of them (19).

Medical ethics today encounters a multitude of issues due to its unique predicament that owes to its special status as an enterprise that negotiates between two interest groups. On the one hand, it is a highly scientific and technological endeavour largely managed by corporate interests. On the other hand, medicine has to deal with people who deserve compassionate dealings and expects justice. The expectations and claims of the people are articulated in the form of ethical norms and codes and many of them are formulated as the laws of the country. However, unlike the ancient world, medical ethics today is a complex field. There are several factors that make it so, such as its continuity as well as skirmish connection with the ethical anxieties of the ancient world, its essential interdisciplinary nature, encounter with phenomena like medicalization and technologization that raise fundamental questions regarding human well-being and its failure in addressing some vital medical needs of a large section of human population.

Traditionally, the ethical concerns raised by the world of medicine were always associated with the medical practices of different cultures. Though these concerns stem out from the religious and cultural lives of different people, there were several common features such as no harm and beneficence that could be found in almost all codes of medical ethics of the ancient world. The transition from ancient to modern bioethics was necessitated by the replacement of traditional medical systems with modern medicine in all cultures. However, the central features of the ancient moral ecosystem remained unchanged and continued to define acceptable physician behaviour till the intensive growth of biotechnology and artificial reproduction technologies and many other technological accomplishments of contemporary medicine that undermined its very nature. Medicine, in its rapid evolution into a techno-scientific and corporate endeavour, began to give rise to new ethical challenges and complex legal problems, which the ancient moral paradigm could not comprehend and address effectively. But the ancient wisdom never became completely obsolete, and hence, contemporary bioethics is not an entirely new exercise but is also a continuation of the old.

However, we should not overblow this continuity and similarity. When Beauchamp and Childress articulated the crux of contemporary bioethics by articulating the four principles, they retained beneficence and nonmaleficence that were central to most ancient medical traditions but also added autonomy and justice in order to address ethical issues relevant in the new world. Autonomy became a fundamental ethical precept only since the Enlightenment, as the emergence of individualism was one of the major features of that age. As mentioned earlier, the individual became the epicentre of moral evaluations since the Enlightenment. This is a complete deviation from ancient wisdom. By emphasizing autonomy, the focus was shifted from society to the individual and this shift has also introduced a conflict between the two.

Another internal conflict that contemporary medical ethics encounters is between altruism and self-interest. As Heather MacDougall and G. Ross Langley (2019) pointed out, the Hippocratic tradition was silent about the payment of physician services. However, during the Middle Ages, the conflict between altruism and self-interest surfaced since only the royalty, the aristocracy or the wealthy upper classes could afford to pay medical assistance and the middle-class merchants, urban workers, farm labourers, peasants, serfs and the poor had to rely on home remedies, astrologers, bone-setters, barber-surgeons and the charity of academically trained practitioners. Medicine then seemed to lose its value as a social institution, as it failed to serve a vast majority of the population.

Medical ethics today is a complex enterprise where experts from a variety of specialized fields and the lay public have important concerns to articulate and anxieties to express from the purview of their respective sphere of engagements. It thus witnesses healthcare professionals, lawyers, philosophers, anthropologists, sociologists, economists, business personalities, biotechnologists, historians, policymakers, politicians and several other people engaging in fierce debates on issues related to health, life and death that interest them. However, it is important to delineate certain fundamental features of the discipline at a time when medicine encounters a number of challenges that our ancestors did not have to face.

2 The History of Bioethics
Learning from Different Traditions

Introduction

Many ancient civilizations have emphasized ethical conduct in the practice of medicine. It is hardly possible to disentangle the ethical from the therapeutic aspects of many ancient medical treatises across civilizations. Whether for the ancient Indian masters Charaka, Susruta and Vaghbhata or Hippocrates, the morality of medicine was no less important than the science and art of healing. All these traditional systems have categorically underlined an impeccable character of the physician. Many of them have their moral views integrated with the broad religious morality of their times. While the Indian classical medical traditions endorse the moral ecology of the idea of *purushartha*, which outlines the purpose of human life and its ultimate destiny, the Hippocratic Oath stresses the importance of integrity and benevolence. The Chinese medical tradition, which is inspired by Confucianism, emphasizes benevolence and universal love. Here, too, in tandem with the ancient Indian medical tradition, the healing practices presume the fundamental unity of nature and the belief in the *yin–yang* dualism (Magner and Kim 2018, 47), which indicates the two halves that chase each other and complete the wholeness. All these ancient frameworks conceive the goal of medicine as primarily a eudaimonic form of life.

In the traditional systems, physicians were treated as guardians of the society, and they have consequently enjoyed immense social trust and respect. As mentioned above, they all have placed healing in the context of a broader social and spiritual context, which insisted upon an exceptionally rigorous regulation of conduct for the ultimate attainment of eudaimonic life objectives. Vaghbhata explicitly affirms that the ultimate objective of medicine is the realization of *dharmarthasukha* (*dharma* means righteous conduct aiming realization, *artha* means material wealth and reputation and *sukha* means either *kama* which is desire for bodily pleasure, or *moksha* which stands for the craving for spiritual realization). Together they—the four of them—constitute the *purusharthas* or the ultimate life objectives of a man. *Ayurveda* or medicine is a form of *Veda* or knowledge. It means knowledge about *ayus* or life. At the mundane level, it aspires to offer remedies for

DOI: 10.4324/9781003312697-2

physical and psychical ailments through medication and other techniques, and at the higher level, it facilitates humans to pursue the path of material and spiritual objectives by ensuring a healthy body and mind.

We may find this stress on the moral objectives of life in other ancient traditions of medicine like the Greek, the Chinese and the Arabic in various degrees. They all emphasize the conduct of physicians, patients and family members of patients. All of them presume the authority of the general philosophical and moral approaches prevalent during their times and therefore hardly engage in any critical examination of their contextual legitimacy. Most of the ethical codes they prescribe are general and universal. There is a stress on a larger process of harmonizing, with society, nature and the universe. They give equal or more importance to the prevention of diseases along with treatment and cure and suggest a lifestyle to be followed by all members of the society to ensure such goals. Therefore, the goal of medicine is not just healing diseases but a harmonious life of the whole of the living creatures in the world. Most of these ancient moral and healing traditions conceive health as consisting of harmonious life that human beings can carry out in their social and environmental surroundings with proper regulation of their conduct and careful dietary restrictions. Since the idea of harmony was emphasized, the focus was on the whole and hence, individuals were primarily treated as constituents of a whole that needs to be preserved and upheld. In their evaluations, medicine never remained an independent institution but was integrated with other social practices that fostered meaningful human life in society.

Most civilizations across the world have developed their unique healing traditions based on a mix of magical, religious and ritualistic practices, which are also rooted in their understanding of other natural substances, including plants, animals and minerals. Religious and rational therapeutic approaches are found entangled in many such traditions in such a way that separating one from the other is impossible. This feature is prominently present in the most ancient healing traditions of the Mesopotamians and the Egyptians, the two ancient civilizations where religion played a vital role in shaping people's life. In these civilizations, the supernatural authors of disease were the gods, the dead or demons (Ferngren 2014, 16). The Mesopotamians, in whose writings the first recorded references to medicine could be found, regarded sin as the root cause of sickness and hence, they considered confessions as a vital feature of therapy (16). In the Egyptian tradition, the same person used to practise the roles of the priest, sorcerer or exorcist and physician (16). Apart from the Mesopotamian and Egyptian civilizations, such an association with religious practices is visible among the ancient Babylonian, Indian, Arabic, Chinese and Hippocratic healing traditions as well. The origins of the ancient Indian medical art can be traced in the healing practices of the Indus Valley people and the Vedic scriptures suggest how religious and mythological concerns were integrated with scientific pursuits, as the scriptures deal not only with scientific pursuits but also with moral prescriptions, magic, ritualistic practices and many other intellectual, religious and social concerns (Nellickappilly 2010, 32).

However, despite these commonalities in their ethical approaches, many aspects make the traditional medicine of each civilization unique, as the social, cultural and climatic conditions of the places they have originated are all different from each other. While China developed its medicine art along with its development of agriculture, in India, the diverse geographical patterns facilitated the development of a variety of healing traditions, including *Ayurveda*, *Siddha* and many other local practices, over a period of time. Taking into account India's peculiar scientific account of the human body and its organic relationship with the environment, most of the indigenous healing traditions in India gave equal importance to medicine, diet and control of the mind. Arabic medicine and particularly the Islamic medicine emphasized dietary restrictions.

As indicated above, despite such differences in the therapeutic strategies, the ethical approaches proposed by most of these ancient traditions sound similar and they all highlight a common set of virtues and principles. They all emphasize a set of personal virtues to be possessed by the physicians and occasionally the patients as well. Their approaches largely accentuate the obligations each stakeholder has to the society, which needs to function as a unit. Many of them—the Indian and the Chinese traditions more prominently—underscore the essential unity of nature and man. They, therefore, affirm that it is imperative to be in harmony with one's social and natural environments in order to maintain proper health. Hippocrates too embraces this insight, as he believes that health consists of striking a balance between man and nature through a natural lifestyle. The human body itself should attain a balance among its various components and this bodily equilibrium needs to be supplemented with a more substantial equilibrium with nature and environment. The body continually endeavours to attain such harmony, and the art of medicine is expected to aid this process. This is much in tune with the idea of *dosha samyam*, or balance among the three *doshas* or bodily bio-elements of *vata*, *pitta* and *kapha*, advocated by *Ayurveda* and *Siddha* traditions in India. These bio-elements or *doshas* are the essential constituents of the body. *Vata* is understood as the vital force that is responsible for the motion of bodily processes, represented by air, *pitta* stands for the heat symbolised by fire and *kapha* is responsible for bodily stability by balancing the bodily fluids. *Ayurveda* and *Siddha* hold that the three, though oppose each other, need to maintain an equilibrium for attaining health.

From the outset itself, it is evident that most of the ancient healing traditions do not advocate any distinct moral perspective but fundamentally try to assimilate the society's general moral outlook. Since most ancient societies espoused a duty-based and eudaimonic moral outlook, indigenous medicine in many cultures was explicitly oriented towards such a duty-based moral ecosystem. Though practising and adopting some of these moral prescriptions are not feasible today with the essential changes that happened in human societies and also with the emergence of more scientific approaches towards diseases and cure, many aspects of these systems are still valid and relevant.

While considering the bioethical insights of traditional societies, the predominant influence of religion and philosophy needs to be accredited. As indicated above, in most ancient societies, healing and well-being were not just medical phenomena but were also matters primarily related to religious beliefs and convictions. It is essential to understand how religious morality influenced bioethical deliberations in different societies.

Religion and Moral Considerations about Health and Healing

In his book *Medicine and Religion: A Historical Introduction* (2014), Gary B. Ferngren observes that to the educated mind, the association of religion with healing seems to be an anachronism that is incompatible with scientific medicine, though he acknowledges that medicine and religion have had a close association throughout history. According to Ferngren, the only role belief in God has today is that it may motivate physicians to provide compassionate care for those who are ill, or to help the sick to endure pain and suffering or to give spiritual consolation to the dying. He reiterates that when made public, the association of religious beliefs with healing is ridiculed as hopelessly anachronistic (1–2).

This perspective is, however, not necessarily true and particularly in non-Western societies, such an association between healing and religious beliefs is still robust. It is true that medicine today is a highly advanced techno-scientific activity and evidence-based research in various fields of science contributes to its further growth. However, healing is not necessarily a process that science alone can bring forth. It has solid and evident social, emotional and spiritual dimensions. Moreover, there is no necessary contradiction between science and religion. Wittgenstein points out how religious beliefs and language games coexist with the language game of science. While the latter provides descriptions of reality, the former does not, as it has no factual content. Nonetheless, it is an independent language game and has validity for those who believe in it. He affirms that in a religious discourse we use expressions as: "I believe so and so will happen" differently to the way we use them in science (Barret 1966, 57).

The ethical framework of ancient medicine, therefore, never remained independent of the religious beliefs that regulated individual and social lives and the values derived from them. The situation today is different. There is less focus on the contribution of religious traditions to bioethics and the religious approaches to bioethical issues. There is a strong belief that religious reasoning is incompetent to rewardingly engage with the complex ethical issues that arise due to the new developments in medicine and medical technologies. This is primarily because most of the ancient religious ethical insights were formulated during an age where medicine was predominantly an art espoused by a group of practitioners who were enthused by a strong sense of compassion and social trusteeship. Its practices contained a mix of religious-magical elements along with various therapies, which were based on common knowledge and observation. Medicine was neither part of the industry nor a complete science during that time. Things have changed drastically now and medicine is primarily a science. It is increasingly becoming part of an industry and the general impression is that we require a different set of values to address the new ethical issues arising from such a scenario.

This situation raises several concerns. Daniel Muller (2008) points to one such significant anxiety that arises due to the aggressive secularization of bioethics. He traces the development of two contradictory tendencies here. One is the sidelining of the contributions of religious ethics to public debate and the other consists of the efforts directed at the political recovery of bioethics by conservative religious forces that attempt an active re-theologizing of ethics (280). Further, when ethicists and professional medical bodies at the global level and in different countries advocate this secularization, it may end up raising many worries and dilemmas. Many countries outside Europe and the United States, where modern medicine is practised today, do not share a conducive cultural environment for secularization. While engaging with bioethical issues, complete neglect of the indigenous moral assumptions, which are rooted mainly in the respective religious traditions of those societies, will not yield any positive results. More importantly, there are specific problems related to health and human well-being like suffering, caring, aging, etc. that traditional and religious moral values can address more effectively than modern bioethical principles.

Religious insights are indeed of very little relevance to many ethical anxieties modern medicine raises in our highly technology-reliant society. The scope of bioethics seems to be extended far beyond what traditional medical ethics or for that matter, what the biomedical ethics of the 20th century thought it would deal with. As Muller (2008) observes, it now raises biopolitical questions connected to biotechnology and the life sciences, and by addressing ethical issues arising in the domains of the most cutting-edge life sciences like genetics, genomics, proteomics, etc., it is distanced more and more from the realities of daily medical practice which we encounter for the most part as normal situations and as involved individuals (283). These are more significant questions that deal with political and ideological issues and questions related to social and global justice. Many such issues require broad rational and secular frameworks to deal with and hence, traditional approaches prove to be inappropriate.

But at the same time, it could be argued that such complexities and diversities point to the necessity of adopting a multidisciplinary approach, deriving insights from multiple perspectives, including religious and ancient medical traditions. Today, the practice of medicine takes place in hospitals, clinical and pharmacy laboratories, clinical research centres and many other locations where practitioners at different levels encounter people from diverse backgrounds. In all such situations, individuals at various capacities meet each other and confront varied perspectives. They encounter multiple values and belief systems and may have to negotiate with all such diverse perspectives. An approach that is purely argumentative and discourse-oriented does not provide sufficient room for this plurality of convictions (Muller 2008, 283). This is particularly the case in countries like India, which prides a culture that celebrates immense cultural, linguistic and religious diversities. Medical decision-making is not always a rational process that takes place from a secular and argumentative angle but often involves perspectives that are emotional, cultural and religious. In the oriental world, it derives insights from the indigenous medical morality as well. There are quite lively conventions—that interfere with peoples' life decisively—among physicians in the *Siddha* and *Ayurveda* systems in India, the indigenous medical practices in China and the traditional healing practices in the different African societies. Hence, any important debate about bioethics needs to address the religious and indigenous medical moral perspectives.

Religious Values and Bioethics

Most religions in the world instruct their followers to be compassionate and duty-bound and regulate their behaviour, following the values that highlight individual purity, integrity and loyalty to the divine will. There are a few religious traditions in the world that do not endorse such values. However, most of them do. And, in ancient societies, social values were not differentiated from professional values. Before the spread of religions to other cultures, most religious values were indistinguishable from the cultural values of the place of its origin. Christianity is arguably the first major religion that spread to other cultures and played an important role in shaping the cultural values of different places, where it reached with its evangelical mission. In many places it went, it highlighted the message of Jesus; to love and to be compassionate to everyone, including the sinner. There are references in the Bible of Jesus curing the lepers and the sightless. Hence, the churchmen took some interest in alleviating the sufferings of the sick with proper medication and therapies.

But the fact that medicine was primarily meant for addressing the well-being of the body has created some confusion within the Christian church, as it always considered the body or matter as unimportant. One important way in which many religious traditions situate illness is by associating it with the divine will or punishment. All sufferings are understood to be retribution and rebuke for the sins. In other words, patients' illness and well-being are connected with the moral character of her actions. Further, some religious traditions, like Hinduism and Buddhism, believe in rebirth and they link the roots of a person's sufferings to her past births. The orthodox Hindu religion and philosophies believe in the concept of *samsara chakra*, or the cycle of birth and death, to which the individual is attached with the chains of past and present life *karmas* or actions that have moral implications. This chain of *karmas* is the cause of all sufferings, including diseases, and the individual is bound to them, so long as she continues to be chained to the cycle of birth and death. In general, the internal link between human sin and diseases is recognized by almost all major religions.

Yet, in general, most religious traditions were not completely antithetical to the practice of medicine and many of them considered healthcare as an important enterprise in the spiritual journey as well. Buddhism, for instance, had given extreme importance to healthcare and there are references to the Buddhist kings establishing hospitals and clinics in various parts of their kingdoms. While the caste system and the *Brahmanical* emphasis on the *Vedic* rituals dominated Hinduism, the science of *Ayurveda* witnessed a decline, and Buddhism liberated the science from its total decline by promoting its practice in various ways. The author of *Ashtangasamgraha* and *Ashtangamarga*, Vaghbhata profusely tenders his salutations to Lord Buddha and calls him *apoorva vaidya*, or rare physician, who could ultimately liberate humankind from its sufferings (Vidyanath 2013, 3 & 280). Later, the Brahmanical tradition, too, has revived its tradition of healthcare. The *Siddha* tradition, which developed mostly in the southern parts of India like Kerala and Tamil Nadu, was a unique system of medicine that specializes in the usage of heavy metals in medicinal preparations besides plant and animal products. The *Siddha* system believes that it was none other than Lord Siva who had instructed the science for the benefit of the human and animal world. Though in *Ayurveda* and *Siddha*, there is an underlying belief that sufferings due to diseases are the consequences of our unrighteous past actions, they never resign into quietism, attributing its origin to human fate. They endeavoured to overcome the sufferings due to diseases and constantly reminded the importance of keeping a healthy body for the sake of a healthy mind and for the attainment of our goals in life.

Though religions are based on faith and most of them also breed several superstitions, they, in general, cared for human betterment and well-being and hence could not neglect the hindrances diseases could create in human life. Initially, in many societies, people attributed diseases and their cures as direct divine or evil engagements. But many religious traditions later seemed to have altered such a firm conviction and preferred to accept immediate material causes like climate conditions and diet as causing diseases. They had accepted the view of the more advanced evidence-based science of medicine. However, this would not be a contradiction to their original belief, as they could still believe that though the immediate cause of a disease can be external material factors such as microbes and viruses, the ultimate cause of disease—why an individual fell ill at a particular time—remains the divine will. Most of them now have endorsed the critical role medicine plays in liberating humanity from pain and suffering, which they too consider as crucial from a religious point of view.

The General Ethical Framework of *Ayurveda*

A strong spirituality is ingrained within *Ayurveda*'s healing practices and philosophy of science. It advocates a philosophy of life that suggests a form of living for man, which is essentially in harmony with the society and also with the rest of the universe. Its comprehensive eudaimonic perspective not only encompasses the field of the administration of medicine but also the regulation of the whole of a man's life for the prevention and cure of diseases. Humans harmonize with the universe in a process of living that is achieved with a moral regulation of their life. Ayurveda, therefore, is not just a science. It is rather "a way of physical, mental and spiritual living, which aims at the eradication of all kinds of sufferings including diseases" (Nellickappilly 2010, 32).

The major objective of medicine is no doubt the healing of the sick. In the traditional context, this involves a direct relationship between the physician, the patient and the person(s) who assists the patient. Ayurveda's practical ethics revolves around this relationship, which is built upon the firm foundation of physician trust. Physicians used to command immense trust among the public in general and their patients in particular. In this context, the ancient masters of medicine in India prescribed several behavioural codes all these stakeholders were expected to follow.

Charaka Samhita has an elaborate code regarding the training, duties, privileges and social status of physicians in order to ensure exceptional composure of character and high moral integrity, both in the personal and professional lives of the practising physicians. Those who aspire to be physicians should have the capacity for sustained effort and single-minded devotion to the science, besides being practising celibacy (Ray and Gupta 1965, 20). The personal integrity of physicians was emphasized more, as besides dedication to a continuous updating of knowledge, the physician is expected to lead a disciplined and unostentatious life, to be pleasant in his manners and to be considerate and gentle in speech (20–21). The four cornerstones of medical practice are friendship towards all, compassion for the ailing, devotion to professional duties and a philosophical attitude to cases with fatal endings (21). Similar moral prescriptions are given to the patients and their attendants as well. All three stakeholders are expected to follow the norms and contribute to the sustenance of the environment of trust, as the healing process functions effectively only in such an ecosystem.

According to *Ayurveda*, illness is a state where the totality of a person's being—her body and mind—undergoes some changes that eventually prevent her from pursuing normal life and consequently, the goals of human life. In this sense, illness is not only a pathological condition that affects a specific organ in the body, but it pervades the whole of our being (*asesa kaya prasrutam*). Contrary to this, health is conceived as our natural state, with which we can perform all essential activities effortlessly. Placed in the context of *Ayurveda*'s eudaimonic conception of life, we may say that with a healthy body and mind, we can perform *dharma* and attain the higher objectives of life (Thirumulpad 2006, 7). *Ayurveda* shares, with most of the philosophical traditions of ancient India, an unshakeable belief in what can be treated as the four fundamental postulates of Indian ethics: the belief in the fundamentality of suffering in our corporeal existence, belief in *karma* theory, belief in an eternal soul and the conviction about the highest spiritual emancipation in life (Nellickappilly 2010, 33). As a corollary to this, the empirical self, or the *jiva*, carries with it the baggage of its past *karmas*, which it has to enjoy or suffer. Diseases are primarily born out of such baggage of lingering *karmas*.

Ayurveda's conceptualization of diseases, as well as the healing methods and processes they suggest, is unique in many ways. It essentially visualizes both disease and health from such a broad context. According to *Ayuskameeyam* #41 of *Ashtangasangraha*, three constituents determine the state of health: climate (*kala*), sense objects (*artha*) and actions (*karma*). Climate is the external natural condition that changes periodically. Climate has important bearing upon the generation of diseases. To different climatic conditions, the body and mind respond differently. Disease or *roga* results from the wrongful (*heena*), inappropriate (*mithya*) and excessive (*athi*) combination of the three, while their right union causes health or *arogya*. The combination is a psycho-physical process and hence, on many occasions, diseases are caused by wrongful practices (*ahita charya*). Therefore, the right regulation of the senses and intellect is important in the process of cure as well as prevention of diseases. This starts from knowing to discriminate between appropriate and inappropriate behaviour (Thirumulpad 2006, 31–32).

Further, from its philosophical perspective, *Ayurveda* conceives diseases or *rogas* as ultimately caused by bodily passions or *ragas*, which are treated as the great poisons [*maha visha*] in the Indian tradition. All diseases are ultimately born of these passions, declares *Ashtangasangraha, Ayushkameeuyam* #1, which comprise attachment, hatred, greed, delusion, pride and animosity (1). These passions determine our character to a great extent and they are inherent in us. *Ayurveda*'s spiritual and religious therapeutics link them with the residues of our past-life actions. In other words, they reside in us in causal forms due to the *karmas* performed in the past, both in this life and in the past lives. Hence, medicine and food may help to get rid of them only temporarily. For an ultimate cure of diseases and a lasting peaceful life, the spiritual path has to be followed and the practice of detachment needs to be perfected (4). This begins with the regulation of mind and body, which is an essential aspect of traditional Indian morality across different traditions. Here Ayurveda is intimately related to *Yoga* philosophy, which stresses on *Yama*, *Niyama* and *Prathyahara*, which visibly aim at regulation of the body, mind, conduct, interactions with other human beings and other living creatures and also the strict adoption of moderate consumption of commodities.

The administering of medicine and proper diet constitute only one aspect of the healing process as the effectiveness of the treatment depends on physical, mental and supernatural causes of the disease (Nellickappilly 2010, 37). As shown above, the *karmic* residue plays a significant role in the generation of diseases, and its removal is not accomplished with medication alone. For this, one needs to proceed from the *karma* itself, as the *karmic* residue incites the agent to respond in specific ways that it may find gratifying. The residual *karma* functions as inner dispositions (*vasanas*) that manifest in the form of various tendencies that stimulate one to act and make oneself morally accountable for what one does (38). Hence, the agent's present *karmas* are kindled by the residue of her past *karmas*, which perpetually clings her to the *karmic* cycle that is the source of all enjoyments and sufferings, including diseases. The eradication of diseases involves not only administering proper medicines but also rupturing the *karmic* cycle. One needs to dig deep from the immediate physical and psychic causes of diseases until one accomplishes the complete removal of sufferings. The complete cure from diseases ultimately leads to the attainment of *moksha* or according to Buddhism, *Nirvana*.

The intimate association of medical well-being with spiritual well-being is asserted repeatedly by various Indian systems of medicine. As mentioned above, for Vaghbhata, the goal of medicine is the attainment of *purushartha*. Various ailments hinder human beings from pursuing these goals, which under normal circumstances they would be able to do effortlessly. When diseases prevent their normal life by creating dissonance both within the body and with the environment and society, the art of medicine could be of aid. Medicine consists not only of therapies that directly address the symptoms but also prescribes a total transformation of the individual with alterations in her lifestyle, food habits, the ways she thinks and behaves, etc.

Vaghbhata says that only the knowledge imparted by the Buddha would alleviate man from all diseases. As mentioned above, according to Vaghbhata, the Buddha is the most exceptional physician because his teachings ultimately remove the individual's ignorance and lead her to spiritual enlightenment. This spiritual enlightenment is well-being in the ultimate sense of the term, for both Buddhism as a religion and *Ayurveda* as an art of medicine.

Indian systems of medicine and healing practices go beyond the boundaries of *Ayurvedia*. The Siddha tradition itself is significantly different in its approach and style, though the philosophical and moral aspects remain more or less the same. There were also a variety of micro and local traditions and systems that existed such as the tribal. Although the practice of *Ayurveda* was founded upon grand spiritualist ideals, its actual practice took place in a highly hierarchical and stratified society, where certain groups invariably enjoyed unequivocal monopoly over all knowledge. This made the services of specialized physicians inaccessible to a large section of people in the society. Although many physicians and their families rendered selfless services, they hardly reached those sections of people belonging to the lower strata of the society due to caste impediments.

Chinese Medicine and Its Moral Fabric

Shen Nong Ben Cao Jing, who is regarded as one of the celestial emperors—the second one—in Chinese mythology, is also revered as the father of Chinese medicine. He is believed to be the author of the *Divine Husbandman's Classic of Materia Medica*, the first Chinese pharmacopeia that catalogues 365 medicines derived from minerals, plants and animals, and also the inventor of the technique of acupuncture (Zhao et al. 2018, 2). In a sense, Chinese medicine and medical morality have their roots in the life and works of this mythical figure. What is highlighted in the popular accounts about Shen Nong is the emperor's extremely compassionate nature and his devotion to the well-being of his subjects. Apart from inventing the fundamental techniques of agriculture and animal husbandry, the compassionate emperor had resolved to end his people's suffering from illnesses and poisons. He taught them to sow five types of grain and personally investigated 1,000 herbs to test their medicinal value and to distinguish the therapeutic from the toxic. Shen Nung died after an unsuccessful experiment, which itself testifies his extreme kindheartedness to fellow human beings and unselfish devotion to medical research (Magner and Kim 2018, 48).

Virtues like compassion, dedication and caring constitute the foundations of ancient Chinese medical morality. The Chinese healing tradition was influenced by certain religious and philosophical assumptions that shaped Chinese life since antiquity. The fundamental moral paradigm was primarily governed by Confucian outlook with substantial influences from Taoist and Buddhist insights. Many ancient Chinese physicians were Confucian scholars as they considered healing of the sick as one of their moral duties towards humanity.

Among those mentioned above, three crucial religious and cultural streams of Taoism, Confucianism and Buddhism that governed the ancient Chinese polis for several centuries, the influence of Confucian philosophy and religion were more profound. Confucian philosophy decisively determined the nature of government and the social fabric in ancient China. This philosophy affirms the underlying link between man, nature and the cosmos and consequently concludes that since the universe exhibits an order, there ought to be an order in the society as well among humans.

One of the striking features of Confucian philosophy is its recognition of the family, which comprised certain fundamental forms of relationships, as the primary social unit and the various types of relationships that constitute the family as archetypal to all other forms of social relationships. Underlying this assumption is the belief that the entire human society is a family. The family and society as units constitute various relationships where people are intimately related to each other in terms of certain obligations. Every relational unit is a micro social unit that is in several interrelations with other similar units. The mutual obligations of the members decide each unit's status in the society, as several such units constitute the society in terms of obligatory mutual commitments. The role each individual plays in such a relational unit is defined in terms of duties each of them have to the other.

Chinese physicians were expected to achieve the high moral standards of a Confucian person and they treated humanness as the supreme medical virtue. The Confucian moral outlook has deep roots in the Chinese culture as for more than two millennia the Confucian scriptures were essential teaching materials for students and Confucian ethics was its dominant moral philosophy and ideology (Tsai 1999, 316). Hence, reflecting the essential principles that shape the Confucian moral paradigm, the ancient Chinese physicians were advised to be compassionate, devoted to their profession and their duty as healers towards the sick. Daniel Fu-Chang Tsai (1999) delineates the important moral insights of ancient Chinese physicians by summarizing the important common principles they all seem to be endorsing. He affirms that the physicians needed to master Confucianism before learning medicine. Apart from a commitment to sincere learning and maintaining very high professional standards, physicians were expected to avoid greed for wealth, fame, selfishness and lust and be sincere, decorous, devoted and respect confidentiality. They also needed to be modest and prudent towards other physicians (316).

Though the Chinese tradition insists that physicians be professionals by dedicating themselves to a constant improvement of their trade by an incessant commitment to continuous learning, the Confucian human values were something they had to imbibe necessarily. In a sense, these values are more important to the Chinese tradition and also for anyone who tries to attain the supreme good in life.

The Hippocratic Tradition and the Ethics of the Oath

The practitioners of modern medicine all over the world refer to the Hippocratic ethical tradition even today. The methods and procedures Hippocrates adopted are hardly espoused by anyone today and modern medicine has a fundamentally distinct character from this classical Greek system. The Hippocratic tradition was appropriated by subsequent traditions in Europe differently. The only therapeutic aspect the new medicine seems to have adopted from the Hippocratic tradition is its commitment to conceive and explain ailments from a rational point of view. As far as the ethical framework is concerned, modern medicine embraces its spirit, but omits many of its detailed prescriptions. As a custom, almost everywhere in the world, the new physicians are initiated to their profession with the oath the master had formulated more than two millennia ago.

Echoing the Greek pagan beliefs of those days, the Hippocratic system broadly alludes to certain fundamental assumptions about the divine character of nature. However, the Hippocratic art of medicine was different, as it was predominantly rational and removed the moral, religious and supernatural elements from its diagnostic and therapeutic processes (Pai-Dhungat 2015, 18). Diseases are, therefore, explained rationally with the four humours theory. Similar to *Ayurveda*, which propagates the *thridosha* theory—the doctrine of the three *doshas* of *vata*, *pitta* and *kapha*—the humours theory explains that the four humours of blood, phlegm, yellow bile and black bile jointly design the constitution of the human body. While *Ayurveda* conceives diseases and their cure in terms of the balance and imbalance of the three *doshas*, Hippocratic tradition conceives the four components as constituting the human body while their imbalance is conceived to be amounting to diseases and their harmony designs health. However, unlike the system of *Ayurveda*, the Hippocratic art of medicine never alludes to any supernatural causes for human diseases. All diseases are simply explained by means of the four humours and their excess and deficiency.

One limitation of the Hippocratic tradition of medicine is its failure to develop cures to many diseases. Here the Chinese and Indian systems evidently surpass their Greek counterpart. It is often stated that Hippocratic tradition was more credited for its approach to medicine and treatment, where the commitment to a rational explanation was discernible, rather than its discovery of drugs. As pointed out by Pai-Dhungat (2015), the Hippocratic School achieved greater success by applying general diagnosis and passive treatment. Its focus was on patient care and prognosis, not diagnosis. It could effectively treat diseases and allowed for further development in clinical practice (18). Hippocrates should be credited for discerning medicine from religion and paving the way towards the development of more scientific contemplations on healthcare. But more importantly, his ethical inscriptions ensured a very high social status for the physicians. Pai-Dhungat adds, "Hippocratic medicine was kind to the patient. Treatment was gentle and emphasized keeping the patient clean. He was reluctant to administer drugs and engage in specialized treatment that might harm the patient" (18).

However, Hippocratic medicine is a medical system of antiquity. Neither his methods of diagnosis nor his medication are appropriate today. Physicians across the world hardly allude to the humoural theory of the master, which constituted the core principle of his system. In this sense, the Hippocratic tradition is a dead medicine art and the only living component in the system is its ethical module.

Hence, what makes the Hippocratic system really relevant today is not its distinctive therapeutic principles or theoretical foundations but the oath the master physician had formulated, which contain the principles all physicians across the world have to follow while practising their trade. The oath is still highly relevant and the principles cited and the virtues highlighted in it are germane even in the world of highly sophisticated medical technologies and advanced procedures and practices followed by hospitals and practitioners to arrive at correct diagnosis and suggest appropriate therapies. In a sense, the principles of beneficence and nonmaleficence have universal validity, as some versions of these principles are followed by almost all traditional healthcare systems.

The Hippocratic Oath and Its Moral Framework

The physicians' oath is believed to be the composition of Hippocrates, who is also hailed as the father of western medicine. The oath highlights some of the important virtues, society by and large expect to see among the physicians. However, some of the principles mentioned in the oath are not relevant today, as the oath in its original spirit is the product of a society that was governed by values that are predominantly religious. The oath was modified several times and the Catholic church used it with sufficient alterations during the Middle Ages, in many parts of Europe. At least since the 18th century, the English medical schools started using it and subsequently the oath became popular in other European countries and the United States where its different versions were used during the graduation ceremonies (Bhatnagar and Gupta 2013, 668).

As mentioned above, the Hippocratic oath is not a completely secular document. It is sworn in the name of Greek gods and its scope is limited to the conduct of the physicians. Nevertheless, it represents the most secular ethical document of the ancient age. The unique political and social environment prevalent in ancient Greece was responsible for this exceptional feature of Greek medicine. Among all the ancient civilizations, the Greeks had one that reinforced free-thinking and speculation and the priestly class was not very strong and powerful in their society. Hence, the polis provided sufficient room for rational thought to flourish. The moral contemplations of the Greek philosophers were also not predominantly religious. The oath was the product of such a social and cultural environment. It highlights the following principles (Augustyne 2019):

1. The physician swore to look after his teachers, who taught the art of medicine, and their families. The physician here invokes the family values that most ancient societies considered as paramount.
2. Further, the physicians summon to the commitment to the art of medicine, which he swears to teach his sons and his teacher's sons.
3. The physician expresses his determination to ensure his patient's well-being by following the system of the regimen that would benefit his patients and abstain from whatever is deleterious and mischievous. He swears to keep away from all that would be harmful to his patients like administering any deadly medicine or giving a woman a pessary to produce abortion.
4. The physician takes a resolution to pass his life and practice his art with purity and holiness.

5. The physician will do things that will be beneficial to his patients, consciously avoiding all acts of mischief and corruption.
6. He will maintain patient confidentiality.

It is important to note that the Hippocratic oath emphasizes specific principles like no harm, patient confidentiality, commitment to professional competence, etc. as well as personal virtues like gratitude, purity of character, integrity and righteousness. Though the Hippocratic moral framework does not separate the personal morality from professional ethics, it nevertheless refrains from alluding to supernatural beliefs. No wonder modern medicine could appropriate the Hippocratic Oath to its system with ease and with minimal modifications.

The ethical codes of Hippocrates have survived the passage of time with few modifications and this testifies the universal acceptability of its moral perspective. Even during the modern era of bioethics, the Hippocratic principles have been repeatedly invoked. This is visible in the preparation of the Nuremberg codes, the Declaration of Helsinki by the World Medical Association and the formulation of the four principles of bioethics notably by Beauchamp and Childress.

The Arabic Bioethics

Because of the nomadic nature of the unsettled tribes and the desert environment they lived, the pre-Islamic period in Arab history is not very glorious as far as scientific and medical knowledge is concerned. Their medicines were mainly produced from plants and leaves of trees, certain pods, animals' bones and incense (Ead 2016). Islam brought a new light and direction in the Arab understanding of health and diseases. Qur'an, the holy book of Islam and Prophet Mohammad's teachings, plays a key role in shaping the Islamic view about medicine, which was dominated by ideas related to hygiene and better healthy living (Akanni 2013, 176). Again, there are many *hadiths* where the Prophet mentions about health and medicine. It is believed that the Prophet once said: "There is no disease that Allah has created, except that He also has created its treatment" (al-Almany 2009, 1271).

Medicine in the Arabic world began to flourish during the Golden Age of the Arab-Islamic Empire, which spanned since the middle of the 7th century to the end of the 15th century. During this period, Arabic became the most important scientific language of the world, as many important works in philosophy and medicine were translated into it (Azeem 2005, 1486). With this assimilation of knowledge from different parts of the world, Arab healthcare system was transformed into an advanced body of knowledge and practice. It then gradually became independent of its religious origins, while retaining the moral spirit of the religious foundations. Unlike its European counterparts, the Arab system had established hospitals, which also functioned as centres for medical education, modernized healthcare with the introduction of separate wards for men and women, and established new medical protocols that ensured personal and institutional hygiene, medical records and pharmacies (1486). During the Golden Age, medicine was deemed with very high esteem in the Islamic civilization. The great 11th-century Islamic scholar Al-'Iz Ibn Abd Al-Salaam observes that medicine is like legislation, as along with the latter, medicine was also instituted in order to ensure the safety and well-being of people by removing the harms caused by various diseases (EM/RC52/7 2005, 3).

Notwithstanding these facts, the foundations of Islamic medical ethics are to be found in the three fundamental sources of the religion; the *Qur'an*, which is the holy book that is believed to have revealed to the Prophet, the *Hadith*, which represents the sayings of the Prophet and the *Shari'a*, or the Islamic law, that constitutes the divine commands that regulate a believer's life. Analogous to most of the other ancient traditions of medicine, the Islamic approaches to bioethics adopt a predominantly duty-based perspective. Although these duties are explicitly directed towards stakeholders who are human beings, they are devoted to Allah, the almighty. There are many insights present in these three sources of Islam and such fundamental insights are appropriated by different Islamic societies variedly.

The Qur'an emphasizes the importance of health and its maintenance and also the need for treating ailments. Like Christianity, respect for life and human dignity are very important in Islam as well. It is being asserted that God has bestowed upon man the basic knowledge required to distinguish between what is (morally) good or bad. Human beings are the most precious and special creations of God and it is important to respect and protect them. Hence, the holy book affirms that both seeking treatment and providing treatment constitute the duties of patients and physicians, respectively. Moreover, unlike many other religious traditions, Islam never conceives ailments as a punishment of God's wrath (Akhmad and Rosita 2012, 9). Hence, as mentioned above, it is categorically asserted that there are hardly any diseases without treatment and it is obligatory to seek it (by patients) and provide it (by physicians).

Physicians used to enjoy a very high social status in the ancient Islamic societies as their profession was considered to be sacred. Islam firmly believes that it was Allah who is the true healer and thus one of the names of God is "the Healer" (9), and by virtue of his profession, the physician is very close to the divine power. The virtues expected to be present in a physician are compassion, care and respect, as he has to be an instrument of God's mercy (9). As mentioned above, the basic principles of the revealed religion of Islam remain the foundations of Islamic bioethics. Like other traditional systems, Islam, too, propagates an ethical view that highlights a set of values based on certain fundamental assumptions regarding the value of human life and its essential sacred nature. More than what people do and the consequences of their actions, the intention of the doer becomes morally significant in Islam. This is because Allah is all-pervasive and knows everything.

The modern-day Islamic scholars are, therefore, able to find answers and solutions to many bioethical issues we face today, sacrificing neither the essential spirit of their religion nor compromising on the modern-day values and needs.

Features of Traditional Bioethics

We saw in the previous chapter how the ancient contemplations on medical morality differ from the modern-day bioethics with its preeminent focus on the isolated relational contexts where individual physicians encountered their patients. To be more precise, traditional medical morality in most civilizations were emphasizing the obligations of different individual stakeholders. Hippocrates, for instance, insists that a physician should refrain from giving a deadly drug to anybody who asked for it and should not make a suggestion to this effect (Miles 2005, xiv). Vaghbhata, too, prevents physicians from giving women abortive remedies and Charaka emphasizes the need for physicians exhibiting remarkable moral integrity and cultivating good character. Such virtues and convictions are necessary to ensure the society benefits from the efficient services of the physicians.

Many of the ancient systems of medicine share certain common features. The most prominent among them is the entanglement of religious with rational therapeutic approaches. It was common to many ancient societies to assume that the causes, as well as remedy for illness, are related not only to natural causes but also to spiritual and moral factors and they tend to believe that supernatural beings like gods, demons, quasi-divine beings and other positive and negative forces make their presence known through diseases. Consequently, their therapeutic procedure involves several ritualistic practices like chanting, dancing and sacrifices along with medication. It is therefore difficult to separate the rational aspects from other non-rational and irrational components of the healing practices of many of these traditional approaches. In spite of such difficulties, some of these traditional systems have endeavoured to discern the rational therapeutics from the religious therapeutics and have succeeded significantly in this process. *Ayurveda*, for instance, has considerably modernized and is still prevalent in India in a significant way. It has an elaborate pharmacopeia, which outlines the specifications of drugs and the diseases for which they have to be used. The Chinese system of medicine also has accomplished remarkable triumph in this regard. As mentioned above, the contribution of the Hippocratic system is limited to its ethical prescriptions.

Ironically though, the Chinese and Indian traditions of medicine still make headways even in this age of evidence-based science and advancement in technology, many of the moral guidelines and directives put forth by them are not given any significant consideration. The patient–physician relationship is no longer controlled by the codes of ancient medical morality but is primarily regulated by legal provisions and protocols. Though modern bioethics is not entirely impervious to traditional moral wisdom, it is not proactively attentive to its decrees either. The main reason is, as mentioned above, its approach to morality is grossly inadequate in dealing with the multifaceted ethical issues and uncharacteristic moral dilemmas of the modern age. There are three important dimensions to this problem. On the one hand, bioethics today deals with much more significant issues than its ancestral discipline, which focused mostly on issues related to the conduct of individuals involved. There are complex geopolitical, biopolitical and ideological issues along with problems related to non-compliance to norms and codes, corporate crimes, etc., which do not fall within the scope of traditional medical morality. The third category of issues may arise due to cultural diversity and individuals holding to very different moral perspectives. The limited framework of traditional bioethics cannot negotiate with people who come from such diverse backgrounds and who subscribe to multiple worldviews and value frameworks.

A few central features of ancient bioethics are the following:

1. The importance given to the dignity of the profession; often treated as a divine occupation.
2. Physicians' social status as social trustees and custodians of the health of people.
3. Physicians' impeccable moral character; being caring, compassionate, not greedy, unselfish, advocate of simplicity and humility, honesty, integrity, etc.
4. Patients' unshakeable trust on the physician's ability and intentions.
5. Belief in the system of medicine.
6. Treatment of medical morality as a component of the general moral framework.

Throughout these ancient rubrics, we find a strong emphasis on duty and character of individual physicians. The image of a benevolent physician is central in most ancient medical traditions. As a corollary to this, patients and the society as a whole trust the phyicians and consider them as their well-wishers and guardians of their well-being. The key role trust played in ancient healing traditions is discussed above. It was believed that in the absence of trust, medicines fail to work.

In the intimate relationship between the physicians and their patients, the former are professionally and personally related to the latter. Hence, it is not a mere detached professional association. The physicians know their patient's social and emotional life, which enable them to decide the right therapeutic remedies for psychosomatic problems. Owing to the long personal relationship, the patients bestow complete trust upon their physicians and will have the conviction that the latter would warrant their well-being. All therapeutic interactions happen in the context of such an environment of trust and warm relationship.

The prevalence of trust and the sacred nature of the patient–physician relationship are further reiterated by the exceptional moral character of physicians and the latter carrying out their profession with a spirit of social trusteeship and professional acumen. Ancient societies did not develop independent moral codes for individual professions, which is a common feature of modern societies. Hence, the moral codes of the healthcare system reflected the spirit of the general moral framework of the society and they responded to all the anxieties of the moral community. In other words, there were very few specific moral demands and concerns the healthcare system raised during those days that were not present in other domains of life. This aspect is discussed in the first chapter, when the process of societal modernization was discussed. With the advent of modernization, the different functional spheres in the society began to raise very distinct and unique moral demands, which the unitary moral framework of a homogenous social group found challenging and difficult to negotiate. This situation led to the proliferation of ethical inquiries and deliberations in different functional spheres in society, including medicine.

A comparative look at the medical morality of the two ages reveals how important are moral values in the very conception of health and illness. While most of the ancient systems conceive these principal concepts in terms of an idea of harmony, modern medicine hardly alludes to such a belief. Harmony has both micro and macro dimensions. Health is here primarily understood as a result of the bodily components functioning in a harmony, which results when the humours (Hippocrates) or *doshas* (*Ayurveda*) are in harmony. All forms of diseases cause bodily disharmony. Systems like *Ayurveda* and *Siddha* may go further and affirm that the cause of such a disharmony could be the failure of the individual, who is a psychosomatic conglomeration in harmonizing with her natural and social environment. This conception of health and illness eminently evokes a moral outlook, which recommends the individual to regulate her internal and external life with strong moral values.

However, modern medicine presents a unique scenario, as the new innovations and discoveries in biomedical sciences and the success of the new medicine across the world changed its face. The way modern medicine developed deriving its nourishment from the novel discoveries, biological and other natural sciences incessantly made enabled it to effectively address many health issues that were fatal and incurable earlier. In its evolution as a complex scientific and technological enterprise, modern medicine has drastically changed the way it was practised earlier where apothecaries and doctors controlled everything right from diagnosis to medication and cure. Modern medicine involves a large number of professionals at different levels contributing to the various stages of the healing process. Hospitals, laboratories, research centres, pharmaceutical firms, diagnostic centres, insurance companies, etc. constitute the complex network that gives modern medicine its contemporary shape. Healthcare is provided at different levels—primary, secondary and tertiary—by professionally qualified individuals at different places and such a network determines the origination, prognosis, diagnosis and cure of a disease. Many hospitals function like corporate organizations and relate to their patients mainly as customers. An individual, who falls ill, practically loses all control over herself, although modern medicine profoundly asserts the value of patient autonomy and considers the patient as the ultimate decision-maker. In traditional healthcare, the physician is the decision-maker, which makes the system paternalistic. However, often in the contemporary scenario, along with the physician and the patient, the market forces also play a vital role in regulating the entire dynamics of the decision-making process.

The Social Context of Ancient Medicine

In many of the ancient societies, the social order was regulated by a moral outlook, which was shaped by a mix of religious beliefs, societal rituals, conventions and a multitude of other factors. Generally, individuals were treated as members of certain communities and by virtue of their membership in their respective communities, their corresponding moral behaviour was specified. In other words, morality was largely determined by the role and occupation of individuals. Society functioned as a single interconnected unit, determined by the various complex interrelations between the communities. This moral order was ultimately regulated by a eudaimonic ethics, which benefitted both the society and the individual. The society was benefitted from the contributions of the dutiful individuals and, in turn, the individual realized her potential within the social context of action, which granted her a position in it, an occupation with which she found her subsistence and served the society. The concept of virtuous obligations of the ancient Greeks and the idea of righteous dutiful obligations or *dharma* of the ancient Indians reflect this idea. In both these contexts, the emphasis was more on obligations. An undeniable ego-centrism is inbuilt into these frameworks. But, it is not an individualistic egoism that focuses exclusively on the benefits of the agent. Instead, the agent realizes her eudaimonic goals within a broad socio-economic and political context that inevitably involves her fellow beings.

In Europe, with the spread of Christianity, the Catholic clergymen practised altruistic ethics rooted in their religious tenets and built clinics to serve the community. They even used an amended version of the Hippocratic Oath. There was a predominant view, which considered the suffering related to the contracting and treatment of a disease as a corrective process, which would ultimately benefit a man spiritually. But since love is the central message of Christianity, the early Christians could not neglect those who suffer from various diseases. The early Christian hospitals in Europe thus reflected this central message of Jesus and tried to alleviate the sufferings of the common man. The medieval Christian approach towards diseases and their cure surrounded a few beliefs such as the conception of disease as an admonition, disease as an opportunity to correct ourselves and hence helpful for our moral development. It was the duty of a Christian to help those who suffer and many physicians were motivated by charity.

The identification of diseases with suffering and their causes to the sinful acts of the patient was a common belief in many cultures. Ayurveda emphatically states that diseases are caused by lust and other human attachments that cause indignations and rages (Thirumulpad 2006, 2) This conviction is in tandem with the general religious ecosystem that believes in the theory of *karma*, according to which one reaps the fruits of one's actions. The entire *dharmic* traditions share this view and thus, it constitutes the central precept of medical morality in India. However, at a practical level, patients expect physicians to behave, reflecting the spirit of guardianship, trusteeship and professionalism. The social context of ancient India envisaged a unique relationship between the public and their professionals. Physicians, like the rulers, were perceived as guardians; the rulers regulate their social life and physicians their health. In some places, there were village physicians, which was an official designation. For example, ancient Kerala had 64 *gramam*s, or villages and one physician family was in charge of each one of the villages. This physician's family used to enjoy certain rights and privileges. In turn, they offered dedicated service, often being indifferent to the fee.

The social and economic structure of most of the societies before industrialization was predominantly agrarian and feudal. Wealth was concentrated in the hands of a few during the pre-industrialized era, and people's identities were determined by their class belongingness, such as peasants, nobles and knights in Europe and the *Brahmins, Kshatriyas, Vaishyas* and *Sudras* in India. Here the ethical responsibilities of any individual were defined in terms of her class identity and the individual's independent subjectivity was not significant. Medical ethics in this scenario reflected this class dynamics. The public expected the physicians to be a certain kind of person delivering services to the society with certain obligations. The obligations in return from the public to the class of physicians were also predefined. Each individual, regardless of class, was expected to fit into the moral mould.

The characteristic feature of the traditional model of physician–society relationship was the resilient trust that not only made the physician's profession unique and peculiar but also superior to many other occupations in society. People had conviction in the physician's abilities in diagnosing the disease and recommending appropriate therapies. The conviction was emphatically firm so that the physicians' decisions were hardly doubted or questioned. This was mainly because of two factors. First, the extent of medical knowledge available was limited in those days. There existed hardly any specialization within the healthcare profession and there was limited standardized corpus of knowledge. Instead, there were different schools where the practitioners were adopting similar but different styles of diagnosis and treatment. In India, for example, some physicians rely entirely on pulse reading for diagnosis, while some others arrive at a diagnosis by examining the colour and other properties of the patient's urine. The diversity was not confined to the methods of diagnosis alone; rather, the medication and therapies offered were also different. Physicians heavily depended upon practical wisdom, which they gain as part of their education. There were physicians who excelled in diagnosis and had attained better success rates in curing and people had high regard for them. There are stories of several legendary physicians whose fame crossed boundaries. But, hardly anyone doubted the sincerity of any physician, nor there was any doubt about their competence. There are barely any stories about physicians who were quacks. If people found a physician ineffective, they would never go to them and those who had good practice were physicians who have earned their confidence and trust.

Second, physicians earned trust not only through efficiency but also with their selfless, dedicated service, which often did not care for any financial returns. The readiness of physicians to offer free service was an evidence, not only of their selflessness and integrity but also for their competence and authenticity. It is also a proof for their regards for the highest values of their profession that posits service as its prime motto. Medicine in those days was not an impersonal professional institution but was constitutive of a group of individual physicians who offered private services in an individual capacity to patients whom they knew. The patient–physician relationship was more than a professional association, a personal relationship. Such relationships used to last for a very long period and the success of the practice of any physician depended upon the extent of personal relationships each physician was capable of making.

Ancient Bioethics: Some Common Features

Healing practices existed virtually in every civilization, and though they share a few common features, they differ from each other in important ways. In some civilizations, they existed as magical practices, as the cause of illness remained a mystery for a long time. The ancient healers of Mesopotamia were primarily religious men. In some cultures, people believed that the priestly class knew about the surreptitious dealings happening in the human world and had access to the unknown mysteries of nature and human destiny. They postulated diseases and their cure as signs of divine or evil messages to the mortal world. These religious therapeutics relied mostly on revelations.

A few cultures, however, developed rational therapeutics which relied more on observation-based diagnosis and medication. The Greek medicine, which initially considered diseases to be divine punishment and healing as a gift from gods, gradually moved towards rational explanations of diseases and turned its attention from supernatural causes and began to focus on the vital elements in living creatures such as the four humours (Taher, Mannan and Dulal 2018, 1096). This paradigm shift constitutes the basis of scientific inquiry in medicine, though such inquiries confined to the searching for the causes within the body itself. The idea of associating bodily imbalance and harmony with the diseases and their cure could be found in the Hippocratic writings. Here the Hippocratic physicians were attempting to locate material causes for diseases—and not supernatural ones—but they were unaware of the microbes that cause diseases and also about infectious diseases (1096).

We may trace the evolution of Indian medicine from religious to rational therapeutics in the development of the Vedic age, from medical aphorisms to the medicinal treatises of the *Brihat-trayi* (the three books of medicine by the three great masters Charaka, Susruta and Vaghbhata). Here too, there was a search for material causes of diseases rather than the supernatural causes and the *thridosha* theory was developed in this context. The masters of this tradition developed a detailed pharmacopeia and they possessed deep knowledge about the medicinal properties of various plants, herbs and metals.

Ancient medicine in all civilizations began to decline due to several factors. The notable exceptions are the Indian and Chinese medical traditions, which are still in existence. The development of scientific inquiries and the spread of more effective western medicine was the primary reason for the decline of indigenous medical traditions in most cultures. With the growth of industrialization and urbanization, several infectious diseases began to threaten the very survival of human societies in the urbanized settings. Traditional indigenous medicine failed to offer effective cures for many such diseases. The emergence of modern medicine and its integration with the new sciences during the 19th and 20th centuries made the Hippocratic medical tradition and its theoretical foundations completely obsolete. However, a few traditions like the *Ayurveda* and Chinese medicine still survived, though with adaptations and modifications. *Ayurveda's* theoretical foundations based on the theory of *thridoshas* are considered to be still valid by practitioners. Nevertheless, the modern *Ayurvedic* practitioners are trained in accordance with the new medical knowledge developed by modern medicine and they arrive at diagnosis using many modern techniques and with the assistance of laboratories and diagnostic centres.

Though the triumph of modern medicine in our contemporary world is conclusive, the moral beliefs associated with the traditional healing practices did not diminish as quickly as the therapeutic side. People's expectations about physicians' behaviour remained the same for a long time and even today in many non-Western civilizations, the medical morality of antiquity is still endorsed by both patients and physicians. However, this environment is rapidly changing due to several factors. In many countries like the United States, the practice of medicine has already adopted a business model in order to ensure professionalism and efficiency. Many other countries tend to follow this model as it favours the interests of medical professionals, hospitals, pharmaceutical firms and insurance companies, besides offering the patients superior care. But what dominates in this framework is a business model of physician–patient relationship, which gives very little space for traditional medical moral values like compassion and personal care. Hence, it finds resistance in many non-Western countries, where communitarian values still dominate social and cultural lives.

As mentioned above, the medical moralities of different cultures are drastically different from each other. Nevertheless, they exhibit certain parallels as some common aspects are visible in many of them. There are similarities in the socio-economic conditions as well. The following are a few such common aspects, which we may find in many ancient traditions.

First, most of the ancient healing traditions are a complex mix of religious and rational therapeutics. Hence, it is not very easy to separate them. Ancient medicine in large had its origin in the religious practices of the community where they had originated. Consequently, many of the therapeutic practices of ancient physicians were hardly distinguishable from religious rituals. Ayurveda, for example, ever since the great treatises or *Samhithas* of Charaka and Susrutha and *Ashtangasamgraha* of Vaghbhata began to move towards finding out rational explanations for the causes of diseases. Climate, objects and our deeds, says Vaghbhata, are the causes of our well-being and diseases. Nevertheless, according to Vaghbhata, the root cause of all diseases is our lust (Thirumulpad, 01). Here the master refers to a spiritual vision integral to Buddhism. He thus says that only Lord Buddha, the exceptional physician, can offer an ultimate cure to our diseases with his spiritual knowledge (4). The implication is that only the Buddha's vision and wisdom can alleviate human suffering.

Unlike contemporary societies, where specialized professional domains have developed their codes of conduct, ancient medical moral expectations never fundamentally differed from the general moral ecosystem. The whole of society constituted a single moral community, and all constituents of the society shared the same moral sentiments and aspirations. Both the physicians and the patients subscribed to a set of common moral principles as well as beliefs about human life and human destiny. Hence, their values were necessarily not different, and their association jointly aimed at accomplishing something which neither of them has any hesitation in envisioning as well-being. The ethical commitment of the physician was not fundamentally different from that of a professor or a warrior. Aristotle explains this with the notion of virtue. Though the virtues that define each profession may be different, the ultimate accomplishment and gratification derived from the virtuous performance of actions by the professionals contribute to the same goal: individual happiness or *eudaimonia* and the flourishing of a just society.

Most traditional healing systems considered the relationship between physicians and society as forming part of a deeper ecosystem that affirms the internal links between society's various components. Society as a whole is related to the community of physicians for the satisfaction of an essential need. It is a truism to say that the rich could always buy better facilities. But as far as ancient healing traditions are concerned, this was not necessarily true, as the fact is not that healthcare was economically inaccessible, but it was not available to anyone beyond a point. One major factor that makes modern medicine inaccessible today to many people is the cost of treatment. Though more and more technological innovations make healthcare further effective, they also make it more expensive and inaccessible to a vast majority. Ancient medicine hardly faced such a scenario. The element of financial transactions was not an inevitable aspect of the physician–patient relationship. What mattered was honour and personal integrity. As mentioned above, physicians offered their services with a spirit of public welfare and deontological disposition. They mostly behaved like trustees of the health of people and were like the guardians of their patients.

In some cultures, several social, political and economic changes made the ancient moral frameworks irrelevant. In the European context, such changes were compellingly present during the 18th-century Enlightenment era, which had witnessed a complete change in its moral perspective. It was during this time, along with several other vicissitudes, the social ethos came to be significantly determined by an emerging scientific temperament. The incipient new economic order made such changes inevitable. The domain of medicine had also undergone remarkable changes during this time. It got transformed from a set of healing practices based on inherited experiential knowledge and life-world assumptions to a science, which adopted the empirical observational method in understanding the functioning of the human body. Modern medicine has thus emerged initially as a science and then developed into a highly complex techno-scientific activity.

Along with the sociopolitical and economic changes during the Enlightenment, the philosophical and moral outlooks had also undergone astonishing changes. The notable modern ethical frameworks like contractarianism, deontology and utilitarianism have emerged during this period and they have insisted on evaluating moral behaviour not purely on the basis of customs, conventions and religious beliefs, but from the pedestal of universal rationality. Ethical deliberations about the practice of medicine in this new scenario necessitated the adoption of new approaches and frameworks. Such changes were not confined to the realm of medicine but suggested radical revisions in our ethical outlook about every phenomenon. They virtually prepared the grounds for the transition from traditional medical morality to modern bioethics.

3 Passage to Modern-Day Bioethics

Introduction: From Traditional to Modern Bioethics

Albert R. Jonsen (1990), who was professor and chairman of the Department of Medical History and Ethics, School of Medicine, University of Washington, outlines a fascinating account of modern-day bioethics. He says:

> As an ethicist, I am professionally concerned with ethical problems and the issues of the moral life. These can be found wherever human beings are found. ... In medical care such topics abound: life-support systems, abortion, artificial hearts, genetic engineering, neonatal intensive care, and research with human subjects, euthanasia. And these are only a partial index of the moral problems in medicine.
>
> (3)

Many of the issues Jonsen referred to are typical of modern-day medicine and even those issues like abortion and euthanasia, which were not the creations of advances in the new biological sciences and biotechnology, the way they are perceived and debated is characteristically different today. During ancient days, these issues were never debated, as society by and large held to one single moral standpoint, which was unquestionably accepted as right. Modern-day medicine is practised in an environment where there are multiple perspectives, and every issue is viewed and weighed from different angles. Jonsen's primary concern boils down to the replacement of altruism with greed. It further points to the more significant issues related to biopolitics and power. Though the moral problems raised by ancient and contemporary practice of medicine significantly differ—an issue which we have already discussed in the previous chapter—Jonsen traces a continuity, which according to him is inbuilt in the very practice of institutionalized medicine.

Jonsen talks about a central axis in the world of medicine and affirms that in medicine's moral history and present, that axis forms at the point where altruism and self-interest meet, and at that intersection a profound moral paradox pervades medicine. This opposition is built into the very structure of medical care and woven into the very fabric of physicians' lives.

DOI: 10.4324/9781003312697-3

The particular moral problems encountered in medicine are symptoms of this paradox (5). He further observes that there can be no question that self-interest and altruism are elements in all moral life, and they may even be seen as basic principles of the moral life. He traces the history of altruism to the Judaeo-Christian tradition where the theological belief about God's love manifested in His healing powers. Jonsen adds that both traditions still exist as deep moral foundations of medicine, and it is impossible to eradicate the traces of these ancient traditions. It is a skill that is acquired with the effort, it promises great rewards such as income, prestige, reputation and gratitude. It is therefore a skill so rare that it can be sold at a great price and like any other skill can be shamefully and dishonestly used (10). However, every society values this skill and desires it to be used for its benefit. Jonsen argues that even physicians who are indifferent to Hippocrates and who have never heard of monastic medicine have these traditions stored deep in their consciousness. Hence, while permitting them to learn and use their skills in order to earn a living, the society insists that those skills be used for the benefit of society. According to Jonsen, the Western society has invented the medical licence in order to safeguard this dual goal. He adds that this licence thereafter reinforced the moral paradox of self-interest and altruism (10).

The conflict between altruism and self-interest has several aspects in the present scenario. As reminded by Jonsen, it is not a modern phenomenon but would have marred the practice of medicine at all times. This is essentially the case with most of the non-Western cultures also. The image of physician as a social trustee that dominated the pre-modern societies is not completely forgotten. However, with the emergence of new medicine, the self-interest and greed that had infected the profession have multiplied in strength and scope. Rather than individual physicians, the patients have to negotiate now with institutions, which have multinational interests and are guided by the ideology of global capitalism. Many of these institutions have the power even to fight against governments and they eventually make individual patients helpless.

As mentioned in the previous chapter, ethical issues emerging today, therefore, require new approaches and techniques. Modern bioethics responds to such requirements. Hence, bioethics today requires new definitions and descriptions. Bioethicists today no longer engage with formulating norms that determine the right behaviour. They rather battle with multiple perspectives, which include not only issues related to clinical correctness and patient–physician relationship but also broader questions that have cultural, religious, political, legal and social dimensions.

However, the shift to modern bioethics was not a sudden one. Nor has it happened everywhere in the same manner. In many places, the traditional approaches still exert strong influences. Nevertheless, the methods and protocols of modern medicine demand a different moral paradigm to conceptualize and implement regulatory measures. It is not easy to outline this shift due to these reasons at the global level. In the United States, which is the birth land of modern bioethics, the secularized modern approaches have gained wide acceptability, and they have been implemented with policies and legal stipulations. However, this is not the case with most Asian and African countries. Even in the United States, ethnic minorities pose some challenges to the secularized framework. However, to understand the shift that has been happening across societies, it is important to understand the dynamics of change that occurred in the United States and the important historical and other factors that accelerated such changes.

Modern bioethics, as we understand it today, has originated in the United States during the 1960s and there are several historical, cultural, social and economic reasons for this. The term "bioethics" was coined in 1927 by the German theologian Fritz Jahr in an article where he analyzed the relationship between human beings and other living creatures and plants (Jahr 2010). However, Jahr hardly finds any serious mention in the vast bioethics literature produced since the 1970s in the United States and other places. Since the 1980s, the discipline of bioethics has witnessed remarkable growth both from academic and practical points of view. Scholars have ventured to publish, exploring different aspects of the discipline from different disciplinary perspectives such as medicine, ethics, philosophy, history, anthropology, sociology, law, political science and economics. Such multidisciplinary contributions have given modern-day bioethics a distinct character. Hence, it ceases to be a mere continuation of the traditional contemplations on medical morality.

As discussed in previous chapters, the traditional healing systems in different societies espoused their moral regulatory norms and the Hippocratic tradition in the West is credited for the famous oath for the physicians. Many insights in these systems are hugely relevant even in the modern age, as the principles of beneficence and nonmaleficence are pertinent to all times. However, modern bioethics is not a mere continuation of the moral deliberations of ancient medicine art. The former is primarily different, as it is predominantly secular and is fundamentally argumentative. It perceives medicine not just as a system of healing but as a body of knowledge, which has theoretical and practical features, and its practice has a wide range of social, political and economic implications in the lives of people and nations. Hence, it is absolutely essential to understand it from diverse perspectives.

Multiple factors kindled such drastic changes, which ultimately resulted in the evolution of a practically intricate and theoretically complex modern-day bioethics. As stated above, patients' trust in their physicians constituted the core of ancient bioethics, and the former always believed that their physicians knew better and would always do what is right for them. The doctor always knew what is best for the patient, and hence, medical ethics was primarily their concern. This situation changed since the 1960s, particularly in the United States, after several social, political and historical factors, including the revelations about unethical human experimentations and political upheavals that happened during the Vietnam War. The judiciary began taking a proactive stance in litigation issues involving medical professionals and pharmaceutical firms. The potential harms many new medical technologies could cause to patients, growing awareness about human rights, etc. have fostered a strong scepticism towards physician paternalism and their status as custodians of patients' good. Health and well-being ceased to be concepts that were unreflectively taken for granted by society and were debated as concepts that need to be understood from different perspectives. Consequently, philosophers, lawyers, political theorists, theologians and many other experts from different domains engaged in contemplating the idea of patients' good from their disciplinary perspectives. This ultimately led to the birth of the interdisciplinary field, bioethics. There are certain obvious factors that necessitated the shift from traditional medical morality to modern-day bioethics. A few of them are listed below.

1. Biotechnological innovations raising certain serious ethical challenges.
2. Unethical clinical research.
3. Changing conceptions of life and its values due to changes in the socio-cultural, political and economic domains.
4. The recognition of the diverse implications of the practice of medicine in the Modern Age, and hence of the multiple disciplinary angles from where any issue related to it can be explored.
5. Medicine and poverty. The benefits of science hardly reach the poor who constitute the majority.
6. Questions about social justice.
7. Economic globalization and also globalization of medicine.
8. Increasing democratization and secularization of societies across the world.
9. Corporatization, medicalization, etc.
10. Bioethical approaches becoming increasingly adopting a utilitarian spirit.

Biotechnological Innovations and Ethical Concerns

Ever since the Cartesian revolution that separated the world of the thinking mind from the mechanical world, there existed a strong tendency to understand the human body as a machine. This mechanistic view had not only changed our age-old assumptions about living creatures and life as such but also changed our basic convictions about the values that constitute the basis for our understanding and our behaviour towards the rest of the living creatures. Bioethics can be understood as representing the concerns and sentiments against such a mechanistic understanding of nature and life. In this sense, Charles Darwin's theory of evolution and natural selection presents the idea of evolution in order to explain the biological phenomenon (Lima and Cicovacki 2014, 269).

Lima and Cicovacki suggest to organize the field of bioethics in terms of "traditional" and "emerging" scenarios of bioethical concerns, where they categorize issues related to abortion, assisted suicide, euthanasia, organ donation, eugenics and clinical investigation under the traditional scenarios and ethical issues occurring due to technologies like cloning, stem-cells research, genetic engineering and reproductive technologies under emerging scenarios and new fields of research (271). Modern biotechnology finds its applications in various fields directly related to health like food production, agriculture, various therapies, pharmaceutical, etc. They have immensely contributed to the betterment of human well-being and have the potential to further make remarkable improvements in health through the practical and relatively cost-effective diagnosis of a range of diseases, better drug development and the production of vaccines, novel therapeutic approaches and nutritionally enriched genetically modified crops (Afzal et al. 2016, 1). Abdallah S. Daar and Peter A. Singer (2009) summarize the important uses of modern biotechnology by the five Fs—food, fuel, feedstock, fibre and pharmaceuticals (171–172). The biotechnology revolution, fuelled by developments in information technology, according to them, will have a profound impact on humanity in this new century. They continue:

> It will challenge our understanding of ourselves and the etiology, manifestation, progression, and management of physical and mental diseases. The new era will witness a profound change in traditional healthcare delivery and public health, and in the pharmaceutical and agricultural industries.
>
> (172)

This is not a new phenomenon altogether. Humans have been using biotechnology since ages for aiding improvements in agricultural practices and even for medicinal purposes. However, the application of modern biotechnology in manipulating human life raises unprecedented moral challenges. Many such challenges require new paradigms of evaluations to understand them properly and to evolve effective solutions to the problems they give rise to. Nevertheless, all interferences made by biotechnologists are not necessarily ethically problematic. As stated above, humans were engaged in processes like selective breeding for better performance of crops and even animals for ages. One may argue that it is unfair to disapprove when similar things are done at a faster rate with more efficiency and certainty with the employment of biotechnology. After all, the main issue involved is interference with nature, which happens in both cases. There is very little evidence that suggests that genetic modification done using modern scientific techniques aided by sophisticated laboratory equipment is more dangerous than conventional methods adopted by farmers and other people when they breed selectively.

However, the numerous uses of biotechnology in various human societies raise some genuine moral concerns. Subsequent chapters will address a few of such specific uses and their potential ethical challenges. The ethical concerns and crises that evolve here result from the inability of our conventional moral frameworks in effectively responding to the issues such technologies potentially raise. For instance, the acquisition of embryonic stem cells—which may find many uses in regenerative medicine—demands the destruction of the embryo, which represents life in a rudimentary form. Research in this domain may immensely benefit humanity. However, its acquisition requires the consent of the parents. Many parents are now reluctant to permit this, as they think that the destroyed embryo has the potential to be their child. Nevertheless, there could be significant differences between the moral status of the actual human child and the moral status of an embryo. But, from certain perspectives—such as Catholicism—such differences are blurred, which may cause confusion in such cases and may lead to several inconveniences.

Biotechnology is an advanced sphere of technology, which involves the application of highly sophisticated scientific principles and the use of cutting-edge technological innovations, and there is a great deal of ambiguity about most of its applications among the general public. Such ambiguity and people's ignorance about the procedures involved and the outcomes expected jointly raise several ethical concerns. Since it is a domain that experiences rapid growth and its potentials in benefiting humanity are substantially huge, the ethical issues it raises have severe repercussions on the lives of people. On the one hand, humanity cannot outrightly denounce the use of this technology because it raises ethical issues. On the other hand, we cannot cite substantial human benefits as a justification for violating the values related to human life.

Unethical Clinical Research

At the social and cultural front, the overtly individual-centric values of the modern era have made the overarching moral environment in the society irrelevant and each sphere of activity in the society has developed its peculiar norms and principles. The newly evolving science of medicine, therefore, functions with a new set of norms and practices. This would aid constant development through research and application of scientific and technological knowledge to the betterment of health and well-being as defined in terms of new values of the age. Wherever these values conflicted with the old set of morals, they forced the latter to either change or became obsolete.

Traditionally, the patients' unshakeable trust has been the foundation of medical ethics. This trust is normally understood in terms of the patients trusting their physicians. However, patients in reality bestow their trust in the system of healthcare that existed as a socially regulated exercise primarily monitored by the overarching moral framework that governed social life in all its departments. With the development of modern medicine and the integration of medicine into the purview of modern science, particularly in biological and chemical sciences, many physicians found this environment of trust conducive for experimenting with new drugs and medical procedures. On many occasions, this ensued exploiting the patients. Ultimately, this has resulted in the erosion of trust, and it further has led to a moral crisis in the field of healthcare.

As a science, medicine offers numerous promises about improved care and ensures quality life to millions worldwide. However, to explore all its potentials, medical professionals, biotechnologists and pharmaceutical firms have to engage in research and generate continuous technological innovations constantly. This may need the participation of human subjects and such participation in research may often harm the latter. There is hardly any benefit that comes without a risk. The participants in clinical research need protection both from any intentional harm of the researchers and from harm due to the latter's negligence. The researchers, therefore, will have to take the utmost care and there should be an appropriate mechanism to monitor and regulate the process. Hence, the focus is to minimize the risk and proceed with further experiments following newly formulated ethical guidelines. The ideas of informed consent, confidentiality, respecting persons, caring for the health and well-being of the participant, etc. are a few essential ethical values highlighted in such contexts. There are also rigorous legal requirements formulated at both national and international levels. These issues will be discussed further in the subsequent chapters.

Clinical research and experiments involving human beings need to take utmost care and precautions in order to avoid irreparable harm to the patients or participants. However, human experimentation is an inevitable component of clinical research. The triumph of global capitalism after the end of the cold war has annexed healthcare as one of the significant sectors of global economic development. Huge investments were available for further research and development in the sector and the strict regulations in many advanced developed countries prompted many multinational companies to channelize their funding to developing and underdeveloped countries. Such initiatives have introduced an array of ethical problems. The economic and educational backwardness of the people in these regions made them vulnerable to the exploitation of profit-seeking pharmaceutical and other medical technology-manufacturing firms.

Historically, several incidents incited public conscience to be aware of and resist harmful clinical experiments that physicians and other scientists conduct in different parts of the world completely disregarding the ethical aspects. Though such unethical experimentation and research abuses have happened in many places ever since the advent of modern science and the initiatives to integrate scientific methods with healing practices, a few of them are hallmark cases that proposed the immediate need for stringent regulations. The human experimentations conducted by German physicians during the Nazi regime; the Tuskegee Syphilis Study conducted to study the progress and effect of untreated syphilis by American physicians on 400 African American men in the state of Alabama from 1932 to 1972 (where the participants were denied medication even after penicillin became available); the US government-sponsored secret research on the radiation effects on human beings which involved the participation of cancer patients, pregnant women and military personnel during 1944–1980; and the hepatitis experiments on mentally disabled children at the Willowbrook State School, which had the approval of the New York Department of Health, where the participants were deliberately infected with the virus to study the natural progression of the disease during 1956–1980 are some crucial cases.

The Nazi Inhuman Experiments

During 1933–1945, the Nazis lashed out several social and political atrocities against the Jews, gypsies, their political opponents and prisoners. The Nazis subjected them to unparalleled cruelties and killed millions of them in concentration camps and gas chambers. Germany was one of the most scientifically advanced nations before the war. The political scenario before the war offered the Nazi scientists and physicians the opportunities to conduct scientific experiments involving human subjects that involved enormous risks to them. The Nazis suspended all political and civil rights of the Jews, their political adversaries and the soldiers and civilians of their occupied territories. They used them as subjects in scientific experiments, completely disregarding all safety concerns. For instance, they conducted experiments on concentration camp inmates in order to study the effects of and treatments for high-altitude conditions, such as freezing; malaria; poisonous gas; sulphanilamide; bone, muscle and nerve regeneration; bone transplantation; saltwater consumption; epidemic jaundice; sterilization; typhus; poisons; and incendiary bombs (Anilkumar and Anitha 2015, 262). Besides, the Nazis subjected sick and disabled civilians in Germany and their occupied territories to euthanasia by employing physicians.

The inhuman Nazi experimentations were not just part of a political programme. It was channelled by the idea of rebuilding the society guided by certain laws of biology. Ideologically, the Nazi idea of racial purification inspired scientists to envision achieving the goal, with the applications of some possibilities biological science guarantees. They were captivated by the idea that human behaviour is determined by their biological constitution and therefore genes play a crucial role in one's lives. The Nazi totalitarian regime, which espoused the ideology of racial purity, created an environment where the scientists who were interested in addressing such questions pursued their research work with hardly any hindrances. Under normal circumstances, such research works that require the participation of a large number of human subjects are not feasible. The biological experimentations to be conducted on them did not guarantee their safety, and in many such experiments, the chances of harm were very high or even certain. But the Nazi Law for the Protection of German Blood and Honor conceived all others among the population, except the Germans as racially inferior and having a biologically minor value. Hence, they had no claim to civil rights and were easily available as research material (Roelcke 2004). The political and ideological environment thus provided the scientists with a conducive environment to pursue their unethical and inhuman research without any obstacles.

After World War II, the Allied forces seized many records and documents, which undoubtedly established the direct involvement of many physicians in such human experimentations and cruelties. Subsequently, they prosecuted the physicians for their activities after the Charter of the International Military Tribunal, establishing the laws and procedures on 6 August 1945, which eventually came to be known as the Nuremberg trials. Thirteen such trials were carried out in Nuremberg, Germany, during 1945–1949, which examined the accusations raised against Nazi military officers, government officials, some German industrialists, lawyers and also physicians who conducted abusive human experimentation. They were all accused of charges of crimes against peace, war crimes and crimes against humanity. The trials were followed by the formulation of the Nuremberg codes, which had outlined some important ethical parameters, researchers are required to follow when they involve human participants in their research. The United States played a significant role in the Nuremberg trials in ensuring that the proceedings follow strict norms of justice and law. In this sense, it can be contended that the birth of modern bioethics took place in the United States. However, physicians, policymakers and ethicists of many other countries share the general sentiments as well.

It will be ironic to note that, though the United States was at the forefront of all these ethical and legal initiatives, it failed to regulate and prevent from happening one of the most heinous examples of research abuse in the modern era. The Tuskegee Study of Untreated Syphilis, conducted by the US Public Health Service and the Tuskegee Institute, Alabama, is a historical case conducted to study and record the natural history of syphilis.

The Tuskegee Study of Untreated Syphilis

The Tuskegee Study, began in 1932, was envisaged to be a medical study that would monitor to discover the effects of untreated syphilis and it was called "Tuskegee Study of Untreated Syphilis in the Negro Male." In the course of the study, the very idea behind it became ethically questionable with the invention of penicillin, as it was intended to observe syphilis patients who remained untreated while treatment became available! In other words, the patients were denied available treatment, which eventually subjected them to pain and suffering that could have been avoided. But, what makes it more unethical is its racial orientation, as all the subjects were recruited exclusively from the African American community. Moreover, the consent of the subjects was never taken prior to conducting the study. The participants were told that they were being treated for "bad blood." This was the local term used to describe several diseases, including anaemia and fatigue, along with syphilis (CDC).

The US Public Health Service initiated the study programme by converting a treatment programme into a non-therapeutic human experiment. The fundamental objective was to collect data on the progression of the disease when it was untreated. The study was particularly conducted among the African Americans in order to understand how it manifested among them with respect to their biological differences. With the cooperation of the Alabama State Board of Health, the Macon County Health Department and the Tuskegee Institute, the programme began by offering free blood tests and free treatment for "bad blood" by County Health Department and government doctors along with free meals and free burial insurance. The subjects were in the second stage of syphilis. Initially, the study recruited 399 black men with syphilis and 201 black men who did not have the disease. The study was initially planned for six months but ultimately it continued for 40 years, till a public outcry stopped it in 1972.

Though since 1943, the Division of Venereal Diseases was treating syphilitic patients with penicillin, the Tuskegee men were considered an exception, as they were not considered patients but viewed as experimental subjects. By the same token, the authorities harmed them recklessly. In 1965, Irwin J. Schatz, who was a physician, and in the following year a public health service investigator, Peter Buxtun, wrote to the PHS authorities raising serious moral concerns about the study. Though the agency ignored such concerns, Buxtun continued his efforts to stop the study and eventually leaked information about the study to Jean Heller, who was an Associated Press reporter. *The New York Times* carried Jean Heller's story on the front page of its 26 July 1972 edition, which ultimately brought the study to a halt (Brown 2017). Following this, a lawsuit was filed on behalf of the men in the study in 1973 and finally, an out-of-court settlement of $10 million was reached. In the following year, the Congress passed the National Research Act, which had provisions that would prevent the exploitation of human subjects for research purposes. On 16 May 1997, President Bill Clinton issued an apology to the remaining survivors of the study.

The ethics of the Tuskegee Study has to be evaluated with the strictest measures possible for several reasons, and it also reminds us about the constant threats the vulnerable people in a society face with respect to the violation of their rights and exploitation, however much there is public awareness about the democratic and constitutional rights of people in the society. The fact that the study had a racial orientation would ever remain shameful to the US government. Several men met with premature death by being subjects in the study. The data assembled was not very useful as they could contribute neither to prevent the disease nor to find a cure for it.

Further to these aspects, the study unswervingly violated the constitutional rights of the participants both by not providing the required information and by not taking proper consent from them. The United States was at the forefront of framing the Nuremberg codes that underline the need for respecting human dignity. Even after 20 years of framing the Nuremberg codes (1949), the US physicians conducted inhuman experimentation without any visible remorse and continuously defended its rationale. Only when the press brought it out in front of the public, the professional community felt the need for retreat. It thus reminds us of the need for keeping a constant vigil against rights violations and exploitation.

The Tuskegee experiments were unethical and illegal to the core. Besides violating the constitutional rights and human rights of the participants, it involved cheating them, as they were not informed that they were actually "used" as experimental subjects. This violated the fundamental deontological dictum that insists that no human being should be treated as a mere means but should always be considered as an end in himself/herself. Instead, the participants were given the impression that they were being properly treated for their diseases. Another fundamental ethical precept concerning the safety of the participant was never taken into account, as the scientists literally "pushed" the participants into death, which was undoubtedly avoidable had they been adequately treated. However, above all other factors, the Tuskegee Study exposed another dark face of scientific experimentation; racism. The study was racially motivated, as it was conducted only among African Americans and no whites were part of the study.

The Willowbrook State School Hepatitis Experiments

During mid-1950, Dr Saul Krugman and his colleague Dr Robert Ward joined as consultants in infectious diseases in the Willowbrook State School in Staten Island, New York, which was an institution for mentally disabled children. The school had been reporting repeated occurrences of the epidemic and endemic diseases as measles and hepatitis. They eradicated measles by vaccinating the children, and for controlling hepatitis, Krugman and Ward decided to gather knowledge about the natural history of the disease. They initiated their studies in 1955, which made the children in the school experimental subjects. The study continued for the next 15 years. Over this period, the doctors collected 25,000 serum specimens from 700 patients. The researchers understood that most of the hepatitis infections found in the school were acquired after children were admitted to the institution. Certain studies and observations confirmed that the cause of infection was contact with infected children and not food. Intending to get more precise data, they deliberately infected some newly admitted children with the strain of the hepatitis virus.

The doctors were aware of the ethical issues involved in the process, especially in deliberately infecting them with the disease for the sake of research.

However, they defended their actions with several arguments. They contended that the susceptible children would not avoid getting infected in the institution, and being a research subject would entitle them to receive special care. Walter M. Robinson and Brandon T. Unruh (2008) comment on the ethical precautions taken by Krugman:

> Krugman designed an experiment that presented the least risk possible for those enrolled. He began with a low dose to observe side effects, created a specialized system for monitoring the children, and used an agent known to produce a mild form of the disease. Krugman then took into account the risks that the children faced in the absence of participating in the research. He considered the benefit to those enrolled as well as to other children facing the same circumstances. He obtained consent from the parents of every child who participated. And he obtained an independent review of the study design from experts in the field.
>
> (82)

Further, the study was approved by the New York State Department for Mental Hygiene, the New York State Department of Mental Health, the Armed Forces Epidemiological Board, and the human-experimentation committees of the New York University School of Medicine and the Willowbrook School. The study also met the World Medical Association's Draft Code on Human Experimentation (Munson 2008, 39).

However, any research that involves children as subject raises certain inherent ethical issues, since the intellectual maturity required for giving informed consent after evaluating the risks and benefits of the research experiment to which they are subjects is absent in them. They are physically and psychologically not to be equated with adults in whom we believe autonomy and the ability to consent are manifested to their fullest extent. They are the most vulnerable among human beings and it is relatively easy to exploit them. As far as the Willowbrook research study is concerned, the subjects were not ordinary children but mentally retarded children who, by all means, cannot understand what process they were undergoing and the risks and benefits involved in it. The researchers, of course, have taken the consent of the parents for enrolling in the research study. However, it was found that "[M]ost parents consented to this experiment on their children when the researchers told that the children, even if not the subjects of experimentation, would develop more serious cases of hepatitis once they mingled with the institution's general population" (Holder 1988, 141).

Some other factors also make the Willowbrook hepatitis study problematic. Though it may not be feasible to stop all research on children, since they are more vulnerable than others, the case of mentally disabled children definitely demands special attention. On the one hand, they are unable to give consent, and on the other, their status in the society and in their family may place them in the group of children who are in need of special care.

Krugman's experiment deliberately infected them with the virus and this scenario raises questions like whether the researchers treated them as persons or as mere objects of an experiment.

According to some critics, Krugman's experiment hardly benefits the participants. Instead, it harmed the mentally defective children by carrying out artificial induction of hepatitis. This is evidently against the World Medical Association's resolution. There is no right to risk any injury to one person for the benefit of others (Beecher 1966, 371). Again, selecting children, especially mentally disabled children, can hardly be justified, while conducting the same research study among adults who could exercise voluntary informed consent. The adults who work in the institution and who were exposed similarly to the disease were never used as subjects (Holder 1988, 142). However, these two criticisms cannot be justified as the study ultimately benefitted the children participants. The research was conducted primarily to control the endemic disease, which was found in Willowbrook School.

However, there is one important point which many critics have pointed out, which carry with it significant weight. As Krugman himself says, the primary reason for designing the research study and conducting it in Willowbrook is to control and eradicate hepatitis, which was endemic among the inmates of the institution. However, it was evident that the primary reason for the infection spreading at an alarming rate was the overcrowding and unsanitary conditions in the institution. The authorities and healthcare professionals had the responsibility to improve this situation since they knew that this was the primary cause of the problem. A research study should have been conducted elsewhere and not necessarily among children who are mentally disabled. The researchers seem to have taken advantage of this unhygienic scenario for conducting their experiment.

Krugman published a special article in the journal *Reviews of Infectious Diseases* in 1986, elaborately discussing the ethical aspects of the experiment he and his colleagues conducted in the Willowbrook School for about 15 years. He asserts that he remains as convinced as he was at the time the studies were conducted that they were ethical and justifiable and adds that this judgement is based on knowledge of the extraordinary conditions that existed in the institution as well as on an assessment of the potential risks and benefits of the participants (Krugman 1986, 157).

I have outlined only these three landmark cases, which expose a set of factors that may act as detrimental to ethical practices in clinical medicine and medical research. Several other examples can also be cited that took place during this time. However, these three events have drawn much public attention and forced the international community to rethink about the steps to be taken for ensuring moral practices. The Nuremberg trials, of course, mark the beginning towards formulating codes that could regulate human research. The codes delineate a set of broad bioethical principles that any research involving human experimentation needs to follow. The idea of consent is introduced here, along with other principles like no-harm and beneficence in their rudimentary form. A shift from the traditional approaches is visible in the formulation of the codes, even though the latter lacked any legal authority. The Tuskegee syphilis study brings out the need for being sensitive to the specific ethical problems that may surface when experiments are conducted among disadvantaged populations. It warns us about the possibilities of exploitation and coercion. The Willowbrook study, though, was ultimately beneficial to the society, enlightens us about the distinctive ethical problems concerning the experiments conducted on children and mentally disabled people. These two incidents also remind us how the vulnerable population is easily exploited in spite of several regulations and legal provisos in force. All these cases problematize the notion of consent and highlight the importance of respecting the status of individuals as persons and valuing their basic human rights. The Nazi experiments happened under a totalitarian regime, which had no respect and regard for human rights and other democratic values. But the Tuskegee and Willowbrook studies were conducted in a society, which prides on its democratic commitments. This factor reveals how exploitative scientific experiments can be, despite the presence of constitutional assurances about the protection of rights. This affirms the need for constant vigil and more initiatives at the national and international levels for the protection of individuals, particularly those who are disadvantaged. The Belmont Report published in 1979 has restated the importance of fundamental values that need to be evoked while human beings are being used as subjects in biomedical and behavioural research.

Changing Conceptions of Life and Its Values

The changes that have happened in the medical world during the past few decades, particularly since 1990s, are literally phenomenal. Such changes have enabled humanity to eradicate many life-threatening diseases through effective medication or vaccines. The life expectancy in many countries has substantially increased over the past few decades. While in 1990, the average life expectancy at birth for the world was about 64 years, in 2015, it had risen to more than 71 years. Though this was primarily viewed as one of the indicators of development, it more specifically points to one of the phenomenal advancements that have happened in the medical sciences in terms of new discoveries and technologies.

However, the consequences of the innovations in the medical field are not confined to the increase in life expectancy alone. There are more far-reaching impacts. The new medicines, clinical procedures and technologies that are available today have changed the way we conceive our own life and they have very deep impacts on our values. For example, the gender reassignment surgeries that are very commonly performed today among transgender people to change their primary and/or secondary sex characteristics. With such clinical possibilities, doctors now perform both male-to-female and female-to-male gender reassignment surgeries, where the procedures may include genital reconstruction, cosmetic surgery, voice modification surgery, mastectomy, etc. With such procedures, an individual may overcome his/her gender dysphoria, which refers to discomfort or distress that is caused by a discrepancy between an individual's gender identity and the gender assigned at birth (GRS 2020). Thus, a new clinical procedure has the potential to change the personal identity of individuals in society, both from biological and social perspectives. Such possibilities have suggested revolutionary changes in our self-image as we cease to treat our body as it is—natural and sacred. It is no longer a mere "given," as we can manipulate it and make alterations in accordance with our wishes. With such revolutionary changes happening to our engagements with our own body and identity, many of our long-established values were replaced with a new set of values and this scenario calls for new assumptions and possibilities.

Again, many diseases, which were believed to be fatal and life-threatening, are easily treatable today. Plague and smallpox are examples. TB, which was incurable and has killed a large number of people a few decades ago, is entirely curable today. The eradication of some of these diseases has led to the closure of many sanatoriums around the world and changed the lives of millions forever. Modern medicine thus adds different meanings to human life, kindling the hopes of millions of people, but it also raises several social, cultural, economic and moral issues. Some of them will be discussed in subsequent sections. The longevity revolution, along with the drastic changes in the family structure that happened in many societies, has engendered a moral crisis in such places. With the breaking of joint families in many societies, caring for the aged now needs to be outsourced. But the supply levels are inadequate to meet the high demand on this front. Medication and medical technologies, though are available, often are very expensive and many find it difficult to afford them. Many families turn bankrupt after the illness of a member. Though these are not typically ethical issues, they create several moral dilemmas and also a moral crisis in society by impacting relationships.

The Multidimensionality of Ethical Issues

Contemporary bioethics presents a range of issues, and in this sense, it drastically differs from traditional medical morality, which confined its scope to physician behaviour. The latter primarily addressed patients' expectations about their physicians, the way they are treated, the quality of care they receive, the reasonableness of the fee, and the effectiveness of the treatment. Since in traditional healing systems, patients and physicians are related to each other more intimately, patients make judgements about physicians' character from their behaviour in their professional and personal lives. Such judgements were critical in the whole process since those physicians who did not fit the image of the anticipated ideal failed to gain acceptance from society.

Moreover, contemporary bioethical issues like consent, confidentiality and patient autonomy had not surfaced in ancient medical ethics discussions. They became relevant only with the emergence of post-enlightenment ethical sensibilities, which began to acknowledge the individual as the focal point in moral evaluations. However, many traditional ethical concerns were retained by contemporary approaches as well. For example, patients' benefit and not harming the patient are equally important at all times. However, the traditional image of a physician as an honest and compassionate individual whose personal bond with his patients is a crucial element in his association with them is fading fast in the contemporary era. Physicians in many places now keep only a professional and impersonal relationship with their patients.

In short, the focus of contemporary bioethics is no longer the physician. On the one hand, bioethics ceases to be an exclusive business of the physicians. As David Rothman (1991) observes, "it was clear that the monopoly of the medical profession in medical ethics was over. The issues were now public and national – the province of an extraordinary variety of outsiders" (189). It thus becomes fundamentally interdisciplinary. Professionals from diverse backgrounds such as philosophy, law, medicine, biotechnology, political science, history, sociology, anthropology and policy studies contribute to its development and bring in diverse viewpoints to its evolution.

On the other hand, bioethical discussions are no longer confined to physician behaviour. They are expanding further rapidly to the consideration of other issues like the definition of life and death; the status of the embryo; legal, moral and safety considerations in the use of medical technologies; artificial reproduction; euthanasia; cloning; and procuring and using of stem cells. These issues have vast implications in many areas of human life and are in need to be explored from multiple perspectives. Hence, the sphere of bioethics derives its nourishment from different domains of human engagements. Social, political and economic considerations are equally important in understanding the real nature of the ethical issues involved. The sphere of contemporary bioethics is therefore drastically different from the domain of traditional medical morality.

Health, Medicine and Poverty

Major national newspapers in India report on 21 June 2019 that 142 children have lost their lives since 1 June 2019 due to Acute Encephalitis Syndrome (AES), popularly known as brain fever that has afflicted more than 600 children across 16 districts of Bihar. In Muzaffarpur district itself, 117 children died. The disease is linked to a toxic substance found in unripe litchi fruit, which was consumed by malnourished children from underprivileged backgrounds (India Today 2019). Incidents like this point to a very strong link between poverty and diseases. There are several other health issues like those caused by malnourishment, which is directly related to poverty. However, there are certain other facets to this troubled relationship between health and poverty.

Poverty is an important determining factor in a person's prospects for health, observes Susan Sherwin (2010), as it may negatively impact health, since it affects our access to adequate nutrition, housing, heat, clean water, clothing and sanitation. Again, the poor suffer higher rates of mental illness and addiction than others, and their financial situation may prevent them from seeking professional help before their disease reaches an advanced state (283). She adds that those who are oppressed by virtue of their gender, race, class, sexual orientation or disabilities will experience a disproportional share of illness and will often suffer reduced access to resources (284). Sherwin discusses the issue from the background of the North American society, which according to her is characteristically sexist, racist, classist, homophobic and frightened of physical or mental imperfections. However, such descriptions fit many other developing countries in the world today. In India, they are particularly true, as the society is truly multi-cultural, multi-religious and multi-lingual. The situation is further complicated by the presence of caste system.

Referring to the WHO and Word Bank data, the "MSF Access to Essential Medicines Campaign" of the Drugs for the Neglected Diseases Working Group publication, titled "Fatal Imbalance: The Crisis in Research and Development for Drugs for Neglected Diseases" (Berman and Moon 2001), observes that people in developing countries, who make up about 80% of the population, only represent about 20% of worldwide medicine sales and the imbalance between their needs and the availability of medicines is fatal. Quoting various other sources, this document further observes:

> There is a strong link between poverty and health. People from low- and middle-income countries carry a disproportionate burden of disease, particularly with regard to communicable diseases. Those living in absolute poverty (on less than one dollar per day) are five times more likely to die before reaching the age of five and two and half times more likely to die between ages of 15 and 59. Infectious and parasitic diseases account for 25% of the disease burden in low-and middle-income countries, compared to only 3% in high income countries. According to the World Bank, eliminating communicable diseases would almost completely level the mortality gap between the richest 20% of the population and the poorest 20%.

(10)

Hence, when we examine the ethical problems related to modern medicine from the perspective of factors like socio-economic backwardness, all such issues need to be considered. Besides, the cost of treatment makes many people poor or significantly adds to their poverty.

The scenario seems to be involving a vicious circle. Despite their ineffectiveness in treating many diseases, traditional medicine and indigenous healing systems were not inaccessible to any section of people in the society. They were not very expensive and physicians hardly prioritized charging a fee from their patients. Hence, poverty never prevented people from gaining the healing benefits offered by medicine. The situation is different in the case of modern medicine as institutional infrastructure is essential for its practice. The medical institution is constitutive of various other corporate institutions, including the pharmaceutical firms, research institutions, developers of various products and technologies required for the functioning of hospitals and laboratories. They gather the capital investment required for the sustenance of such a multifaceted institution from the end-users, i.e., the patients. The quality of care is, in a sense, proportional to the availability of better infrastructure and medicines, which, in turn, makes it expensive. The strict regulations governing pharmaceutical firms make new drug discovery a costly affair. The R&D is elaborate and time-consuming, which makes medicines costly and sometimes even prohibitively expensive.

The situation in developing countries is even graver as most developing countries lack facilities, where innovative scientific research in healthcare can happen. Therefore, they depend mostly on imports to meet their requirements. Since they are manufactured and imported from abroad, they are not always available unless there is a massive demand in the indigenous healthcare sector. Hence, much advancement in healthcare is not readily available or accessible to a large number of people who require them. This issue raises significant concerns regarding justice in healthcare delivery and accessibility.

Questions about Justice

The remarkable advancements in modern medicine have benefitted many in different parts of the world, and this is visible in the steep increase in the life expectancy of populations across different countries. However, it is ironic to note that a large section of people is not benefitted from such advancements and remains deprived of the benefits they could bring. Some countries in the world have benefitted more by such developments due to their advanced economic status and better healthcare management systems and infrastructure. On the other hand, some other countries are severely affected, as they are unable to afford the high purchasing cost involved in the delivery of modern healthcare and technologies. In many developing countries like India, the income disparity among its citizens is substantial and this makes a large section of people finding it hard to afford quality healthcare, even though it is available in these countries. In both these scenarios, the sad situation is that despite the availability of the resources, access to them is denied to people owing to economic factors. Income disparities are reflected as health disparities.

The United Nations Policy Brief on Social Justice and Participation brought out by the Economic and Social Commission for Western Asia (ESCWA 2013) defines social justice as a "normative concept centered on the principles of fairness, equality, equity, rights and participation." ESCWA further defines the principles of equality and equity. While equality refers to equal access to the public goods and resources of the society, such as education, information, healthcare, employment and job opportunities, equity assures fairness and equal opportunity for all by "striving to remove or overcome the barriers that hinder certain individuals and groups (e.g. people with disabilities and the poor) from fulfilling their potential, by maximizing their opportunities for advancement" (ESCWA). The principle of equality cannot secure this. Rights are divided into legal and moral rights, where the latter include human rights either incorporated into the legal system or like human rights are protected by adequate procedures, norms and rules. Finally, the principle of participation implies the involvement of people in the decisions that govern their lives for achieving better distributive outcomes and strengthening democracy. Among the various areas of inequality, the UN Policy Brief addresses the distribution of health services. It designs policies to improve health and life expectancy, the decline in infant mortality and reduction in the vulnerability of poor people. All these are done with the objective of reducing the inequalities in healthcare (ESCWA 2013).

Charlene A. Galarneau (1998) observes that justice, rights and obligations constitute the central ethical concepts invoked to address access to healthcare. According to her, the few common ethical questions regarding access that reflect these diverse elements are:

> Is there a right to health care? What does justice require regarding access to health care? What standard or level of access is appropriate? What is a just health care community and who belongs? Is there a societal obligation to provide access to health care?
>
> (306)

She adds that one approach to the ethics of access examines the implications of general theories of justice for healthcare, which understands justice as distributive and asks the question: according to which criterion—need, ability to pay, or merit—should the benefits and burdens of healthcare be distributed (307)?

Norman Daniels (2003) argues that the right to healthcare is a positive as opposed to a negative right (317). Hence, other people are required to contribute their resources or skills to benefit right-bearers, rather than merely refraining from interfering with them. Healthcare forms a part of a broader family of positive "welfare" rights that include rights to education and income support. Therefore, this right is more complicated, and it is hard to characterize its scope and limits. Daniels adds that society has the duty to its members to allocate an adequate share of its total resources to health. It has to ensure the just allocation of different types of healthcare services, taking into account the competing claims of different types of healthcare needs. According to him, each person is entitled to a fair share of such services, which includes an answer to the question, who should pay for the services (317)?

The scientific and technological constituents of medicine are making incredible progress, and this trend is likely to continue in the future as well. On the one hand, a steep increase in the creation of new technologies, the development of new medicines and establishing new infrastructure are anticipated. On the other hand, several social factors may create more demands for the facilities and resources available. However, such developments need not necessarily conclude in proper distribution of its benefits and drawbacks to everyone in society. Several inequalities exist in many human societies, particularly in developing countries. Several vulnerabilities too exist, as many developing countries have a significant number of disadvantaged people. Hence, it is important to form and establish proper structures and frame proper policies for the just distribution of healthcare in the society, which is inevitable for people to participate in several activities that design their life meaningfully.

In many developing countries, several factors contribute to social inequalities and injustices that exist even today. For example, in India, the caste system is still practised in many states, especially in the rural areas, which contributes to the inequalities and inequities that threaten a just scenario. However, the vision that recognizes health as a fundamental human right, which is getting popular in many democratic countries, makes inequalities in healthcare deplorable. Health, thus, becomes an essential component in deciding social justice.

Medicalization and Its Ethical Concerns

Medicine arts and systems across civilizations have always responded to various health problems people encountered. With the growth of medicine, more and more human problems received medical attention. For example, in India, *Ayurveda* has developed several specialized therapies for infertility. However, this has never been successful beyond a point and childless couples have depended mainly on other means like adoption. Infertility has always been a painful experience, which appeared to have no effective solution beyond a point, although many indigenous medical systems attempted remedies for it. But modern medicine began to address it in a huge variety of ways. Subsequently, infertility treatment now offers multiple options to individuals who desire to have their own children. Besides medication, there are several artificial reproductive technologies and other technological means. A large number of infertility clinics have mushroomed in different parts of the world, which employ a variety of technologies such as artificial insemination (AI), in vitro fertilization (IVF), donor conception, gamete intrafallopian transfer (GIFT), intracytoplasmic sperm injection (ICSI), and surrogacy. In addition to this, ART offers couples a variety of choices like gene editing, employing which they could eliminate several diseases, pre-implantation genetic testing (PGT) for reducing their risk of passing on a known genetic condition, etc. All aspects of reproduction, beginning from the sperm-egg union to childbirth, are now highly medicalized events that happen within hospitals under the supervision of physicians. However, these possibilities raise several ethical issues.

The fact that these technological possibilities are increasingly making human reproduction a medical event may have severe consequences for future generations of human beings. Reproduction may cease to be a natural event, and when required, people approach the hospitals for "producing" their children as per their aspirations. Sex will also cease to be an act that is essentially related to reproduction, as it becomes not inevitable for the latter. A couple can bring out their offspring without sexual intercourse and even by not being in the same place. This may be seen as an impact of medicalizing human reproduction.

Medicalization is a phenomenon that is common today with the remarkable growth of medicine in general and medical technologies in particular. Certain inconveniences are associated with many events in life, which humans hitherto have treated as natural and normal. Menstruation, pregnancy, menopause, obesity, anxiety, childbirth, ageing and death are some of them. There are certain habits—like adult thumb sucking and nail-biting—that cause concern and embarrassment. Traditionally, humans have addressed them and occasionally tried to overcome them, adopting several means. However, they were hardly approached as medical problems that called for therapeutic interventions. Modern societies attempt to tackle them by conceiving them as medical problems and seeking therapeutic solutions for them. This process is termed medicalization and this tendency is an integral feature of modern medicine. It redefines many phenomena, which were earlier regarded as the natural results of ageing or as part of the normal range of human emotions and reactions as diseases that require medical intervention (Kohli 2012, 255).

With medicalization, medicine establishes its authority over many non-medical events and features of human reality. Peter Conard (2007) observes that "the point in considering medicalization is that an entity that is regarded as an illness or disease is not *ipso facto* a medical problem; rather, it needs to become defined as one" (5–6). Conard adds that the medicalization of deviance includes alcoholism, mental disorders, opiate addictions, eating disorders, sexual and gender differences, sexual dysfunction, learning disabilities, and child and sexual abuse. It has also spawned numerous new categories, from ADHD to PMS to PTSD to CFS (6).

Several factors make our understanding and evaluation of medicalization difficult. In the course of their evolution, humans made several attempts to overcome their various constraints and these included physical and psychical deviations and deformities. One effective way in which this has been attempted is by medicalizing them and then finding out appropriate therapeutic remedies. However, this may add many of our habits, individual bodily features and emotional reactions to the list of medically problematic phenomena. This is done by positing a standard for normalcy and treating any mild deviation from the latter as a disease that demands medical attention. It substantially takes away our autonomy by labelling us as patients as it demonstrates the growing authority of medicine in our lives. The more we depend on medicine for solving our problems, the more we deprive ourselves of our autonomy and freedom. Peter Conard states:

> Critics have been concerned that medicalization transforms aspects of everyday life into pathologies, narrowing the range of what is considered acceptable. Medicalization also focuses the source of the problem in the individual rather than in the social environment; it calls for individual medical interventions rather than more collective or social solutions. Furthermore, by expanding medical jurisdiction, medicalization increases the amount of medical social control over human behaviour.
>
> (7–8)

However, while medicalization is a disquieting phenomenon, which concurrently happens with the triumphant progress of modern medicine, demedicalization too happens by which some problems, which gained medical attention earlier, ceased to be defined in medical terms and subsequently deemed no medical intervention. Conard thus argues that medicalization is bidirectional. Several phenomena that were treated as abnormal and were medically treated or socially stigmatized were later demedicalized and destigmatized. Examples for these include masturbation and homosexuality (8). Masturbation is no longer considered by the medical world as a medical problem that requires treatment. Further, phenomena like homosexuality which was once considered an "abnormality" and was stigmatized and even criminalized is no longer treated so. It is now decriminalized as well. Many such reversals are the result of the growing political awareness and democratization and secularization of society.

As discussed in the first chapter, in most ancient civilizations, an overarching moral community was present engrossing all members of the society and its shared moral environment facilitated the assessment and evaluation of the moral behaviour of all members. The active membership in this community made members responsible for its sustenance and obligated each of them to come together and function with a collective moral agency, rather than as individual moral agents of modern societies. Patients and physicians are components of this collective moral agency, albeit with different sets of obligations and commitments.

The absence of such an overarching moral community and the lack of any shared moral convictions made the practice of traditional medicine and the functioning of its obligatory moral framework difficult in today's social environment. With society becoming a system constituted of autonomous functional spheres, the notion of collective moral agency becomes archaic and irrelevant. Moreover, the nature of healthcare itself has undergone drastic changes, as from a set of healing practices based on customary norms and experiential procedures, medicine, in most societies, is radically transformed into a complex scientific and technological exercise. The scope of moral prescriptions is extended far beyond the ambit of patient–physician interactions. Consequently, the ethical concerns about the practice of medicine in the modern-day encompass issues that may arise not only in clinical practice but also the problems surfacing the whole medical ecosystem.

One general feature of modern life is its heavy reliance on scientific knowledge and technological know-how. This has made human life better in many ways. However, the use of medical technologies precipitates several complexities as well, as it engenders a manifold of ethical concerns.

Modern medicine widely employs state-of-the-art technologies for diagnosis, treatment and many other therapeutic purposes. However, they are often used for corroborating a model of the human body defined in terms of a machine. This machine metaphor has been dominant in European civilization, at least since the Cartesian revolution. Subsequently, any variation from the medically accepted standards is viewed as "abnormal" conditions that call for therapeutic interventions. Such "standardization" and "normalization" have become foremost medical concerns. This culture of medicalization further strengthens the rift that already existed in the society ever since the advent of enlightenment in the European world, as a consequence of societal modernization.

The modernization concurrently happened with the scientific revolution and changed the way medicine was conceived and practised. Medicine redefined itself as a complete science with very intricate methods and procedures of practice. This science needed to continually refine itself with better understanding and knowledge and the development of novel techniques and devices. The traditional model of a wise, compassionate and benevolent physician did not any longer fit into this framework. The institution of medical science finds it necessary to cooperate with the scientific institutions, pharmaceutical firms and other technology developers to meet the demands it encounters from within and without. On the one hand, it needs to explore and realize its immense potentials in contributing to human well-being, and on the other hand, it has to engage in those activities that will ensure the advancement of its knowledge base. The institution eventually is forced to function mainly as a corporate body. Redefining the role of physicians and other healthcare professionals, as well as patients, becomes inevitable in this context. Here, the professionally developed institution of medicine has to function as an autonomous entity with its interests and concerns. This is a consequence of the fragmentation of human life into different autonomous spheres due to societal modernization since the 18th century onwards. Such an autonomous status was inexorable for medicine as an institution to deliver its professional function in an increasingly modernizing society. The framework of values that regulated this paradigm of professionalism could no longer hang on to the medical morality of the traditional model.

In tandem with such developments, the society in large started realizing the need for conceptualizing its relationship with the medical institution, which was aggressively asserting its sovereignty. The conflict between the interests of the medical institution—which becomes identical with the interests of the medical professionals and organizations that create the infrastructure—and the varied interest of the members of the society needed to be amicably resolved. It was important to realize the total change in the relationship between various stakeholders and redefine it in terms of professional standards in order to accomplish a win-win situation. Members of the society had to be protected from possible coercion and exploitation from an autonomous institution. The rights of patients had to be protected since the old patient–physician relationship, where patients were related to their physicians, had become obsolete. Now they need to negotiate with a whole institution, which was economically and politically powerful. It is in this backdrop that biomedical ethics needed to be institutionalized, employing principles and well-articulated codes based on the new challenges.

The institutionalization of medical ethics focuses more on the ethical issues in the context of institutions than in relations between individual physicians and their patients. Hence, the emphasis shifts from individuals to institutions. The paradigm of medical ethics has now changed from the "guardianship model," where physicians served as guardians of patients' medical well-being or as trustees of their health, to a "corporate professional model" where physicians serve multiple interests by actively negotiating with them. On the one hand, physicians and other medical professionals have to act following the values of their organizations—hospitals, labs, research centres—and on the other, as professionals, they are obligated to their patients. They often encounter the clash between the market forces and the concerns for the well-being of their patients.

Another significant feature of the modern world is the globalization of modern medicine and issues related to this phenomenon. Though it originated in the West, the practice of modern medicine is now no longer confined to the Western world. Consequently, all the infrastructure ranging from hospitals to state-of-the-art laboratories and the industrial houses that produce technological equipment and other materials needed for the sustenance of the institution need to be established in all the places where it is practised. In many such cultural contexts, the philosophy of modern medicine conflicts with the philosophies of the indigenous medical traditions. Such conflicts may lead to several ethical issues. Medical institutions can no longer function as mere trustees, as the sustenance of the infrastructure needs substantial financial investment and their maintenance and management also need continued financial support.

Moreover, different cultural contexts may have different moral outlooks. Hence, it is practically and theoretically not feasible to advocate one single ethical perspective. The practice of modern medicine, therefore, will have to negotiate with different moral frameworks in different places. Hence, while adopting and accepting the validity of certain ethical principles as vital, modern medicine may have to find different means to apply them in different contexts.

Medicine and Bioethics in the Changing World

In the rapidly changing world, medicine is both a science and an industry. Hence, it needs, on the one hand, a solid knowledge base, which needs to be created and constantly renewed through research, and on the other hand, it has to generate profits consistently. It faces the challenges, which both science and industry face in the contemporary world. What makes it different from other industries is the fact that it is an enterprise, which actively deals with the lives of human beings. Its practice has to negotiate with the values that exist in society continuously. Hence, the usual standards followed both by science and industry are to be applied to healthcare with extreme caution. In its research endeavours, medicine requires the active participation of human beings as research subjects. However, unlike the inanimate and non-human animate world, there is the requirement that the subjects take part in research voluntarily, without even a trace of coercion, as many clinical research processes involve risks in various degrees. Nevertheless, these standards are often hard to comply with and very frequently conflict with other interests that are key to scientific research and industrial subsistence.

One important reason for the greater advancements and achievements of medicine in the past few decades is due to the integration of technological know-how into its practice at various stages. However, the flip side of this phenomenon is the fact that the integration of technology will also necessitate huge investments, which can be ensured only with a profit-making model. This makes the healthcare sector inaccessible and unaffordable to a vast majority of people. Consequently, the enormous benefits of this science remain a distant dream for a vast majority of people in society. The huge expenses for healthcare may also contribute to widening the rift between the rich and the poor.

The Changing World and the Change in Values

The changes in the contemporary world and the subsequent vicissitudes in the ways medicine is conceived and practised today have strong implications on values. These changes have pungently redefined the values that regulate the practice of medicine today. Such changes in values have altered the role of every stakeholder in the healthcare sector, namely patients, physicians, family members, hospitals and others who make up the entire healthcare ecosystem today.

However, the value environment of society is essentially a mix of religious beliefs, customary practices and conventions along with political awareness. They are not entirely disentangled from the social and cultural spheres in society. These social and cultural spheres jointly mould an intricate network of rituals, customs and conventions, which exert a regulatory power over social life as a whole. However, the fragmented contemporary life demands different moral evaluations, as it witnesses new issues that are made possible by the growing authority of science and technology. For instance, the technology for assisted reproduction available today introduces a set of novel challenges for the moral community to ponder. The possibilities of sex selection may allow families to maintain sex balancing, but may simultaneously raise serious questions about the processes of reproduction and childbirth. Again, with technological help, it is possible to know about disabilities, and after that, prevent "undesirable" childbirth. Here the concept of "undesirable" is problematic, particularly if it is perceived from a religious perspective. The concept of designer babies has attracted much attention today, and it also raises several moral quandaries. Surrogacy is another highly contentious issue. With the surrogate mother, a child can now have three mothers; the intending mother, the woman from whom the egg comes, and the surrogate woman who biologically carries the child in her womb for nine months. Such possibilities raise challenges to the accepted notions of parenthood and family. Can we treat the surrogate mother as a family member? Can the single parent and her cloned child constitute a family? Since many societies now accept same-sex marriage, can we consider such a couple constituting a family? All these are questions that we may ask when we consider the scientific and technological possibilities medicine offers today.

Perhaps, the most pertinent ethical issue that surfaces in biomedical ethics is in the context of patient–physician interactions. Traditionally, many significant moral concerns related to patients' well-being were addressed within the models rooted in the ideas of "social trustee professionalism" and "patients–family physician intimate bond." Conversely, what marks the present-day physician is not just an empathetic mind, as he/she may have to play several roles in the multifaceted healthcare institution. Beyond merely saving the lives of his/her patients, the physician may have to negotiate with the latter and facilitate what they consider is their well-being. The physician may have to accept certain choices her patients make, which she finds difficult to agree with. For example, abortion. Sometimes, the physician may not morally agree with the idea of abortion in the absence of any medical risk. However, in modern medicine, the views of the patients gain priority. Again, in some places, the physicians may even assist her patient's decision for passive or active euthanasia. She may have to make difficult decisions on resource allocation, disclosure of errors of self and colleagues, organ donation and maintaining confidentiality.

We thus see that the model of patient–physician relationship based on the idea of a "benevolent physician" is becoming increasingly obsolete and we now have to take into account the newly emerging professional health-care context, which witnesses a play of multiple interests—institutional, corporate, bureaucratic, patients'—that may often conflict with each other. Hence, the moral framework to be adopted today in order to address the ethical issues needs to be comprehensive enough so that it will be able to accommodate the concerns of various stakeholders and interest groups. More than codes, what is needed is a set of well-articulated regulations and protocols and their observance is to be ensured by law.

From Principles, Regulations and Law

The ethical codes of physicians emphasize the responsibilities of the physicians and they are mostly self-regulating in nature. The Hippocratic Oath is an example. The primary objective of the oath is to make the physician a person with a compassionate heart, integrity and character. In the present context, the oath has only a ceremonial value. It may boost the morale of the young graduate by instilling in her a sense of pride and solidarity. Most colleges use some versions of the oath, but hardly anywhere, the old Hippocratic oath is used verbatim. Moreover, even the content of the oath is inadequate to deal with the present situation, as it was not designed to address the scenario where modern medicine is practised. The focus of ancient medicine in most societies was physician behaviour and was suggesting the physicians a set of obligations. Modern medicine is not exclusively physician-centric. It ideally aims to be patient-centric and is concerned about the rights of the patients. Nevertheless, it brings together a large number of stakeholders, each pushing their interest in an open market system of free trading.

The oath and other medical codes practised in most ancient societies are inadequate in addressing the complexities involved in contemporary medical practice. There are important issues related to the use of modern technologies; the procedure followed; substances used in clinical research; legal and social requirements; and safety issues, which ancient codes of medical ethics cannot adequately address. Many modern societies witness a growing sense of individualism and the emphasis is more on the rights of individuals and groups. As mentioned earlier, one of the principles that found the normative concept of justice is rights. Most ancient ethical codes are more or less silent about the rights of the individuals. Again, an important feature of modern medicine is the constant updating of knowledge and improvement of technology with continuous research. The context of clinical research is marred with controversies and, therefore, is characteristically different from the context of clinical medicine, where the relationship between a physician and their patients comes into the picture. Research is primarily concerned with the development of new drugs and this sector regularly witnesses fervent competition between different pharmaceutical firms. Huge investments are made in this sector and now we witness a grand bargain between the pharmaceutical industry and society, where it is in tatters and public mistrust and resentment of the industry run feverishly high (Santoro 2005, 1).

All such factors that occurred as part of the historical development of human societies have induced radical changes in our ethical perspectives. However, the most important and immediate provocation that led to a paradigm change in the ethical approaches in medicine has emerged from the domain of medical research. A number of research initiatives in medicine conducted by physicians in different parts of the world disregarding fundamental moral aspects have ultimately led to the formulation of significant ethical principles in the 20th century. After the formulation of the Nuremberg codes, public uproar and criticism against the experimentations in Tuskegee and Willowbrook led to the preparation of the Belmont Report. All these documents have underlined the need for taking extreme caution and care while conducting research experiments on human beings. These documents can be regarded as global initiatives to arrive at commonly accepted norms and regulations.

These ethical norms and the principles that were developed later have been regarded to have some validity across different countries. But these ethical principles do not offer anything more than broad frameworks within which important ethical concerns can be addressed. They may not help us to adopt concrete steps towards finding solutions to the problems we encounter in actual situations. Many of these principles need to be further interpreted in the light of values that shape the lives of people in different places. The principle of respect for persons, for example, may find different applications in different places, as the moral status of a person in an individualistic culture substantially varies from that in a collectivist culture. Again, the meaning of autonomy varies drastically from culture to culture. We may find that virtually all principles have different intents in different cultural contexts.

Hence, it is not helpful to rely on ethics, which is entirely based on broad principles, as we may need to take appropriate actions in concrete contexts of life in society. We need more concrete suggestions and guidance, and here the need for translating the ethical concerns into legal frameworks becomes apparent. While conflicts involving bioethical issues are presented before the courts for adjudication, the judiciary usually consults the broad ethical norms and explores the feasibility in applying them in actual contexts. This journey from principles to regulations and from there to the law is nevertheless a difficult accomplishment. Despite overlaps, ethics and law have different concerns and applications. Hence, translating ethical concerns to the law is not always feasible, as a law is often well-articulated, intersubjectively intelligible and is enforceable through a legal process (Hazard Jr 1995, 458). Ethics, on the other hand, is not enforceable in this manner.

Contemporary bioethics focuses on the whole biomedical institution, the people who make it function, its norms and rules, procedures, and its relationship with society as a whole. It is also sensitive to the requirement of identifying a set of norms that would be shared by a large number of people. The principles of bioethics and several other bioethics concepts discussed today jointly encompass a vast domain of professional activity. Though they are not enforceable as the laws of a country, their regulative status is recognized even by courts of law of several countries. Many of them reflect the spirit of some fundamental democratic ideas and principles. For example, when courts in India adjudicate cases involving the issues of medical negligence or improper consent, they refer to the regulations and litigations existing both in India and other democratic countries like the UK, Canada and the United States. Though the principles themselves lack any legal authority, the behaviour of individual professionals as well as professional institutions is evaluated in the light of these principles and adjudicated accordingly. Contemporary bioethics primarily deals with such broad principles and their effective and intelligent application in actual situations.

4 The Focus of Modern-Day Bioethics

Introduction

An important feature that distinguishes modern medicine from traditional healing practices is its global acceptability and remarkable effectiveness. Modern medicine in most societies is delivered as a unified and standardized system of care. Though different countries have different ethical frameworks and different legal structures that guide and regulate its delivery, all these diverse forms of practice follow a universal system of healthcare science and philosophy. Though they situate in different cultural contexts, they all practise the same science of medicine with the same assumptions and presuppositions. The philosophy of modern medicine is entirely different from the indigenous systems of healing. It endorses the fundamental assumptions of modern science, which is evidence-based and is guided by observations and experiments conducted in advanced laboratories and is heavily dependent on modern technology. Unlike many traditional healing systems that advocate a holistic philosophy of life, modern medicine is enormously instrumental. Unlike the former, it never envisages an overall psychical and moral development of the patient. Instead, it tries only to find remedies to their immediate health problems.

Discussions in the previous chapters show that traditional medicine in most societies was a mix of religion, spiritual practices, magic, customs and several other practices. Religious beliefs played essential roles in the healing process in most of the ancient traditions. However, with the development of modern medicine, where medicine became a complete science, the religious, spiritual and other aspects of the healing process became irrelevant. Consequently, they were completely separated and discarded. Even today, the rift between science and religion is absent in the practice of traditional medicine in many societies. However, religion has hardly any role to play when it comes to the practice of modern medicine. Individual practitioners as well as patients may still believe in God, but the institution of medicine has no legitimate link with the religious beliefs and practices.

However, this rift is not the result of natural evolution. Modern medicine in the present day is not just an evolved form of traditional European

DOI: 10.4324/9781003312697-4

medicine. Instead, it owes its emergence almost entirely to the scientific investigations and theories that were developed with the advent of modern science in Europe after the Renaissance. Since Renaissance, the influence of religion over the European society started weakening gradually and with the advent of the Renaissance in the 15th century, this scenario changed drastically when the state took over the responsibility of granting certification to doctors. However, the church was still in control of the management of hospitals and it continued to institutionally care for the sick in the hospitals it established in different parts of Europe. After the Enlightenment period that had witnessed remarkable progress in natural sciences, medicine changed its approach towards various diseases. The new knowledge about nature and the deeper scientific understanding of the human body brought a revolution in the science of medicine. It developed new methods for diagnosis and treatment. Ultimately by 1802, with the end of the French Revolution, the separation between medicine and religion was nearly complete (Koenig 2000, 387–388).

The traditional moral frameworks prove inadequate in many parts of the world in dealing with the multiple ethical challenges evolving from the practice of modern medicine as the most effective healing system in addressing health issues. As a science, modern medicine has enormous potentials in making human life better. However, the scope of abuse is also abundant. Since the traditional moral frameworks do not have sufficient tools in addressing such aberrations, society will have to develop new regulatory mechanisms based on certain moral principles that human societies, in general, have been holding high. Chapter 3 discussed a few examples of systematic abuse of selected human populations employing modern medical knowledge. What was characteristic of such abuses was that those who were socially, politically, financially and physically disadvantaged and hence vulnerable invariably found themselves at the receiving end. In Nazi Germany, the Jews, mentally retarded and captured enemy soldiers; in the Tuskegee trials, the financially and educationally backward black Americans; and in the Willowbrook study, the mentally retarded children. In all these cases, they were victims of inhuman and unethical scientific experiments conducted by well-qualified scientists and physicians. Their in-depth knowledge in the respective disciplines never prevented the scientists from being unethical. They were highly accomplished scientists, but human beings with questionable moral esteem. This separation of good science from a good human being is at the root of the modern-day moral crisis.

The principal means by which modern medicine develops its knowledge base is through experimental scientific research. Research work that contributed to medical knowledge was carried out in different ways. Research in biochemistry has immensely contributed to the development of new drugs. Many medical innovations, such as novel methods in surgery, transplantation, reproductive technologies, stem cell research and cloning, have inaugurated several critical improvements in the world of medicine. Modern medicine, with its immense potential for biomedical research, suggests remarkable advancements in the ways humans conduct their lives today. The domain of modern medicine recurrently keeps expanding its frontiers and is triumphant in suggesting novel methods of cure for many ailments. Nonetheless, there are many common and rare health issues for which the contemporary world of biomedical science does not offer any effective remedies. This makes research an inevitable component of medicine, as new drugs, procedures and methods have to be discovered to meet this challenge. In many of the medical research projects, the participation of humans as research subjects is essential in proving the efficacy of their end product. No experimentation in modern medicine would be complete without human participation at some level and every human experimentation involves/poses a significant risk to the participants. This scenario presents a complicated situation, leaving abundant scope for coercion and exploitation of the vulnerable among the population. The three incidents discussed in the previous chapter are classic examples of such exploitation. They have become hallmarks in the history of bioethics, as they intensely evoke the public conscience by making people aware of the potential damages that scientific experiments can cause to humanity. Following considerable protests, there have been several formal initiatives to contemplate the moral requirements to be followed while conducting scientific research involving human participation. The Nuremberg codes, the Belmont Report and the Helsinki Declaration are a few such initiatives that have global significance. All of them attempt to articulate the fundamental prerequisites and requirements of ethical practices in modern medicine. Now, most countries have developed their ethical guidelines that specify the requirements researchers have to follow while conducting research that involves human participation. Most of these national guidelines fundamentally reflect the spirit of these global initiatives. The Indian Council for Medical Research (ICMR) also has come up with such guidelines. ICMR's revised ethical guideline document of 2017 has adapted important guidance points from several international guidelines such as the Federal Policy for the Protection of Human Subjects as the "Common Rule" published by the Department of Health and Human Services (DHHS), USA, in 1991 and revised in 2017; the Good Clinical Practice Guidelines E6 (R1) brought out by the International Conference on Harmonization (ICH) in E6 (R1) in 1996 and revised as E6 (R2) in 2016; and the recommendations/guidelines relevant to research in developing countries by the National Bioethics Advisory Commission, United States (2001), the Council for International Organizations of Medical Sciences (CIOMS), Geneva, in 2002 and revised in 2016, and the Nuffield Council of Bioethics, UK, in 2002.

The Nuremberg Codes

The International Military Tribunal at Nuremberg faced several challenges. The trials were controversial when they took place, but no one doubted the need for a substantial moral and legal reparation from the wrongdoers. The Chief Prosecutor for the United States at a war-crimes trial, Robert Jackson's states, "[T]he wrongs which we seek to condemn and punish have been so calculated, so malignant, and so devastating that civilization cannot tolerate their being ignored because it cannot survive their being repeated" (Jackson 2005).

This statement of Jackson reflects the general sentiment shared by everyone in the civilized world. There was a lack of clarity on the modus operandi of the trials, which had no precedent in human history. The allied forces who were to decide on the alleged perpetrators themselves had come from diverse ideological backdrops and the world leaders held differing opinions on what should be the fate of the offenders. Some of the world leaders, like Winston Churchill and Josef Stalin, wanted them to be summarily executed. However, the US Secretary of War, Henry L. Stimson, and the Supreme Court Justice, Robert H. Jackson, were in favour of a fair trial based on the principle of universal justice (King Jr 2003, 264). Finally, the decision was to follow the broad judicial framework of the British-American law. Accordingly, both prosecutors and defence attorneys were appointed to carry out the legal proceedings. The panel consisted of judges from all four Allied powers. Such standard procedures emphasized the importance of documentary evidence in the trial proceedings, and the defendants were declared acquitted wherever it was not present. They got the opportunity to appoint the attorneys of their choice and to present evidence. Ben Ferencz, one of the US Nuremberg prosecutors, observes, "the trials were just" and set "a precedent" for the ad hoc tribunals that would be established much later (Pitts 2001). Robert Jackson was also of the view that Nuremberg would have greater historic credibility if the cases were based on the defendants' sown documents (King Jr 2003, 264). In the Doctors' Trial that took place between 9 December 1946 and 20 August 1947, total 23 defendants were trialed, among whom 20 were doctors and 3 were administrators. Nuremberg is the genesis of the concept of universal jurisdiction (267).

Since 1931 in Germany, there were government guidelines which were required to be followed when therapeutic and scientific research on human subjects were conducted. However, it was evident that the defendants did not honour them. Further, as Brig General Telford Taylor, the Chief of Counsel for the Prosecution, noted in his opening statement for the prosecution that the Nazis had passed a law in 1933 itself to protect animals from being cruelly treated and to ensure their judicious use in experiments, but the defendants behaved with less humanity towards fellow humans than what was demanded by the animal protection law (Ghooi 2011).

The trial did not proceed smoothly, as the judges were addressing the question of human medical experimentation in which no one could guarantee the absolute safety of the participants. Moreover, a trial like this was unprecedented and it had no clear international guidelines available before it. Despite the inherent risks involved, human participation is an essential aspect of clinical research. However, at the same time, such research experiments should be very strictly regulated, and it was evident that the Nazi experiments never followed any such guidelines, even though they were available in their own country. The racial hygiene ideology created an environment in which they could treat any human being outside the German race as inferior. Hence, they refused to apply the norms and principles which they applied in the case of the latter to such inferior people.

Towards the end of the trials, the American physicians who were associated with the prosecutors submitted a few recommendations that would define ethically legitimate research involving the participation of human subjects. The tribunal ultimately developed certain guidelines that researchers have to follow while conducting what are known as "permissible medical experiments." These guidelines had no precedents and these guidelines formulated are significant as it was the first time such an attempt was made at the international level.

The tribunal articulates ten principles to be followed by all those who practise human experimentation, besides justifying "their views on the basis that such experiments yield results for the good of society that are unprocurable by other methods or means of study" (Mitscherlich and Mielke 1949, xxiv). Such principles are essential for ensuring legitimacy from moral and legal perspectives. These principles, laid out by the tribunal, are known as the "Nuremberg codes," which represent the first attempt at formulating ethical and legal codes that govern human research across the world. The ten principles can be summarized as the following (xxiii–xxv).

1. Voluntary consent.
2. The experiment should be such as to yield fruitful results for the good of society, unprocurable by other methods or means of study, and not random and unnecessary.
3. The experiment should be based on prior scientific knowledge about the disease and animal experimentation.
4. Avoid all unnecessary physical and mental suffering and injury.
5. If it is certain that death or disability will occur, researchers should refrain from experimenting.
6. The humanitarian importance of the experiment should exceed the risk involved in the experiment.
7. Ensure the protection of the subject.
8. The experiment should be conducted only by scientifically qualified persons.
9. The subject has the liberty to end the experiment at any time.
10. The researcher should be willing to terminate the experiment if he is convinced that its continuation may harm the subject.

The notion of voluntary consent, which is modified as voluntary informed consent, is central to the present-day medical practice, and from the perspective of contemporary medical practice in many advanced democratic countries, it is perhaps the most important one among the standards verbalized by the tribunal. Because scientific experiments may involve substantive risks, it is essential that it should be based on the previous results of animal experimentation and prior scientific knowledge. Moreover, they should yield fruitful results for humanity and aid common good. Reflecting the spirit of the age-old medical wisdom contained in the "no harm" principle, the codes categorically stressed the need for avoiding unnecessary pain, suffering, injury and the importance of weighing risks against expected benefits. It is imperative to stop the experiment at any stage, if its continuation is likely to cause harm to the participants. In order to ensure these aspects, the codes insist that the experiments should be conducted only by qualified professionals and the participants have right to withdraw at any point of time from the experiment.

The Importance of the Nuremberg Codes

The initiatives behind the formulation of the Nuremberg codes are remarkable, and the codes represent an important milestone in the development of modern-day bioethics. However, before acknowledging the importance of the Nuremberg codes, we need to understand some distinct features of the codes and their special status in the development of bioethics in the modern era. As indicated above, the tribunal's proceedings were marred by several controversies from the very beginning, and the prosecutors encountered several challenges that required elaborate negotiations.

Firstly, among the four nations that constituted the allied forces, there were several cultural, ideological and political disagreements. The US and the UK mostly shared the same Anglo-Saxon judicial system. However, the Soviet Union and France subscribed to different systems. The Soviet Union mainly found the Anglo-American idea of a court as an independent agency responsible only before the law as fundamentally problematic. For them, the court was one of the organs of government power and a weapon in the hands of the ruling class to safeguard its interests (Jackson 1949, vi). However, such differences were reconciled to a great extent and the trials proceeded intending to deliver justice. The trials roped in a large number of experts from different professions like law, military, medicine and the bureaucracy.

The codes were formulated towards the end of the trials reflecting the spirit of the moral and legal principles that were agreeable to the international community. In this sense, they represent the first initiative at the global level towards the formulation of ethical and legal norms that guide medical research involving human participation. Participants representing different traditions and cultures arrived at a broad consensus in the formulation of the codes. The surviving victims of the Nazi human experimentations and several physicians from the allied nations have significantly contributed to the process.

The importance of the codes can be summarized with the following three points. First, they represented the first full-fledged international effort with some authority—as it grew out of the trials that were jointly conducted by the four nations that constituted the allied forces that won World War II. Hence, though the codes lacked any legal status, they still enjoyed an unprecedented authority. Second, the authors of the code deliberately attempted to go beyond the Hippocratic Oath, which underlines the maxim of *primum non nocere*, meaning "first of all, do no harm," a principle that finds place in bioethics literature worldwide as nonmaleficence. In this sense, the codes represent the first modern-day initiative to articulate a framework of bioethics that goes beyond traditional medical morality. Third, with the articulation of voluntary consent, the codes inaugurate a new approach in bioethics. The notion of consent gives importance to the individual participant and his/her decision. Though the idea of "informed" consent was yet to be formulated, the notion of voluntary consent was recognized. This subsequently refers to the rights of the individual and later affirms his/her autonomy. Henry T. King Jr's (2003) observation about the Nuremberg trials in general is applicable to the medical trials as well. He says:

> Justice was triumphant at Nuremberg. The world is better for it. Nuremberg's impact is universal. Civilization took a giant leap forward at Nuremberg and now we have the opportunity to institutionalize Nuremberg permanently through the establishment of the International Criminal Court at The Hague. This is, indeed, a golden moment in history and we must make the most of it.
>
> (271–272)

The Nuremberg trials were the precedent of all the subsequent debates and initiatives on human rights and justice on the one hand, and on the other, the codes formulated following the Doctors' Trials constituted the precedent for all global initiatives in arriving at commonly accepted norms and regulations.

After Nuremberg: The Helsinki Declaration

Following these developments, the Third General Assembly of the World Medical Association (WMA) in London in October 1949 adopted the International Code of Medical Ethics, which outlined the duties of physicians, in general, to patients and to other physicians. The WMA codes emphasize certain principles such as maintaining the highest standards of professional conduct; patient's right to accept or refuse treatment; physicians not being influenced by personal profit or unfair discrimination; moral independence, compassion and respect for human dignity and honesty; respect the rights and preferences of patients, colleagues and other health professionals; educate the public; respect the local and national codes of ethics; respect human life, caring for the best interest of the patient; respect a patient's right to confidentiality; give emergency care as a humanitarian duty; and avoid abusive or exploitative relationship with patients.

Again in 1964, the WMA formulated a set of ethical guidelines for physicians and other participants in medical research, which is known as the Declaration of Helsinki. While the Nuremberg Codes focused on the human rights of research subjects, the Declaration of Helsinki focused on the obligations of physician-investigators to research subjects (Shuster 1997, 1440). In its preamble, it says that it is a statement of ethical principles for medical research involving human subjects, including research on identifiable human material and data (WMA 2013, 2191).

The declaration emphasizes that safeguarding the health of the people is a physician's primary duty, and it reminds that in medical research on human subjects, the latter's wellbeing is more important than anything else. It asserts that the physicians who are involved in medical research have the duty "to protect the life, health, dignity, integrity, right to self-determination, privacy, and confidentiality of personal information of research subjects" (2191). Besides, the Helsinki Declaration affirms the importance of minimizing all possible harm to the environment while conducting medical research.

Physicians are often tempted to involve their patients as participants in their research activities. This may not only save time but is also convenient, and physicians may get participants without many difficulties. However, this may lead to several forms of exploitations, considering the power asymmetry that exists in the patient–physician relationship. The Declaration cautions physicians, who combine medical research with medical care, and states that this could be done only if the participation in research is justified by its "potential preventive, diagnostic or therapeutic value and if the physician has good reason to believe that participation in the research study will not adversely affect the health of the patients who serve as research subjects" (2192).

The Helsinki Declaration further urges physicians to make a careful assessment of the risks, burden and benefits involved in a research study. Risks may be inexorable, but it is imperative for physicians to try to minimize its intensity by weighing them against the foreseeable benefits to humans. Extra care should be taken when research is conducted involving vulnerable groups and individuals, as they may not be able to give informed consent. The Declaration affirms that no such study should be conducted, involving vulnerable individuals, unless it directly benefits them. Hence, conducting the study among non-vulnerable individuals is useless. A research ethics committee's comment, guidance and approval is mandatory for all such research studies, as public accountability and scrutiny are essential for ensuring the safety of the participants. Finally, it is the responsibility of the sponsors, researchers and host country governments to make provisions for post-trial access for all participants who still need an intervention.

Paul Ndebele (2013) notes that this point concerning the post-trial access gets added in the latest version of the Declaration of Helsinki, and it is more relevant to countries with limited resources. He argues that the possibility of exploitation in such countries is high as

> communities may be used for testing interventions that will not be accessible to their citizens because of high costs and other reasons such as logistical challenges in delivering the new interventions outside the research environment. ...This requirement serves to recognize that research can play an additional role in improving access to care in limited-resource settings.
>
> (2145)

Many critics have pointed out several internal problems of the Helsinki Declaration and a few of its limitations as a global document of research ethics. Ezekiel J. Emanuel (2013), for example, argues that there are many problems with the current version of the Declaration such as incoherent structure, confusion of medical care and research, addressing the wrong audience, making extraneous ethical provisions, including contradictions, containing unnecessary repetitions, using multiple and poor phrasings, including excessive details and making unjustified, unethical recommendations (1532). Ezekiel acknowledges the role of the Helsinki Declaration in developing a set of global regulative principles, which not only prevents exploitation but also positively contributes to further the progress and development of modern medicine. He thus argues that the attempt of the Declaration of Helsinki to establish the universal minimum standard for ensuring ethical research is unethical. He says that we should aspire for a universal document that can be tailored to local circumstances by specification in the laws of individual countries. Similarly, to be authoritative, the Declaration must pronounce what might be considered "tentative immortality" (1532).

Belmont Report and the Bioethical Principles

There is hardly any document that has exerted more influence in determining the ethics that regulate research with the human subject than the Belmont Report, brought out by the National Commission for the protection of Human Subjects of Biomedical and Behavioral Research in 1979. The authors of the Report were given certain tasks such as: identify the boundary between research and practice, determine the role of risk-benefit analysis in human subject research, outline appropriate guidelines for subject selection and provide criteria for what constitutes genuinely informed consent (Friesen et al. 2017, 15). The report outlines three ethical principles for conducting research involving human subjects: respect for persons, beneficence and justice. The first principle of respect for persons implies the recognition of every individual as an autonomous human being who has the right to self-determination. This principle further explicates the norm of voluntary consent articulated by the Nuremberg code and other important codes developed afterwards. An individual is capable of consenting to an experiment voluntarily because he/she has autonomy. However, though self-determination is a right, not everyone is equally endowed with the ability to determine his/her own life and is capable of doing so. There are people with incomplete autonomy like children and diminished autonomy like mentally disabled people or people with certain diseases. However, they too deserve to be respected as persons because they are members of the human race.

The Belmont Report affirms that the researchers should positively act towards securing the wellbeing of their research subjects and carefully try to avoid engaging in any procedure that may irreversibly harm the participants. Every research must lead to scientific knowledge that would benefit humans. At the same time, participation in experimental research as a human subject may involve some risk. Hence, the researcher must judiciously perform a risk-benefit analysis before initiating the research process. It is equally important for the researcher to be able to justify the harm that is inevitably involved in the research process. The third principle of justice upholds that there should be equitable distribution of the benefits and burdens of research. Arriving at such a balance is key to any ethical research. Many researchers, such as the Tuskegee syphilis study, were fundamentally unethical because of their failure to strike such a balance. In such cases, the research subjects invariably suffered all the pains and burdens of the research, while others benefitted from the knowledge created from them.

Whether it is the Nuremberg Code or the Declaration of Helsinki or the Belmont Report, all of them represent various vital initiatives aimed at arriving commonly accepted norms and regulatory principles when scientific research is conducted with human beings recruited as subjects. Before I discuss these historic research abuses, it is important to see the context that makes a unique form of moral reasoning possible.

Some Important Contemporary Bioethics Concerns

One way to understand the nature of contemporary bioethics and to know how it differs from traditional medical morality is to analyze and understand the impacts of prominent principles or concepts, procedures, technologies and phenomena that define the practice of modern medicine on our moral sentiments. In other words, the very idea and practice of contemporary bioethics exist around them. Certain issues have surfaced during the past few decades due to the revolutionary progress made by medicine. Some issues that were already existent have acquired new dimensions of meaning in the changed context. The specific concerns of modern bioethics are mentioned in the global documents mentioned above. I try to summarize them in the following table. Although this is not an exhausting list, it nevertheless defines the face of the contemporary bioethics. Most of these are either not relevant in the context of the practice of ancient healing traditions or had different meanings in the ancient contexts.

The Social Environment of Modern Medicine	Principles of Modern Medicine
• Longevity	• Autonomy—due to individualism
• Vulnerability	• Confidentiality
• Exploitation	• Privacy
• Trust and trust erosion	• Consent—as a principle
• Brain death	• Rights
• Medical error	• Respect
• Public health	• Gender sensitivity
• Research	• Paternalism
• End-of-life decisions	• Dignity
• Advance directives	• Brain death
• Artificial reproduction	
• Euthanasia	
Procedures in Modern Medicine	**The technology Used in Modern Medicine**
• Consent—as a procedure	• Organ harvesting/donation
• Decision-making	• Artificial reproduction
• Disclosure and non-disclosure	• Genetics: stem cells, gene editing
• Placebo	• Cloning
• Resource allocation	• Ventilators

It is evident that the environment of modern medicine, mentioned here, was alien to the ancient healing traditions, and they never employed these principles, procedures and technologies in the practice of their profession. All these are phenomena that give rise to a range of ethical dilemmas that the ancient medical morality never had to encounter.

The Social Environment of Modern Medicine

Modern medicine has created a unique social environment, with its vocabularies and protocols that define and understand the social reality around it in a peculiar manner. For example, there are specific ways in which fundamental terms related to medicine are defined. Who a patient is and the ways in which she should relate herself to the world and other people are prescribed. Furthermore, it redefines virtually every human condition as a medical condition and develops a whole world of knowledge around it. It is not that medicine is unidirectionally defining social reality or is creating it. Nevertheless, the peculiar ways in which modern medicine constructs knowledge about the individual and how it is practised generate some fundamental ethical anxieties. For example, unlike traditional medicine, the practice of modern medicine requires an objective documentation of patient's various bodily functions and the peculiar features of her health problem.

The availability of this information in the public domain may hamper the interests of the individual patient in many ways. If this information is made available to others, they may make use of it for various purposes, which may directly or indirectly affect the individual patient adversely.

Such situations make concepts like "individual privacy" and "confidentiality" relevant in addressing the ethical issues arising in this context. Implemented as normative ideals, they become values that regulate behaviour of different stakeholders in the present social and particularly healthcare context. Confidentiality has never been a major ethical concern for ancient physicians. It is not that ancient physicians never cared for the privacy of their patients, but how confidential information matters in the modern social context makes the practice of guarding it extremely important now. The documented patient details may reveal vital information about her personal life and also about how her body functions.

I have identified a set of such concepts that make up the social environment of medical practice in different parts of the contemporary world. Of course, different cultures are not receptive to these norms and they do not try to address the moral anxieties in the same manner. More individualistic cultures like that of the United States ascribe very different meanings to them than countries like India and Pakistan, where the community identities are still active, and families are still influential in taking fundamental medical decisions. Nevertheless, the ideas of confidentiality and individual privacy, particularly about the medical information of individuals, are critical bioethical norms in all cultures where modern medicine is practised.

Another related idea that is central to contemporary bioethics is vulnerability. Vulnerability is the situation where one is unable to protect one's integrity owing to susceptibility to physical or emotional weakness or both. This may fundamentally harm the person who is vulnerable as she finds it unable to defend and protect herself. She may find herself in a situation where she is not able to act in her best interests. Situations of vulnerability may lead to losing control over one's life due to several reasons, and consequently, one may fail to maintain dignity. Several situations may potentially make an individual vulnerable, such as social and economic backwardness and minority status. Diseases can also make individuals vulnerable, as they lose their integrity and autonomy and may be forced to depend on others for their daily activities. In the context of medicine, one primary domain that is concerned with vulnerability is medical research. The controversial research studies discussed in this chapter—the Nazi experiments, the Tuskegee syphilis study, and the Willowbrook study—were all conducted among the vulnerable groups of individuals. Many of the modern medical ethical principles are derived from the concern to protect individuals who participate in medical research.

In the context of clinical practice, the vulnerability of patients is a primary ethical concern, and several measures are adopted in order to overcome it so that patients would be able to retain and maintain their integrity and autonomy, at least partially. The main problem with vulnerability is the dependence it creates. The patient finds herself dependent on the physician and, on certain other occasions, also on her relatives. Ideally, the context of medical interaction should aim at empowering the patient to regain her integrity.

The condition of vulnerability may lead to the exploitation of the patient and may ultimately harm her, physically and/or emotionally. Often medical decisions are imposed upon her, and in that way, it hampers her autonomy as well. Another important ethically relevant concept in this context is a patient–physician trust (PPT). Situations of vulnerability may make the idea of PPT extremely significant in the context of healthcare. Traditionally, PPT has a significant place in patient–physician relationships, and early physicians enjoyed the unshakable and unconditional trust of their patients. One reason for this is the model of trusteeship medical practice that existed during those days. Moreover, healthcare was never a commercial endeavour, and this made the practice of medicine an exclusive interaction between individual patients and their physicians.

Trust is an important virtue even today. By affecting patient attitudes and behaviours, it impacts the effectiveness of treatment (Plomp and Ballast 2010, 262). However, its meaning and function in the context of contemporary healthcare are different. In many developing countries, the environment of trust that permeated medical practice in the early days still holds good. This scenario gives physicians the opportunity to push their decisions on their patients, which provides room for coercion and exploitation. Hence, it is not conducive to the present situation. The modern scenario requires migrating to a different model of trust, which includes the transparency of following procedures and regulations.

Another defining aspect of modern healthcare is research. As mentioned earlier, the evolution of modern bioethics principles is the product of moral concerns raised by several instances of unethical clinical research that took place in different parts of the world. This factor is one feature that makes it distinct from most of the ancient healing traditions. Modern medicine develops with continuous and persistent research, which requires the participation of human subjects. The fact that every research involves some inherent risk to the participants or communities that are involved as research subjects imposes a prerequisite upon the researchers to make explicit provisions for ensuring their protection. Every research study needs to be designed in such a way that the protection of the participants is built into their very scheme. The ethical prerequisites of medical research with human participants are articulated in terms of certain general principles that emphasize aspects like essentiality, voluntariness, non-exploitation, social responsibility, privacy and confidentiality, risk minimization, professional competence, maximization of benefit, institutional arrangements, transparency and accountability, totality of responsibility and environmental protection (Mathur 2017, 3–4).

Confidentiality of information, vulnerability due to susceptibility to physical or emotional weakness, and the necessity of protection from harm are some direct bioethical concerns that give shape to the social environment of modern medicine. Besides, the practice of modern medicine has given rise to certain phenomena, which have definite social ramifications that may raise serious moral anxieties. For example, the longevity revolution happened across different countries, which is the result of various social and economic factors, including improvements in healthcare. It is a fact that the life span of people has increased considerably, and the advancements in medicine and better accessibility to healthcare facilities are the primary reasons for this. Longevity is not necessarily a modern phenomenon. Earlier also some people lived longer than others. However, a steep increase in the life expectancy of the people in a society as a whole is a new phenomenon. The positive interference of medicine plays a vital role in this.

Several factors have contributed to the increase in life expectancy, which include better awareness, better hygiene practices, availability of nutritious food and quality drinking water. Nevertheless, the role of modern medicine in this achievement is incontestable. The development of various drugs, several procedures and better vaccines for contagious diseases has positively contributed to the longevity revolution. The Statement of the United Nations Population Fund in 2002 states that two-thirds of persons aged 60 years and over, approximately 374 million, live in developing countries, compared with around 231 million in developed countries. By 2020, the number of older persons in developing countries is projected to nearly double to 706 million and rise to 317 million in the wealthy, industrial countries (UAPA 2002). This phenomenon is going to pose several challenges to nations as well as to the international community.

As stated above, longevity is, to a great extent, a direct consequence of improvements in the healthcare system. Modern medicine has not only helped people to live longer, but also has significantly reduced the number of child mortality. However, the challenges older people would pose in different countries are not something the world of medicine alone can tackle. Of course, the development of new and better geriatric medicines and other caring facilities can help in providing quality living to millions of aged people in the world. However, a large number of older people would also bring with them more problems associated with disabilities, physical and emotional ailments and cognitive frailties. The challenge to ensure quality life is very great, as it requires enormous resources, careful planning and appropriate policy initiatives. All these challenges raise equally serious ethical issues.

Another set of concepts that has become relevant in this context is unique to the contemporary healthcare system: end-of-life care, palliative care, death with dignity, etc. End-of-life care is not necessarily a procedure unique to modern medicine. Since the olden days, people who reached the end stage of their lives have been cared for differently. However, in modern medicine, this process adopts a different approach than its usual treatment protocols. Here the physicians, relatives of the patient and sometimes, the patient herself are aware of the imminent death, and any further medical intervention proves to be futile. At this stage, the patient requires medical support from the professionals and emotional support from the family. The aim of the medical support, nevertheless, is not for prolonging life, but for reducing pain and other discomforts and enabling the patient to die with dignity.

One crucial ethical decision involved in the process is the decision to limit life-sustaining therapy, which is available in modern medicine in various forms. Life-sustaining therapy is either withdrawn, whereby it is removed, or withheld by not providing any therapeutic escalation. These decisions are to be taken in the best interests of the patient and with the consent of the family (Chakravarty and Kapoor 2012, 203). The idea of an advance directive becomes relevant in such situations. Such directives represent a person's wish regarding what needs to be done if she loses her mental capacity for decision-making. The 2018 Supreme Court judgement in India concerning passive euthanasia recognizes the official validity of such directives.

Palliative care is another procedure, which is gaining immense popularity in the contemporary world. The World Health Organization defines palliative care as

> an approach that improves the quality of life of patients and their families facing the problem associated with life-threatening illness, through the prevention and relief of suffering by means of early identification and impeccable assessment and treatment of pain and other problems, physical, psychosocial and spiritual.
>
> (WHO 2018, 5)

Palliative care is, again, not a procedure unknown to ancient healing traditions. However, modern medicine practices it more systematically, following several procedures and administering proper medication aimed explicitly at specific objectives. It is said to be essentially affirming life, and it regards dying as a normal process, neither to be hastened nor to be unnecessarily postponed (Chakravarty and Kapoor 2012, 204).

The erosion of trust, as indicated above, is also one important characteristic feature of healthcare today. One reason for this is a large number of scams involving physicians and hospitals, which receive enormous media attention. The corporate interests of hospitals and pharmaceutical firms are no longer secrets. There is reasonable public awareness about many such illegal and immoral practices that have contributed to the erosion of trust. However, it is also not very uncommon that physicians and other healthcare professionals do commit errors in their judgements while administering drugs that may often become fatal to the patients. Medical errors are, therefore, a common phenomenon. A large number of medical errors that happen in hospitals across the world and the attempts by doctors and hospitals to cover up their mistakes have further contributed to the erosion of trust.

A medical error refers to a failure in the treatment process that leads to, or has the potential to lead to, harm to the patient (Aronson 2009, 514). Since the drugs administered have to be taken with care and caution, any mistakes in the prescription, dosage and administration of drugs may cause harm to the patient. Many other therapeutic procedures, including surgeries, have to be carried out with extreme care. Errors can happen if due care is not given while carrying out these procedures, and this is one aspect that distinguishes modern medicine from ancient healing traditions. Medical errors were common at all times. However, the fact that modern medicine uses drugs and employs procedures that can potentially harm patients in the absence of extreme care makes its practice more susceptible.

Another aspect of modern medicine that defines the nature of the social environment of medicine is the various endeavours that are carried out for the sake of safeguarding public health. More than the mere practice of individual physicians, modern healthcare infrastructure consists of a massive establishment. It adopts various measures to improve peoples' health, which include planning of public spaces, better sanitation facilities, making available drinking water and nutritious food, controlling the sale and distribution of various products like beverages and cigarettes, etc. The various public health measures adopted by governments and other agencies are significant public health initiatives. Unlike the usual bioethical concerns, where the focus is more on the individual patient and how she is affected by the healthcare infrastructure, public health ethics focuses on the design and implementation of measures to monitor and improve the health of populations. It also focuses on the structural conditions that promote or inhibit the development of healthy societies (Coleman et al. 2008, 578).

Modern medicine has decisively interfered with natural phenomena like birth and death. Besides radically medicalizing these processes and making them medical events, developments in medical sciences have now opened new possibilities and have provided new definitions to all those aspects of human reproduction, pregnancy, birth and death. The concept of brain death has already replaced the traditional conception of death. Since brain death is a condition in which an individual may continue to breathe, the standard procedures we adopt for establishing the death of a person cannot ascertain brain death. It often needs the facilities of ICU and expert healthcare professionals. However, the fact that it serves the interests of organ harvesting makes it more acceptable to the modern world. Moreover, it may be helpful to the family of the patient, who may otherwise have to undergo several agonies and uncertainties associated with determining the death of the person.

Reproduction, pregnancy and childbirth are other natural phenomena which have been medicalized in the recent past. Though the interference of modern medicine in these fields has generated several ethical anxieties, they have also been immensely beneficial to humanity. These issues, related to birth and death, are discussed in the following two chapters.

Technologies

We have already discussed the important ways in which technology constitutes the practice of modern medicine today. Traditional physicians have hardly employed any technologies, and their methods were characteristically different. *Ayurveda*, for instance, confined its diagnostic procedure to a ten-fold examination schedule. They emphasize on three important aspects to arrive at the right judgement; *darshana* or seeing the patient, *sparshana* or touching her and *prashna* or asking her certain questions (Babu et al. 2012, 33–34). With these three means, the ancient *vaidyas* used to make their diagnosis. They would arrive at a conclusion about the patient's bodily deficiency and imbalances (*dosha vaishamya*), and would prescribe appropriate medication and diet in order to regain the equilibrium (*dosha samya*). What modern medicine considers the fundamental causes of diseases are not matters of concern for them. The diagnostic methods adopted by modern medicine enables modern physicians to delve deep inside the body to locate the external microscopic causes of diseases and a scientific understanding of their biochemical constitution facilitates medical science to design remedies for the problems they have caused.

I have already discussed the ethical problems and dilemmas modern medicine generates due to the extensive use of technology. It is a fact that the practice of modern medicine heavily relies on the use of technology and this has very often facilitated accurate diagnosis and flawless therapeutic interventions. This wide-ranging and deeply permeating employment of modern technology raises a very fundamental philosophical problem by making patients' descriptions of their illness virtually irrelevant. It intervenes all physician–patient relationships and replaces those three basic elements of medicine since ages: seeing, touching and conversation that constitute the heart of all healing processes. The physician's primary data ceases to be the description of the patient, which now becomes unreliable due to the subjective elements present in human feelings and descriptions. More emphasis is given to the output from the machine. Instead of the physician's hands, the patient is "handled" by the various sophisticated machines, and conversation becomes unnecessary as the diagnosis is made based on technological data.

This critical note may sound techno pessimistic, which is not only counterproductive but also detrimental. We need to critically engage with technology, which has ubiquitous presence in modern medicine. The problem does not lie in the employment of technology, as the evolution of medicine today does not happen independently of technology. The problem lies with the shifting of focus from the patient, and this is the primary ethical concern modern medicine encounters in the present scenario.

Principles

The principles that define the field of bioethics in the contemporary world respond to a wide range of ethical concerns that are peculiar to this age. I have already discussed how confidentiality is important in the contemporary scenario. Similarly, patients by and large prefer their physicians revealing information about their diseases, and they appreciate better communication practices, where they are treated as equals and are consulted to decide options in the light of their values. The old concept of "physician as a guardian" no longer holds supreme and more participatory models of clinical interactions gain preference over physician paternalism that existed during the early days. This past image of the physician, as the beneficent and compassionate professional, cannot be separated from the image of the physician who thinks that he knows better what is suitable for the patient. Reciprocally, the patients, too, have believed so and trusted their physicians. The paternalist physicians never value truth-telling, and believe that reassuring the patient is always crucial in the therapeutic process. They believe their duty consists of accentuating the positive and downplaying the negative, which are therapeutically efficacious (Wear 1998, 34).

Many ancient healing traditions highlight the principle of beneficence, along with the no-harm principle. Physicians are expected not to engage with anything that may harm the patient, and all therapeutic decisions are ultimately made for the benefit of the latter. The Hippocratic Oath urges physicians to benefit their patients, and here, they have to rely upon their own understanding and judgement. Here it is the responsibility of the physician to determine the patient's best interests. In this sense, beneficence is hardly distinguishable from medical paternalism. It is a fact that, in most healing traditions across different cultures, paternalism was the dominant and accepted model of the clinical relationship (Pellegrino and Thomasma 1987, 25). Since trust and belief played key roles in the therapeutic and curing processes, hardly anyone challenged the authority of the physicians. A paternalistic physician supersedes his/her patient's preferences or choices, as he believes that he knows better what is good for his patient. By imposing his decisions, he is benefitting or avoiding harm to the latter.

In the 20th century, when contemplations began to ascertain the nature of bioethical principles that could respond to the requirements of the age, the idea of beneficence was not completely discarded. In 1978, when the Belmont Report was framed to provide the necessary moral framework for conducting biomedical research, beneficence was included as one among them, in addition to respect for persons and justice. In this context, beneficence had a broader meaning incorporating the ideas of not harm, risk-benefit balancing, maximizing benefits and minimizing harm.

However, with the development of the principlist approach by Tom L. Beauchamp and James F. Childress (1994), the principle of autonomy gains precedence over most of the other ethical principles. Although Beauchamp and Childress affirm that all these principles are equally important, it is not hard to see how beneficence and nonmaleficence were defined in the light of the principle of autonomy. Beauchamp and Childress have also distinguished the "do no harm" principle from beneficence, which they called nonmaleficence. Finally, to map the ethical concerns of the society in general and public health in particular, they have introduced the concept of justice. Beauchamp (1995) describes the context in which the principlist framework was designed in the following way:

> Health professionals' obligations and virtues have for centuries been framed by professional commitments to provide medical care, to protect patients from the harms of disease, injury, and system failure, and to produce benefits that compensate for any harms introduced. These obligations have been expressed through rules of nonmaleficence and beneficence, and our principles build on this tradition. ... But our structure of principles also reaches beyond these commitments by including parts of morality that traditionally have been neglected, especially respect for autonomy and justice.

(182)

The Principlist Approach

Since the Enlightenment, there was greater awareness about individual and political rights, which, with the democratic sensibilities getting prominent, began to permeate and dominate our ethical deliberations in all spears of life. The concept of patient autonomy reflects this spirit within the purview of healthcare. It not only empowers the individual patient to check physician paternalism effectively but also elevates her moral status by recognizing her as a moral agent, who is capable of making choices about her life. Beauchamp and Childress (1994) use the concept of autonomy to examine decision-making in healthcare, and they contend that their account should be adequate to identify what is protected by rules of informed consent, informed refusal, truth-telling and confidentiality (120).

The principlist approach is attempting to develop a concept of personal autonomy, which is distinguished from political self-rule, as the term "autonomy" is generally used in the context of political philosophy. By emphasizing two conditions of liberty and agency, autonomy is conceived as a personal rule of the self that is free from both controlling interferences by others and from personal limitations that prevent meaningful choice, such as inadequate understanding (121). These conditions are a bit misleading. Liberty, particularly, insists that a person is autonomous only when she is free from controlling influences. This idea reflects Kant's idea of enlightenment, in which he defines enlightenment as freedom from all self-imposed tutelages. The question is if autonomy requires freedom from all those factors that may determine a person's choices, is it possible to ever achieve it? Are we not always conditioned by one or other external factors at different levels? Does this condition amount to suggest something like an external platform like universal rationality to be treated as an ultimate arbiter?

Here Beauchamp and Childress adopt not a form of Kantian formalism, which has hardly any place in the practical world. Their criterion never insists on complete freedom from constraint, in which there is a complete absence of any external influence. Therefore, they never treat fully or completely autonomous decision-making by patients as a requirement. Actions only require a substantial degree of understanding and freedom from constraint. The ideal of absolute liberty is a myth, and there need not be any inconsistency between autonomy and acceptance or submission to the authoritative demands of an institution, tradition or community that they view as a legitimate source of direction (124). This aspect is essential in understanding the principlist framework developed by Beauchamp and Childress, as it never presupposes individuals to be completely free from all religious beliefs and social conditioning in order to be able to exercise autonomous choices. They are never presumed to be emanating from any ahistorical platform. Nevertheless, they can be autonomous, and it is essential to respect such choices. While discussing the concept of competence in this connection, Beauchamp and Childress state that it is determined primarily by whether a person can decide autonomously, and not by whether a person's best interests are protected (141).

The principlist framework draws a lot from the liberal tradition of philosophy, particularly from the thoughts of Immanuel Kant and J.S. Mill, in order to ascertain the need for respecting individual autonomy. Kant's idea of the inner worthiness of all human beings and his insistence on treating all human beings as ends in themselves reiterate the importance of autonomy. Mill (1864), on the other hand, has emphasized the importance of individual liberty. He warns against the tendency in the society, "to fetter the development, and, if possible, prevent the formation, of any individuality not in harmony with its ways, and compel all characters to fashion themselves upon the model of its own" (13–14). Mill further adds:

> The only part of the conduct of anyone, for which he is amenable to society is that which concerns others. In the part which merely concerns himself, his independence is, of right, absolute. Over himself, over his own body and mind, the individual is sovereign.
>
> (22)

Perhaps, another fundamental concept discussed by bioethicists since the formulation of the Nuremberg Codes is informed consent. The Codes, at the very outset, state that the person involved should have legal capacity to give consent and should be so situated as to be able to exercise free power of choice, without the intervention of any element of force, fraud, deceit, duress, overreaching or other ulterior form of constraint or coercion. Therefore, in order to make such a decision, he/she should have sufficient knowledge and comprehension of the elements of the subject matter involved (The Nuremberg Code). It becomes imperative for the researcher to get the informed consent of the participants, departing them sufficient information on the research work, and about the risks, and benefits involved. Besides enabling autonomous choices, the informed consent procedure serves to protect the individual participant from harm.

Other ethical concepts that gain prominence in the practice of medicine, such as human dignity, confidentiality, privacy, disclosure, decision-making, etc., are all inherently related to the concept of personal autonomy. They are all related to the principle of autonomy. The person of the patient deserves to be respected because it is a moral agent who is necessarily autonomous. As affirmed by Immanuel Kant, the inner worthiness of man is non-negotiable, since man is a moral agent who is capable of making independent decisions about his own life. This idea is the basis of the notion of human dignity. Moreover, it is widely regarded that on earth humanity is the greatest type of beings and every member deserves to be treated in a manner consonant with the high worth of the species (Kateb 2011, 3–4).

Almost all documents on medical ethics published ever since the Nuremberg codes stipulated in 1947 have underlined the centrality of the concept of human dignity. Rather this idea has been elevated as a central value in the new emerging scenario. As discussed above, the trials reiterate the importance of informed consent. Behind this stipulation is the idea that all human beings are worthy of equal respect and are to be left with doing what they consider is right for them with the minimum condition that they would not harm others. The idea of consent, therefore, reiterates man's status as a moral agent, who is autonomous and self-deterministic, and whose personhood deserves to be respected by the others in the society.

This concept further leads to the postulation of the idea of human rights. Since humans gain inner worth, and therefore, dignity because they are humans, their moral development and self-realization are also significant. Their moral identity implies the importance of privacy and confidentiality. When patients seek professional help from a physician, they may need to share with the latter many things about them which they do not want others to know (privacy and confidentiality). All humans with dignity wish to be the ultimate decision-maker about their own life and they may expect their physicians to reveal to them about their health status (disclosure) and make them a participant in the decision-making process.

James Rachels (1975) points out that privacy is sometimes necessary to protect people's interests in competitive situations (323). One may find it embarrassing for other people to know about some aspects of one's life or behaviour, such as sexual orientation or details about ailments (325).

Rachels further states that there is a close connection between our ability to control who has access to us and information about us, and our ability to create and maintain different sorts of social relationships with different people (326). For these reasons, they may not prefer information about them to be available to those people other than with whom they have shared it. In this sense, privacy is the control over information about oneself, and confidentiality is the assurance they get from the healthcare professional with whom they have shared information about their personal life.

All these new concepts construct a particular moral environment that shapes patient autonomy as an essential concept in present-day healthcare ethics. Nevertheless, these new sensibilities have not discarded the old moral concerns altogether. The emphasis on beneficence and nonmaleficence reflect the spirit of the old medical morality to a great extent. However, the concept of autonomy is arguably at the centre of contemporary bioethical deliberations. Many other important principles and ideals draw upon this fundamental concept. It emphasizes the importance of self-determinism of the individual in clinical and research contexts in the practice of modern medicine. This concept has come to the forefront of ethical deliberations since the emergence of individualism occasioned during the Renaissance and more prominently during and after the Enlightenment. This principle declares the irreducible status of the individual (patient), who is the ultimate arbiter of her own life and whose right to make decisions about her own life is unequivocally asserted. Since the patient is an autonomous individual, other principles like informed consent, rights of the patient, respect for her person, etc. are strongly emphasized. This idea is the basis of the rights-based approach in bioethics, and it categorically underlines the importance of human dignity.

The primary purpose of any form of healthcare is to overcome or reduce the harm caused by diseases and injuries. Traditionally, healers and physicians were treated with reverence, primarily because they help people to achieve this goal. However, some specific actions of physicians have the potential to cause harm to the patient, and most healing traditions consider this to be unacceptable, which consists of defeating the very purpose of the profession. The principle is derived from the Latin phrase *primum non nocere*, which means first, do no harm. The meaning of this phrase is different in the context of the highly specialized and technologized care, which modern medicine offers today compared to the trusteeship model offered by ancient healers in many traditions. Many procedures in modern medicine often involve risks. For example, the success of open-heart surgery is highly unpredictable, as it involves huge risks. Many such beneficial therapies may involve serious risks. In such cases, the surgeon has to weigh the possibility of risk with benefits and arrive at a relatively safe decision by determining whether the benefits would outweigh the burdens. Nevertheless, the chances of misjudgement are unavoidable, and the patient may get harmed. However, then, the harm is not intentional. The ethical obligation of nonmaleficence only insists that the physician should not inflict harm intentionally.

Nonmaleficence is a principle that targets to address the possible harm that may result in therapeutic interventions. Physicians' actions may cause harm to patients due to various reasons. The harms inflicted upon as part of a usual therapeutic procedure such as surgery are to be neglected in this context as they do not pose any serious moral problem. Instances of harm caused intentionally are not rare, as several malpractices happen every day, which are responsible for the erosion of trust in a significant way. Harm is often caused due to carelessness and negligence, which are avoidable. Again, the professional incompetence of the physician may also harm the patient. This factor mainly requires the physician to be aware of their limitations so that they could refer the patient to an expert if required. It is the responsibility of the physician to ensure that all efforts are taken in providing the most appropriate care and inflicting the least amount of pain to the patient.

Nonmaleficence is the most controversial among the four principles proposed by Beauchamp and Childress. Many feel that nonmaleficence, in its strict form, is not practically possible to practice. It demands not to cause harm to the patient intentionally. However, this is seldom possible in critical situations for the reasons mentioned above. Again, this principle seems to conflict with the principle of beneficence, another bioethics principle, which obligates physicians to bring benefits to patients through therapeutic interventions, and this may involve risks. Beauchamp and Childress themselves have recognized some difficulties with the concept in its relationship with the principle of beneficence.

The advancements in healthcare technology and medicine, in general, make the principle more problematic, as it now gives rise to many more ethical dilemmas. There is often a conflict between quality and longevity. Certain therapies may help to increase the number of years one may live but may do it at the expense of quality of life. In such situations, one may wonder whether it is beneficial to continue or withdraw the treatment. Again, there arises a confusion between withholding (not starting a new treatment) and withdrawing (stopping a continuing treatment), and for many physicians, the former is a more morally comfortable option. However, from a moral perspective, there is hardly any difference between the two.

The principle of nonmaleficence shares some similarities with the principle of beneficence. Many ethicists treat them as a single principle, which is misleading. The obligations not to injure others are sometimes more stringent than the obligations to help them (Beauchamp and Childress 1994, 190). Beauchamp and Childress conceptually distinguish the two principles by stating that nonmaleficence requires one ought not to inflict evil or harm. However, beneficence obligates one ought to prevent and remove evil or harm and also to do or promote good. While nonmaleficence here requires only to intentionally refrain from actions that cause harm, beneficence requires taking actions by helping to prevent and remove harm, besides promoting good (192). The principle of beneficence refers to an action done for the benefit of others.

The principle of beneficence refers to the duty to do good. It is a principle that finds a significant mention in the Belmont Report, where it is clearly distinguished from maleficence. Positively, the principle requires to secure the well-being of human research subjects, by maximizing anticipated benefits and minimizing harms. It insists that researchers should design their work in which benefits are maximized and harm is minimized. However, as stated above, Beauchamp and Childress insist on distinguishing non-maleficence from beneficence. They discuss two principles of beneficence; positive beneficence that requires the provisions of utility and utility that requires benefits to be balanced with drawbacks. They remind us that it is essential to distinguish obligatory beneficent acts from acts of altruism and generosity and argue that we are not morally required to perform acts of generosity and charity and list out the following as a few examples of rules of beneficence.

1. Protect and defend the rights of others.
2. Prevent harm from occurring to others.
3. Remove conditions that will cause harm to others.
4. Help persons with disabilities
5. Rescue persons in danger.

A significant confusion regarding the nature of the principle of beneficence surfaces when it is compared with the principle of autonomy. There are occasions when patients make irresponsible choices by refusing a course of treatment, which is essential. Here, more than patient autonomy, beneficence takes primacy and it seems to conflict with the former. The question is: Does this amount to paternalism? Again, if a physician thinks that disclosing certain information can cause harm to her patient and medical ethics requires her to refrain from causing harm, is it alright for her not to disclose that piece of information to the patient, even if that amounts to the violation of the principle of autonomy? There seems to be a conflict between paternalism and autonomy. It may be the case that the society opposes medical paternalism and the physicians themselves try to be non-paternalistic. However, physicians often find that many patients still expect, hope for, and even urge in both subtle and outright ways, the doctor to be paternalistic (Komrad 1983, 40).

There are diverse opinions about this apparent conflict between autonomy and beneficence, where the physician's decision may ultimately place her in the camp of either anti-paternalists or paternalists. Beauchamp and Childress (1994) affirm that, in contrast to much of the literature on paternalism, they would support restricting autonomous as well as non-autonomous actions on the grounds of beneficence (277). If there is no reasonable alternative, even strong paternalism can be justified. Beauchamp and Childress submit a few limiting conditions for granting this:

1. A patient is at risk of significant, preventable harm.
2. A paternalistic action will probably prevent harm.
3. The projected benefits of the patient of the paternalistic action outweigh its risks to the patient.
4. The least autonomy-restrictive alternative that will secure the benefits and reduce the risks is adopted.

(283)

Like nonmaleficence and beneficence, which are principles present in many ancient healing traditions, justice too was an implicit principle observed by ancient healers but acquired new dimensions of meaning in the contemporary world. The Belmont Report refers to justice as the equitable distribution of the benefits and burdens of research. However, the principle has a much broader application in the field of medical ethics. According to Beauchamp and Childress, a situation of justice is present whenever persons have due benefits or burdens because of their particular properties or circumstances, such as being productive or having been harmed by another person's acts. Besides, they also refer to another concept of justice called distributive justice, which arises under conditions of scarcity and competition. Here the emphasis is on the fair, equitable and appropriate distribution of resources (327). Aristotle, to whom all later thinkers refer to, designed a theory of justice, which is understood as fairness or equality of treatment. The idea that equals must be treated equally and unequals must be treated unequally is derived from Aristotle's principle of formal justice.

The distribution of healthcare consistently raises concerns regarding fair distribution in multiple ways. There are pieces of evidence that suggest that healthcare has often been covertly distributed on the basis of gender and race (345). In the Indian situation, the factor of caste further complicates things. The National Family Health Surveys (NFHS) data suggest that there are intergroup disparities in health outcomes such as infant mortality, maternal mortality, nutritional status and institutional delivery, which are unfavourable to Scheduled Castes (SCs) and Scheduled Tribes (STs) (George 2015, 3). Justice, argue Beauchamp and Childress (1994), can be achieved only if radical inequities are diminished (344). They discuss the situation in the United States in detail. The situation in India and other developing countries is either similar to this or worse than this. Besides social and economic backwardness (e.g., caste), several other factors function as barriers to healthcare to millions of people in India. These include economic factors, lack of adequate insurance, inadequate infrastructure, unavailability of facilities in government hospitals and scarcity of experts to provide services. The government hospitals in India provide free healthcare services, but they are not available in many places. Even if they are available, there is a severe lack of experts and required infrastructure.

The ideal of equitable healthcare for all sounds too idealistic in many developing countries. In India, recent initiatives like the Rashtriya Swasthya Bima Yojana (RSBY) aim at achieving such an ideal. Such initiatives envisage a direct intervention from the government and go against the libertarian view, which argues for the "ability to pay" criterion for distributing healthcare services. The proposal for a "right to health care" originates in this context. It argues that since there are similarities between health needs and other needs that are protected by governments, health also warrants such protection. Moreover, the health of a person has direct implications on the delivery of justice. Many disadvantages, such as injury, disability, or diseases, may cause a lack of opportunity and reduce a person's capacity to function correctly. Justice can be ensured only if societal healthcare resources are used to counter these disadvantages. It asserts that collective moral obligations exist to provide healthcare to needing people.

Scope and Limits of Principlism and Going Beyond them

The principlist framework has certain advantages over other theoretical frameworks in ethics in the contemporary scenario. When ordinary people engage in moral evaluations, they employ several insights about human morality. They use multiple parameters and adopt different modes. Consequently, their reasoning may lack the coherence that is usually found in the reasoning process of an expert. They may adopt contradictory approaches. For example, they may treat the importance of following one's duty as perennially important and at the same time may also consider the consequences of the action as ethically significant. They fail to see the apparent contradiction between these two standpoints. However, when the expert makes evaluations, she may either stress the duty element or underline the consequences. As a result, it may exhibit theoretical coherence but may miss the comprehensiveness of the lay perspective. An expert has to trade it off for the sake of consistency.

The principlist framework never proposes an ultimate solution to this but attempts to shift the focus from one-sided theories to principles, which any theoretical perspective may find acceptable. Beauchamp and Childress attempt to arrive at a methodology to resolve ethical problems in different healthcare settings by identifying certain fundamental principles that are themselves based on more general theories and can inform the rules that guide our actions. They are derived from considered judgements in the conventional morality and medical tradition. Principlism maintains that each of these principles is self-evident and is an obligation to be respected without any order of priority. The proponents of this framework do not claim that their approach has any final authority over the adjudication of complex and varied ethical dilemmas professionals face in their day-to-day practice of medicine. They propose the principles only as moral guides. Hence, its application never closes the scope of applying other well-known theories such as consequentialism and virtue ethics. One important feature of these principles is their general nature. They do not furnish any guidance to act in specific cases but facilitate the development of more detailed rules and policies (Beauchamp and Childress 1994, 38).

Principlism is, no doubt, the foremost theoretical perspective available today, and it is widely accepted as an appropriate framework for evaluating moral issues in modern medicine and a workable model in many places across the world. Nevertheless, it has several limitations. While discussing the importance of four principles and their prima facie validity, Beauchamp and Childress do not prioritize any one of them over others. They treat all the four as important. However, given the fact that the principlist approach aligns with a liberal perspective, the preference of autonomy over beneficence is apparent. But Beauchamp and Childress counter all such preferential organization among the four principles. When one tries to apply these principles in the actual healthcare settings, it creates several confusions. Here, one may come across situations where one principle conflicts with another. For example, beneficence could lead to a form of paternalism, as what is good for the patient is often better known to the physician and the patient's choices may sometime actually harm her. This situation may conflict with the commitment to autonomy. It is often argued that Beauchamp and Childress do not provide any solution to this problem.

This criticism has some substance. From the outset, it appears that among the four principles, the proponents of the principlist framework favour autonomy to occupy the top place in the hierarchy. Although Beauchamp and Childress deny any such hierarchical ordering of the principles, their allegiance to the liberal tradition strengthens this assumption. However, a closer look at the principles reveals certain other important aspects of their function in ethical reasoning. Their validity is not absolute, but only prima facie. Again, they are no rules that govern our actions but are general principles that leave sufficient room for the application of other theories. Hence, their application in each situation may vary in accordance with the demands that each situation may pose. Several factors such as the nature of the ethical dilemma, the context in which it originates and the people involved in the situation would suggest which principle is more relevant and which theoretical insights are more appropriate. In other words, a principle gains priority in accordance with the nature of the situation. It is not possible to assign any primacy a priori.

In the absence of any clear guidelines, this may sound a bit arbitrary that the parameters to decide which principle is to be used are left to the individual's preferences. What ultimately matters is the individual's theoretical allegiance. If the individual is a consequentialist or allies with Rawls' theory of justice, then in the interpretation of the bioethics principles and their application, she may make her preferences in the light of such allegiances.

There are several problems in the understanding of each principle. There is an ambiguity in deciding actions that are autonomous and that are non-autonomous. On what basis, say, for example, a physician can override the choices made by her patient? Does she have to override her patient's choices if the latter is incompetent to make choices? Or does she override her patient's irrational choices that may harm her, even though the patient is competent? There could be rational choices made by an incompetent person and irrational choices made by a competent person. Which one needs to be treated as an autonomous choice? Similar confusions exist in the understanding of other principles as well.

A significant objection towards the principlist framework is its doubtful universalizability. Beauchamp and Childress never claim its absolute validity, as they insist that the principles are only prima facie valid. However, they argue that since these principles are derived from conventional morality and other available theories of ethics, they can be applied universally. Moreover, principlism is a formal theory. As mentioned above, it never asserts the a priori validity of any one principle in a specific case, but it is beyond doubt that principlism is derived from liberal theories originated in Europe. These theories presuppose certain social structure and a political environment which is not present in all the places where modern medicine is practised. Autonomy, for example, is a clear liberal value and may not be understood in the same sense in other societies. Asserting an individual's autonomous status and self-ruling abilities is not usually present in many non-Western states.

Farhat Moazam in her book *Bioethics and Organ Transplantation in a Muslim Society: A Study in Culture, Ethnography and Religion* (2007) brings out certain issues professionals face in practising modern medicine in a non-Western cultural context. She highlights the conflict professionals encounter when they interact with patients in clinics after giving lectures to students and residents on the use of philosophical principles like autonomy for framing ethical issues (Moazam 2012). Ironically, the Urdu-speaking general public in Pakistan, a Muslim country, lack any knowledge about the liberal traditions of the West. They make collective decisions when kin fall ill, prefer to address physicians with relational terms used for family "elders" and perceive them as "instruments of God's mercy" to direct them in what they should do (Moazam 2012). Again, beneficence and nonmaleficence too have very different meanings in different societies. The principle of justice acquires very different dimensions of meaning in non-Western societies.

However, despite such obvious theoretical and practical limitations, it is indisputable that these principles have a predominant place in today's world. Different societies and cultures may indeed interpret and apply these principles in different ways. This possibility, however, does not indicate its weakness, but instead, highlights its strength. The principles are adapted to different places in different ways. In India, for example, principles like beneficence and nonmaleficence seem to gain a clear preference among practitioners—and even patients value them more than autonomy. Though principlism opposes naive paternalism and values autonomous decisions of patients, practitioners in India still hold on to this and many believe that they know what is good for their patients better than the latter. Again, it is not known how far researchers use these principles in making ethical decisions and how conversant the members of various institutional review or ethics boards are with these principles (Lawrance 2007, 39).

The domain of the contemporary practice of medicine frequently introduces moral dilemmas for bioethicists to grapple with and find a way out of them. Since bioethics hardly provides them an a priori framework with which they can find solutions to all possible problems, they continuously face the challenge of negotiating with the changing circumstances and the diverse ways in which various human acts impact our social environment. Introduction of a new therapeutic method or a new technology—which is frequently happening in the world of medicine—may pose new ethical challenges to the practitioners. Although the framework of principles and moral ideas they may make use of remains the same, they may have to now think of adopting new methods in addressing them. The primordial values and principles may remain the same. However, people seek different ways to make use of them and apply them to the ever-evolving social environment of medicine that grows around them.

5 Healthcare Technologies and Ethical Challenges

In November 2018, Chinese scientist He Jiankui claimed that he had successfully altered the genes of the twin girls born in October 2018 to prevent them from contracting HIV. In this procedure, genes are either deleted or replaced from the patient's genome. He Jiankui altered the DNA of the twin girls after practising the gene editing on mice, monkeys and human embryos in the lab for several years. He further revealed that one more woman who was pregnant had received similar treatment, and the provincial government investigation confirmed this.

The scientist had forged ethical review papers and had also evaded supervision and carried out this procedure with the assistance of a private project team that had foreign staff and used "technology of uncertain safety and effectiveness" for illegal human embryo gene editing (Agence France-Presse 2019). The Chinese Academy of Engineering which has a Division of Medicine and Health that provides advice on issues relating to health, medicine, health policy and biomedical sciences came out openly against He Jiankui, whose claim shook scientists and ethicists all over the world, and both the Division of Medicine and Health and the Scientific and Ethics Committee of CAE issued a statement criticizing He Jiankui. The scientists who speak on behalf of CAE affirm:

> Academically and technically, the presented work by Jiankui He and colleagues does not provide a new advance in the science, and the application of genome editing technology in human embryos for reproductive purposes is inappropriate.
>
> Ethically and morally, without solid scientific validation and full consideration of the unpredictable safety risks, these researchers have not adhered to scientific integrity and ethical norms in this clinical operation of human germ cell genome editing for reproductive purposes.
>
> (Zhang et al. 2019, 25)

They further condemn him and his colleagues for violating China's policies and regulations on gene-related research and state that their clinical operations are explicitly prohibited. They urge the scientific community and

DOI: 10.4324/9781003312697-5

society to work together to develop a comprehensive strategy to ensure the twin babies' privacy and to provide preventive measures for potential health and social issues related to genome editing. They further call on all science and technology professionals to strengthen the self-discipline of research ethics and strictly comply with all ethical norms, laws and regulations in their research activities.

On behalf of 149 signatories, another group of Chinese scientists who are HIV professionals in human genome editing opposes genome editing of healthy human germline cells and embryos for reproductive purposes from a scientific, ethical perspective (Zhang et al. 2019, 26–27). This procedure involves several complex issues that are to be addressed at various levels— scientific, technological, social, ethical, etc.—and it also calls for the need to adopt a comprehensive approach that has substantial policy implications. Several factors make gene editing of germ cells or early embryos ethically problematic, as all the consequences of gene editing on patients and subsequent generations are not known at this point. Moreover, the process is still in the stage of basic research, and its safety and validity need to be thoroughly evaluated (Wang et al. 2019, 26).

He Jiankui's experimentation raises multiple ethical and legal concerns, which potentially call for a well thought out regulatory mechanism. A few such issues are discussed here, though this is not an exhaustive list.

1. Research involving humans without proper ethics committee approval—which is imperative for any research that involves human participation—needs to be strictly prohibited. The ethical impacts of such research activities cannot be assessed if details about the procedures followed by the researchers are not discussed.
2. It is vital to ensure that the experiments conducted are not indispensable, and if such experiments do not provide a new advance in science, they have to be discouraged. In the example cited here, the researchers have not adhered to scientific integrity and ethical norms in the clinical operation of human germ cell genome editing for reproductive purposes.
3. The policies and ethical guidelines followed by each society are to be treated as authoritative. He and his team have carried out research, which went against China's policies and regulations on gene-related research and were explicitly prohibitive (Zhang et al. 2019, 25).
4. All the impacts and implications of a research work that employs cutting-edge technologies may not be known to the scientific world. Some of its implications and consequences may be unsafe and detrimental to humanity, and how safe it will be for future generations is also unknown. However, this is no reason for turning away from scientific research. We may have to take chances and calculative risks to achieve the necessary advancements in science. It is here the proper role of regulations and ethics committee evaluations become relevant and important.

5. Factors like career advancements, reputation and financial considerations that are related to their research engagements may motivate scientists. However, it is essential to ensure that such non-professional and non-scientific factors are not the sole elements that enthuse research. We need to reiterate that benefit to humanity should be the prime consideration. Research projects that involve risk to humanity in general and research subjects in particular should be avoided.

6. All guidelines and codes on human research affirm the paramount importance of informed consent. However, informed consent presupposes that the participants know all the relevant features and particularly the safety aspects of the research in which they are subjects. If the ethical considerations are not adequately listed out, it will be impossible to gather proper informed consent from the participants. In He Jiankui's experiments, neither the participants nor the experimenting scientists were aware of all the moral implications of the study, mainly because the safety considerations were not well thought out and articulated.

Many such innovative research initiatives raised serious ethical concerns when they were announced to the public. As mentioned before, medicine is now heavily reliant on state-of-the-art technologies and the more we benefit from them, the more we embrace new technologies.

Introduction

Many such concerns are common to the application of all medical technologies, although the genome editing process is at the cutting edge of a series of healthcare technologies that portray the architecture of the science and art of healing in today's world. Again, not all technologies employed by healthcare professionals raise serious ethical issues in the same manner. Even if they do raise such issues and give rise to many disturbing anxieties, we may not be able to afford to give them up altogether. Many of them are part of the usual treatment protocol followed by professionals for long. Again, the healthcare sector cannot shy off from trying out novel methods and new technologies, since humankind benefits immensely from them. Today an efficient and effective delivery of healthcare is unthinkable without the assistance of technology. Physicians and other healthcare professionals use advanced technologies for diagnosing health issues, medication and treating patients. Though the service of technology has always been drawn upon by medical professionals in order to ensure adequate care, the employment of modern technologies initiated a revolution in the process, assuring superior quality of care at all levels. Moreover, the use of technology in the health sector is not confined to the sphere of direct clinical practice alone, as the application of the former extends to many other fields like genetics, disability treatment, drug development, transplantation treatment and animal and human experimentation. Many of these different fields overlap and generate more complex ethical issues. The use of high-technology diagnostic and therapeutic healthcare facilities raises multiple moral issues and dilemmas, as they may often pose severe challenges to our long-held moral beliefs and assumptions. Moreover, their availability may come into conflict with medical necessity, social justice and cost-effectiveness (Tan and Ong 2002, 231).

Since long, humans have been using technological advancements for therapeutic purposes as well as for the manipulation of life in order to serve desired ends. Some indications suggest the practice of surgery by Indus Valley people and there was mention of surgery in the Rig Vedic hymns. Susruta, the ancient physician and surgeon who lived around 700–600 BCE and the author of one of the three great classics (*Brihat-thrayi*) of Ayurveda, *Susruta Samhita* (Compendium of Susruta), is believed to have employed various techniques in order to perform complex surgeries. His compendium details about 300 kinds of operations that call for 42 different surgical processes and 121 different types of instruments (Banerjee et al. 2011, 320).

Ancient medicine had made such advances in many civilizations. However, those advances were not technological advances. Technology, as we understand it today, is the product of modern science, which emerged during the Enlightenment era. It empowered humans and facilitated significant improvements in their lives by stimulating enormous industrial and financial growth. It ultimately transformed human societies across the world. Technological advancements have made tremendous transformations in the fields of industrial production that resulted in the growth of economies, warfare and health. All these fields fundamentally helped humans to have greater control over the external world. Industrial and economic growth helped in gaining control over nature and the constraints it imposes on us due to our limitations. Warfare technologies helped to have control over other people and their resources, which promoted economic and industrial growth in the first world. Medical technologies facilitated control over health and life to a greater extent, which is testified by the increase in life expectancy and visible decrease in infant mortality. Such innovations nevertheless have their undesirable impacts on human life and raise serious moral issues. In the first two fields, the advances have brought consequences that even hamper the prospects of humankind's survival on the planet. Technological interferences with life that is characteristic of medical technologies raise a different set of ethical issues, which will be the focus of this chapter. Some of them even challenge our very identities as human beings and seriously alter the development of the natural course of our social and cultural history.

In modern medicine, technological innovations have always been milestones in the development of science. However, it was only since the 19th century that the use of machines became an integral part of medical practice. In 1833, Jules Herisson devised arguably the first instrument capable of measuring blood pressure indirectly, which consisted of a mercury reservoir covered by a rubber membrane from which a graduated glass column arose. In 1846, John Hutchinson developed the water spirometer measuring vital capacity. Several other innovations followed, and all these changes gradually remodelled medicine from an enterprise relying on the subjective descriptions of the patients and others into an evidence-based science, which relies more on objective data obtained by mechanical and chemical technology devices.

Nevertheless, it was only after the first half of the 20th century that medicine witnessed significant technological changes. Earlier, since the process of change was slow, there was adequate time for proper assessment of the effectiveness of new equipment and techniques, accompanied by careful and moderate use. However, later, when changes became faster, new dilemmas challenged several of the ethical ideas and principles that constituted the moral fabric of society. Today, highly sophisticated technological changes have revolutionized the field of medicine, and advances in technology play a crucial role in determining various healthcare practices. Medicine today is not merely a science and art of healing. It is also an integral part of the corporate world. It is an advanced techno-scientific enterprise that draws upon the cutting-edge research that takes place in other fields like genetics, biotechnology, robotics and artificial intelligence, and proactively interferes with what is given "naturally." The modern-day biotechnologists can manipulate organisms at the molecular level and engineer their genes in order to produce desired traits. Such involvement of technological know-how in the therapeutic process has always raised serious ethical challenges and various agencies strictly monitor them at different levels.

Regardless of such issues, the enabling power in performing many things that were unthinkable earlier makes the present-day technological context in healthcare significant. We can not only perform highly complicated surgeries but also ensure qualitatively better lives to millions of patients by providing them superior therapeutic services, diagnostic methods and medication. These positive developments have contributed to drastic improvements in the healthcare sector. However, the deleterious impacts of technology on humankind can hardly be undervalued. Its inappropriate use has generated much damage leading to a decline in the medical profession and, consequently, patient care (Cernadas 2017, 106). Technological innovations aided rapid commercialization which brought out new possibilities of treatment. However, they also made healthcare prohibitively expensive and therefore inaccessible to millions. Some immediate consequences of the inappropriate use of technology in healthcare include the commodification of the human body, overreliance of society on technology and alienation of patients from physicians. The overreliance on technology redefines the fundamental ways in which society perceives illness and healing. However, it is not feasible to denounce its usage, as we cannot morally avoid technological progress and what is possible is only monitoring and controlling its potential success and preventing its inappropriate use (107).

As indicated above, human societies encounter many issues due to the clash between traditional and existing value systems and new technological scenarios. A whole range of issues related to birth, reproduction, end-of-life issues and death emerge in this context for us to find solutions. The ethical issues in relation to new healthcare technologies are discussed here by dividing them into five broad categories.

1. Challenges to fundamental moral concepts.
2. Technologization and fragmentation.
3. Issues related to decision-making, scarcity, access, resource allocation and distributive justice.
4. Biotechnology and genetics.
5. Commodification, medicalization and alienation.

Challenges to Fundamental Moral Concepts

The potential benefits of medical technologies make them inevitable and ubiquitous. However, they actively challenge some of the fundamental values that epitomize the practice of medicine in many human societies such as:

(a) The values that embody the patient–physician relationship, which impinges upon effectiveness, trust and patient safety.
(b) Those values related to our understanding and the ways we perceive birth, death, family structure and relationships.
(c) Values that facilitate fundamental decision-making in the various healthcare contexts; the role played by patients, physicians, patients' relatives and government authorities.
(d) Issues related to reproduction in the light of new technologies, including surrogacy, sex selection and eugenics.
(e) Issues related to prolongation of life and delaying death.

Patient–Physician Relationship

When technology becomes the defining feature of medical care, it may induce some changes to the fundamental values in terms of which it has apprehended across different cultures. The relationships among the different stakeholders that constitute the care process that is founded on these values make healthcare a unique profession venerable to the entire society. Traditionally, physicians were regarded as caregivers, whom everyone could trust and their decisions were never doubted or discredited. Trust may be understood as "the optimistic acceptance of a vulnerable situation in which one believes that the trustee will care for their interests" (Hall et al. 2001, 615). Here trust and vulnerability are intimately linked, and the necessity of trust points to the psychological reality inherent in the vulnerability created by illness.

The concept of trust has two important aspects. Interpersonal trust, which is the trust placed by one person in another, is distinguishable from public trust, which refers to the trust placed by a group or a person in a societal institution or system (Schee, Groenewegen and Friele 2006, 471). The trust individuals and society bestowed upon physicians had been central to healthcare institutions in many societies for ages. This situation remained intact even after the emergence of modern medical science with several revolutionary changes that defined its modus operandi. Clinicians and hospitals continued to enjoy public trust. However, as indicated in early chapters, with the introduction of innovative technologies, the practice of medicine had witnessed a paradigm shift. Patients are now related to a multifaceted corporate, institutional network that functions at different levels. They can potentially furnish an exhaustive account of the functioning of different organs but may still fall short of dispensing with the requirements of a more comprehensive perspective on care. The intimate interpersonal relationship where the patients trusted the physicians became an obsolete value in the context of the newly evolving professional association between the patients and the healthcare professional fraternity.

Technology interferes with the patient–physician relationship. Though this may very often make the diagnostic and therapeutic processes more and more impeccable, it may also make it more cumbersome and leave the patients more perturbed. The older model of trusteeship medical practice where physicians individually reached out to their patients, either by going to their residences or through personal interactions in their clinics, had to inevitably give way to a more organized form of medical practice facilitated through corporate hospitals. Such changes made available state-of-the-art technology in one place, which ensure professional accuracy by effectively coordinating the various technological and specialized medical services. Multispecialty hospitals become indispensable for people to access the "best available" healthcare services in the age of technology.

The new technological environment has conclusively transformed the patient–physician relationship, which ultimately made trusteeship medical practice that consolidated around a strong personal bond between the two obsolete. The technological scenario has also made healthcare institutions distrustful to the common man. One of the most significant advantages of the traditional trusteeship model consisted of the way it made the different stakeholders, particularly the patients, complacent. Since the relationship was personal and was based on those values that uphold duty-bound dedication, it ensured a variety of moral protections for patients. With a close and long-standing relationship between the patient and the physician, the relationship was rooted in certain values that respected patient autonomy and confidentiality and encouraged shared decision-making (Rajput and Bekes 2001, 870). The care provided was continuous and physicians enjoyed complete trust. Above all, the therapeutic process was initiated with patient descriptions of the illness. The physicians, in turn, used to be careful listeners of what their patients had to tell them. This conversation played a crucial role in understanding the patient, arriving at an appropriate diagnosis and deciding the proper medication.

The new technological contexts in medical practice present an intensively convoluted scenario where the traditional values prove ineffective in dealing with newly emerging ethical challenges. The impersonal technological environment in the hospital may effectively deal with physical ailments. However, it may fail to reinforce the decisive emotional assurance, which is an essential component of caring and healing. All ailments make an individual vulnerable, and every instance of such vulnerability has an equal or more tenacious emotional component. Despite all its odds, the traditional caregiving ambience could adequately respond to this aspect. The doctors knew their patients as persons and also were aware of their emotional and social surroundings. They could, therefore, make decisions—which were very often a shared one that involved the patients and their family members—that were more appropriate and fruitful. In the modern context, the mechanically documented details of the patients are examined by a number of experts, who individually give their feedback and suggest their recommendations. The patient's descriptions of the illness and its reception by individual physicians constituted the core of the earlier process of caregiving. However, such experiential descriptions have significantly lost their value in the current scenarios. As aforementioned, medicine has become more evidence-based, and the new technologies provide physicians the required objective data for their interpretation and diagnosis of the patient's health.

Since ages, the interpersonal relationship between patients and physicians, the trust commanded by physicians as the trustees of public health, and the idea of care built around the above two constituted the backbone of the healthcare institution across different cultures. The transformation of healing systems into a science of medicine, the introduction of technology into it in a big way and the corporatization of the entire healthcare infrastructure have fundamentally altered the value base of traditional medical systems. Personal values are replaced with professional protocols. In this scenario, trust needs to be understood in terms of transparency, which can be obtained with the observance of values such as confidentiality and integrity and adherence to principles such as informed consent and respect for autonomy. In other words, trust ceases to be a personal value and becomes a professional ideal. This professional ideal occupies the cornerstone of the modern healthcare system.

Cost, Exploitation and Other Factors

Apart from the lack of personal relationships depriving the care process of its critical emotional dimension, the new scenario often makes the patient vulnerable to some other vicissitudes. In place of the traditional physician, with a spirit of trusteeship and caregiving, patients now have to confront the hospital and its professionals primarily. Hence, in place of a more intimate personal relationship with the physician, the patients today are forced to enter into more impersonal professional relationships with a host of professionals. This environment redefines the meaning of care that permeated patient–physician relationship rooted in the idea of strong personal bonds between the two. The hospital brings together the most advanced technological achievements that assist the specialist physicians in arriving at the professionally appropriate diagnostic and therapeutic decisions. Consequently, the availability of superior medical care gets increasingly confined to urban areas. This scenario keeps the advantages of modern medicine away from patients in rural areas. Moreover, since the hospitals require a massive investment to support the machinery and other infrastructure needed for providing care, the process becomes exorbitantly expensive. This factor may further contribute to the already-existing rich–poor divide in society. The technological orientation of medicine, therefore, deprives a considerable portion of the population of the astonishing benefits of the science, which would remain accessible only to the urban rich.

Nevertheless, it appears that modern medical technology is not to be blamed for this. The problem obviously lies in the ways we employ and manage technology. However, the situation is a little more complicated than this. On the one hand, the very availability of some technological possibilities suggests and demands changes in our lives. On the other, technologies themselves have originated as various means by which humans have responded to their needs. The expansion of trade, for example, demanded the need for transportation through land and sea, and this promoted the growth of the automobile industry, astronomy and naval architecture. The growth in the transportation industry has steered several other technological developments. Medicine witnessed radical changes in the past few decades. The extensive use of technology by physicians threw better light in understanding the functioning of the human body and assisted better diagnosis and therapies. However, this technologization eventually makes healthcare more expensive and unaffordable to more and more people in the society. The problem of access seems to be a direct consequence of how we organize healthcare practices in our societies. Governments across the world adopt several measures to overcome such issues.

For example, the Government of India has launched the National Rural Health Mission (NRHM) for improving healthcare delivery in rural India. This programme aims to provide equitable, affordable and quality healthcare to the rural population, especially the vulnerable groups. It aims at

> establishing a fully functional, community-owned, decentralized health delivery system with intersectoral convergence at all levels, to ensure simultaneous action on a wide range of determinants of health such as water, sanitation, education, nutrition, social and gender equality. Institutional integration within the fragmented health sector was

expected to provide a focus on outcomes, measured against Indian Public Health Standards for all health facilities.

(National Health Mission 2019)

Even developed countries face problems related to access and design policies to overcome them. In the United States, in 2010, President Obama signed the Affordable Care Act (ACA) into law. The ACA aimed at comprehensive healthcare reform in the United States by not only lowering healthcare costs but also providing better access to healthcare and consumer protections.

The primary concern is to ensure the accessibility to the benefits of scientific and technological innovations to all classes of people. In developing countries, this calls for more direct governmental interference in the health sector and also the health insurance sector. There are numerous issues in the healthcare infrastructure in most developing countries that need immediate attention in order to ensure a just healthcare system. In order to ensure this, we may have to begin with issues related to fair living conditions such as the proper distribution of water, appropriate maintenance of sanitation and nutritious food. Nearly 63% of primary health centres in India do not have an operation theatre and 29% lack a labour room. Again, community health centres were 81.5% short of specialists such as surgeons, gynaecologists and paediatricians (Yadavar 2018). While referring to the several challenges the current health system in India encounters, the Public Health Foundation of India, in its annual report for the year 2017–2018 identifies several issues that demand immediate attention. They include fragmentation of healthcare delivery, insufficient human resources mainly, primary care physicians, long waiting time, visits to multiple locations, inefficient use of information and unaffordable costs of care (PHFI 2018).

With hospitals adopting the practices of corporate houses, they also begin to compete for market share and more profits. Since corporate houses do this by upgrading existing technology and with a consistent escalation of product quality, hospitals too periodically revamp their infrastructure and for accomplishing higher quality levels, employ more technology. All these add to the cost of care, which patients have to shell out. Since hospitals begin to behave like corporate houses, a reflection on the ethical aspects in this context will have to address the implications of corporate decision-making. Hence, in a sense, bioethics requires knowledge of business ethics (Potras and Meredith 2009, 314). This aspect of bioethics presents a whole range of unique convoluted ethical issues.

These are more significant issues that call for drastic policy changes and restructuring initiatives of the governmental vision of healthcare in a country. Other issues affect the general public more directly, such as the unethical and illegal practices that embody the standard practices that shore up the healthcare system in many places. Many such practices have a direct impact on patient safety. While the kickbacks to doctors associated with prescriptions, referrals, laboratory tests and surgical equipment constitute the most direct and standard set of such practices, doctors also receive incentives from hospitals for patients' bills for treatment and surgeries, encouraging them to escalate the bills. Pharmaceutical companies, for more prescriptions, also directly supply incentives. A recent study conducted by medical and health authorities shows that between April 2014 and February 2015, while the government hospitals have referred only 25% of women expecting delivery for caesarean, for private hospitals it was over 65% (Rao 2015). Dr Arun Gardre in his study conducted for the Pune-based non-governmental organization "Support for Advocacy and Training to Health Initiatives" (SATHI) interviewed 78 doctors throughout India. This study has documented that the main aim of the multispecialty hospitals in India is to generate revenue and profits for their investors and in this endeavour conscience takes a back seat. Doctors are encouraged to indulge in unethical practice (Science Daily 2015).

Value Incommensurability

Two sets of values may become incommensurable when they share no common ground of comparison or sometimes even contradict each other. Traditional and shared values are confronted by the use of medical technologies in many other respects. New technologies challenge our fundamental ideas, assumptions and values associated with the treatment decision-making process, the involvement of family members in the care process, ideas about birth, death and last but not least, family relationships. Traditionally, all these have been crucially involved in shaping the core values that constituted the care process in many cultures across the world. In the Indian society where communities enjoy primacy over individuals, the collective decision-making process garnishes the caregiving system where the family plays a vital role and the physician is adored, revered and honoured by all the stakeholders. Though from the outset, this situation seems to deprive the individual patient of her rights and autonomy, the moral values that form the understructure of such societies prudently ensured the balance of power. We have seen how this moral scaffolding has been shaken off by the new developments and technological revolution. They fundamentally questioned the very structure of the relationship contexts in which the care process evolves. Moreover, the new technologized and commercialized context of healthcare has its own moral scaffolding, which drastically deviates in spirit from the traditional values. For example, the former conceives healthcare as a sector in the industrial world that is driven by the motives to garner more profits, while the traditional value environment that envelops healthcare conceives it as a service to humankind.

Technology made huge impacts outside the framework of the patient–physician relationship as well. One area that has witnessed astounding innovations in technological applications is human reproduction. Developments in genetics and biotechnology have eventuated in the formulation of different therapeutic interventions; medical, surgical and a combination of both. The application of such technologies expedites certain accomplishments in these areas where the role of the medical professional appears to be entirely unconventional. They also change the ideas about the human body and the human reproductive process. Many conventional ideas and assumptions about human reproduction, such as parenthood, sexual relationships, life partnership and parent–child relationship, have been replaced with new ideas. For instance, with the emergence of these technologies, a woman can give birth to a child from an unknown sperm donor, and the family values may require radical alterations in such cases along with the ideas mentioned above and the value environment in which they were understood and presumed.

Such technologies may have direct and indirect impacts on the social life of individuals, particularly of women in many Asian societies, where motherhood is often considered to be a unique occupation that defines the status of women in the society. Further, those who benefit from the full range of assisted reproductive technologies (ART) like ovulation induction, artificial insemination (AI) and in vitro fertilization (IVF) are not only those who have reproductive health issues. Such technologies may also be of help to people with a variety of parenthood requirements and who are not necessarily patients in the ordinary sense of the term. Surrogate mothers are widely employed by many couples to realize their dreams of becoming parents. A surrogate mother is a woman who carries and gives birth to the child of an intended parent, who is the person who intends to raise the child. Surrogate motherhood involves carrying and giving birth to a baby for another woman using either genetic or gestational surrogacy methods (Akker 2010, 5). Utilizing this process, couples who are unable to conceive naturally can have children biologically related, either to both of them or at least to the husband. With surrogacy, a woman who does not have a functional uterus or who is unable to bear a child due to some other health reasons, or who does not want to be pregnant, can bear her child. This possibility offers significant reproductive choices to the couple and particularly to women. This process may help gay or lesbian couples also to have children. Further, it may also help couples to prevent their children from inheriting some of their genetic defects.

Despite such achievements and advantages, the use of such technologies gives rise to several moral concerns. Most of them occur because what we medically achieve and especially, the methodology we adopt for achieving those goals may go against some of our traditional beliefs and practices. Our morality is intimately linked with the conventional ways we conduct our lives. Any of those practices that make drastic deviations from such familiar ways may attract substantial moral scrutiny. Such scenarios encounter serious issues related to the incommensurability of moral values. In many such spheres where these new technologies are applied—such as reproduction, medication, organ transplantation, usage of life-sustaining medications and technologies—we use them and exert direct or indirect control over life. Eventually, we may encounter unprecedented moral dilemmas and anxieties. The possibility of prenatal scanning today may give information about the various health aspects of the foetus. This possibility gives parents a choice if the foetus is diagnosed with any severe ailments or deformities. They can now decide whether to go ahead with the pregnancy or to terminate it. Here the choice is between having a healthy child or terminating the life of the foetus, which carries certain genetic disorders that may severely impact the quality of life of the child to be born. However, this scenario poses the moral problem of terminating life, as even the foetus can be technically treated as a living entity. Many parents believe that aborting pregnancy is equivalent to killing their child.

In a different scenario, the relatives of a terminally ill patient may have to address some embarrassing questions like how far they wish to continue the life support system that sustains life. In several such cases, physicians may not be able to make predictions conclusively, and this leaves the relatives in a dilemma. It is not easy to negotiate with the conflicting moral positions in such situations as all such issues are entangled with the moral values of the society. On the one hand, these new technological possibilities empower us with tools and abilities that enable us to cope up with the world in better ways and control it more efficiently. They help us to overcome many of our biological limitations and the social constraints imposed by them. Nevertheless, this is done at the expense of our value system. However, modern life cannot do away with the benefits they offer, and we can only hope to reorganize our society to make optimum use of them.

Cost Escalation and Accessibility Issues

In the United States, new medical technologies are responsible for a 40%–50% annual cost increase in healthcare (Clemens 2017). The technological scenario has made the care process more expensive and often prolonged. New technologies have contributed to an improvement in the care process, and there is a visible increase in the life expectancy of individuals in many countries. However, their advent has made the cost of healthcare significantly high. Since globalization in the 1990s, the Indian healthcare sector has witnessed such changes. While on the one hand, the opening up of the market has brought the new advances in technologies and innovative products into the country, it has also contributed to a steep increase in the money people have to spend for quality healthcare services. This situation has made many families bankrupt. Those who belong to the lowest strata of society have been severely affected in such a scenario.

Since the technologies employed undergo constant improvements and updations, very few companies manufacture these technologies, and a limited number of multinational companies dominate their market. The prime objective of these companies that face intense competition in the market is not to make the technologies more inexpensive and accessible but to ensure profitability through improvement in quality that gathers a competitive edge and an escalation in price.

With the frequent introduction of new technologies and the constant improvement of the existing ones, countries across the globe have witnessed an upsurge in health expenditure. Unlike many other sectors in the economy, technological innovations lead to a rise in prices of medicine. While new technologies may make many sectors like computers, household items and automobiles cheaper, in the health sector, the trend is reversed. Ultimately, patients who are the end users are forced to bear this increased production and operation cost. It is a fact that many of the new features they add during updating of technology are inessential and hardly facilitate improvements in diagnosis and treatment decision-making (Kumar 2011, 86). In other words, on many occasions, people have to pay more for what they do not want. They are helplessly drawn into the scenario.

This situation may affect the developing countries more adversely, as many of them do not have adequate health insurance schemes that cover a substantial number of their population. In the case of India, the government shells out a meagre 1% of GDP on healthcare. Hence, India's health system ranks as one of the most heavily dependent on out-of-pocket expenditures in the world (Keane and Thakur 2018, 435). A significant share in this amount goes for using technology at various levels of the caregiving process.

This scenario may put a considerable number of people under enormous difficulties, and the out-of-pocket expenses to be borne for healthcare may push people to poverty. Given the fact that quality healthcare is often intersected with hospital care and consequently with the use of technology at the different levels of care, those who are unable to bear the expenses required for meeting these demands may be deprived of the former. This may affect a large number of people in a country like India, where over 73 million people live in extreme poverty, which is around 23% of its population. A study by the Asian Development Bank (2011, 3–4) found that if the Asian Poverty Line is defined at $1.35, then two-thirds of India's population or around 740 million Indian people live in poverty.

The Government of India has initiated several measures to solve such issues. In 2008, the Ministry of Labour and Employment, Government of India introduced the Rashtriya Swasthya Bima Yojana (RSBY) to provide health insurance coverage for below poverty line (BPL) families. The RSBY envisaged protecting unorganized sector workers belonging to the BPL category and their family members from financial liabilities arising out of health shocks that involve hospitalization. Recently in 2018, the Government of India has introduced a new programme named Ayushman Bharat (meaning long-life India). This programme is a National Health Protection Scheme, which plans to cover over 100 million poor and vulnerable families, by providing coverage up to 500,000 rupees per family per year for secondary and tertiary care hospitalization. This new programme is the world's largest government-funded healthcare programme, and the beneficiaries can avail benefits in both public and empanelled private facilities (RSBY & NHPM).

Again, many of these innovative technologies require huge infrastructure, and their usage involves massive power consumption. Moreover, since they function on digital platforms and require expert professionals with adequate training for their operation, only those places with adequate infrastructure would be able to ensure such facilities, and eventually, the patients are obliged to pay for them as well. For the people in the rural and tribal areas and also to the urban poor, these factors prove to be detrimental.

The technological scenario has raised several other issues and sometimes has resulted in certain situations that are wholly unanticipated. For instance, some of the new technologies available in the healthcare sector enable people to live longer. Many diseases, which were fatal a few decades ago, are entirely curable now, and in many countries, the battle against poverty has gained significant success. More people now enjoy better sanitation, clean drinking water and other amenities that may contribute to healthy living. All these have positively contributed to life expectancy, which is exponentially high in many countries now. This situation presents a peculiar health crisis, as the society now has to deal with a large number of aged population and their health issues. The developed countries have better infrastructure for providing elderly care, but even in such places, they fail to extend the emotional care that can come from a family environment. In many non-Western countries, traditionally, the family played a crucial role in providing care to the elderly. However, changing social and economic dynamics are rapidly altering this scenario.

The use of life-sustaining equipment generates a different set of ethical dilemmas. People use various types of life-sustaining equipment such as ventilators, suctioning devices, defibrillators, oxygen concentrator machines, dialysis machines, ventricular assist devices and nebulizer machines. It is true that some of them like stents, artificial valves and dialyzer machines are life-sustaining and have to be used life-long. They are indispensable for patients who suffer from certain diseases. Some of them help patients to lead a normal life without frequent hospital visits. However, prolonged therapeutic intervention, regular hospitalization and medication are not only exhaustive to the patients and their families but also very expensive. Some machines like the mechanical ventilator, ventricular assist device and extracorporeal membrane oxygenation machine are widely used by physicians, mainly during therapy as a bridge to recovery. But it is not uncommon among caregivers to use them for an indefinite period, causing multiple difficulties to many people involved. Such patients may become entirely dependent on these technologies, and since they may have to use them for a longer time, it may destabilize their economic base and may turn out to be extremely cumbersome and painful to them. Such patients may sometimes have to spend their remaining lives in the hospital. Just because life-prolonging technology is available, people feel obligated to use them. Here technologies seem to be serving a different purpose other than providing care and facilitating overall well-being. They simply aid the proper functioning of one or other organs in the body. As mentioned above, if they are used as a bridge to recovery, such technologies prove useful in the care process. Eventually, once the patient is cured, physicians discontinue their use. However, their persistent use is detrimental to the patient's well-being.

The ethical issues healthcare technologies potentially raise are becoming manifold, and they rapidly extend to new areas, which were unthought-of a few years ago. Many scientists believe that very soon anti-ageing technologies may become a successful reality, and life-extension technologies are very soon going to have their impacts on a society where individuals will live much longer than they do now. Such possibilities may redefine not only the parameters of human well-being but also provide new treatment options to physicians. They may further reformulate our ideas about "what is natural." They may potentially bring about severe consequences to people who make use of them as such technologies may have very problematic impacts on the relationship between patients and their family members. They may further have repercussions in the society, as such longer living humans may have severe relationship issues, sexual imbalances and emotional issues. Besides, they pose several economic problems as well, since they have an extended productive age and will compete with the younger generation in the job market. Such people may pose a new set of geriatric and general healthcare requirements. Nevertheless, if we take a clue from the history of science, we may find that such technologies are bound to occur regardless of whether we like them or not and whether they lead to desirable consequences for the society or not.

Scarcity, Access, Resource Allocation and Distributive Justice

No technology is risk-free. However, what makes technological innovations significant and even inevitable is their ability to contribute to human well-being. While the benefits accrued by the use of various technologies are evident in most cases, not all situations warrant their use. For instance, while the use of certain technologies may be of great help to young patients, for elderly patients, it may not be so always. Doctors are hesitant to perform some invasive procedures like implant surgeries on senior patients fearing severe health consequences.

The technological context of modern medicine introduces certain other kinds of issues. Technology assists physicians in diagnosing and treating patients, and many health problems can be adequately addressed with its use. The problem is not the lack of technology but their scarcity and accessibility due to various social and economic factors. Scarcity is a problem that exists worldwide. With the availability of new technologies and advancements in different fields, there is a huge demand from patients for those resources that facilitate appropriate technological intervention. Consequently, there is a severe scarcity of organs, equipment and many other facilities. For example, the use of ventilators in hospitals may often raise ethical dilemmas. The number of patients who require the facility may exceed the number of equipment a hospital would be able to supply. In another scenario, the number of patients who require renal transplantation may exceed the available number of kidneys, or the number of patients who require ventilators and dialysis machines exceeds their availability. Under such circumstances, the hospital may have to adopt a policy or strategy by which it can negotiate the conflicting interests, which amount to denying the facility/resource to some patients in order to make it available for others. Therefore, some criteria need to be adopted through which they would be able to justify their decisions in public.

Here the decision-making often cannot be exclusively based on scientific facts. They may have to consider social factors as well. For example, the hospital may have to choose between a young patient and an old one. While the former has several productive years ahead of him, the latter may have very few. Their respective social contributions may also significantly differ. Under such circumstances, to firmly stick to the Hippocratic principles that believe in the intrinsic value of all human life may not help us to arrive at a practical decision. The resource allocation decision-making process adopted by the committee appointed by the Seattle Artificial Kidney Center at the Swedish Hospital in the early 1960s presented a classic example of the steps adopted for arriving at the morally right decision. The committee entitled to selecting the patients came to be known as the "God Committee," as it is stated that the committee members are making decisions that may be detrimental to the lives of many people who were denied the required equipment for lack of sufficient numbers.

Allocating scarce resources has always posed complex moral and legal issues. The main issue is to arrive at a decisive criterion, which is optimally inclusive and agreeable to all. The Seattle Artificial Kidney Center in the early 1960s encountered a situation that was hitherto unfamiliar to the medical fraternity. About 100,000 people in the United States were dying every year of uremic poisoning and congestive heart failure due to end-stage kidney disease. The Teflon shunt, which the University of Washington Professor of Medicine, Belding H. Scribner, has developed, was a new hope to them all. Implanting the Teflon shunt in a patient's arm made haemodialysis much more straightforward, as it provided permanent access to the patient's veins (Alexander 1962, 108).

However, Seattle's Swedish hospital was able to extend the new life-saving treatment to a meagre 2% of its 100,000 terminal patients, due to the scarcity of dialysis machines. The hospital was regularly caring for five patients and by the end of the year, added five more. All these ten patients were part of a trial programme aimed at determining the feasibility of the expensive treatment on a nationwide basis. More hospitals were expected to set up a similar facility enabling a more significant number of patients to get benefitted from the new invention.

The Problem of Access to Healthcare

This scenario reveals some complex issues that we may have to address while dealing with a large number of patients with our limited medical resources. They are not problems, which medical science can effectively resolve but are social problems that involve multiple issues and hence require a different sensibility than that of an expert physician to find a way out. The Seattle incident happened after the development of a novel medical procedure and technology that could potentially save the lives of millions of people. However, such problems arising due to scarcity of resources may happen in any situation where there is a public healthcare emergency, such as the COVID-19 pandemic that has affected the whole world since the year 2020, or the influenza epidemic that commonly happen during the flu season in different parts of the world, or in a place which is unfortunately hit by a natural disaster, as it happened in many places in India and Sri Lanka in the year 2004 in the aftermath of the tsunami. What is common to all such cases is the difficulty in arriving at any simple and compatible criterion in the light of which decisions about how to use limited resources could be taken. What is required is the practical wisdom that enables one to make decisions that synchronize with the community values. In Seattle, the Artificial Kidney Center constituted a seven-member Admissions and Policies Committee and bestowed on it the authority to take the decision in choosing a few from the thousands of deserving candidates for the treatment. Since it had to be based on social and political parameters, except one member who was a surgeon, the rest were from other walks of life; a lawyer, minister. banker, housewife, state government official and a labour leader. The criteria they employed had hardly anything to do with the medical status of the patient. Instead, factors like age, sex, marital status, number of dependents, net worth, emotional stability, educational background, occupation, past performance and future potential of the patients were considered. The selection committee considered the social worth of the candidates pivotal, which goes against the principle of human dignity.

Another major factor that makes healthcare inaccessible is the escalating cost of treatment due to various factors. For example, with the advancements in medical science, novel therapeutic methods are developed and new technologies are introduced. Patients now are more and more dependent on new procedures and state-of-the-art healthcare technologies. As noted above, unlike in other sectors, technological innovations result in an increase in cost in the healthcare sector, and this factor makes healthcare inaccessible to a large number of people. Any public health emergency care scenario may give rise to similar situations. In many such circumstances, the appropriateness of the decision depends not on the patients' health status but other factors. There are other situations like organ transplantation that yield to similar situations. Again, resources may be scarce due to various reasons. Due to improvements in the quality of healthcare and sanitation, many countries have a large number of older people, whose health needs are much higher than the average. This scenario may cause severe scarcity problems. The limitations of the health budget of different countries may also contribute to this problem.

The common element in all such situations is the disproportionate demand–supply equation between resources and requirements, and arriving at a balance between them poses several serious ethical challenges. The scarce resource is the one that faces an excessive demand from the users, outdoing its supply. Besides, patients, physicians, policymakers and ethicists are concerned with the issue of the allocation of scarce resources. They primarily try to understand the relevant values to be consulted while making a decision. The search is for a paradigm of distributive justice by way of which we can ensure the allocation of limited healthcare resources reasonably within society. We need to develop a system of fair distribution that does justice to all.

Thus, the challenge of contemporary healthcare distribution is to design a framework for normative decision-making, whereby the goal of distributive justice is achieved equitably for as many people as possible. The principle of distributive justice distinguishes itself from the naïve concept of justice, which insists on a mere sharing of benefits and burdens among all. Instead, it requires the principle of equal sharing to be conditional. For instance, even though fairness demands that the benefits of healthcare should be equally distributed among all, distributive justice demands that society should be more sensitive towards the "needs" of individuals. Some may have more substantial and unique needs in comparison to others, owing to their physical and mental health status and natural talents and endowments. Some may require emergency care compared to others, and some may need special care owing to their age.

The framework of distributive justice becomes vital due to multiple factors. In many developed countries, there is an excessive emphasis on the rights of the individuals and an increasing tendency to see "access to health care" as one among the rights of the individual citizen. This may take away the focus from the idea of "common good," which is equally or more important in the very conception of society. As discussed above, increasing corporatization of the healthcare institution makes many values traditionally associated with it obsolete. The idea of distributive justice and its value framework emphasize the responsibilities of the individuals along with their rights. It presupposes the values that cultivate belongingness to a community, and also the idea of a "common good."

The need for a fair distribution system is apparent, as there is hardly any better means by which we can ensure justice. A clear understanding of "what is fair" may help us to design a better system and strategies. George P. Smith (2002) refers to the four conditions outlined by Mary R Anderlik (2001, 134) in order to define fairness, which may provide a comprehensive framework. Smith rearticulates Anderlik's four conditions in the following manner:

(1) public accessibility to "limit-setting decisions" and their policies and rationales; (2) clarity in policy rationales which explain how "value for money" is met in distributing health care resources within a society where there are reasonable resource constraints on the resources themselves; (3) a framework for principled decision making which provides a means for resolution of disputes; and (4) a regulatory process which not only assures public access to the initial "limit-setting decisions" but also provides an equitable mechanism for challenging the reasonableness of contested health care distribution decisions.

(429)

Another way to achieve justice or equity in healthcare is through health service rationing. The idea of rationing sounds negative, as it implies the denial of services. However, such denial is inevitable for ensuring proper distribution and equity. In other words, through the rationing of resources, we achieve its planned distribution. Hence, it is not a harmful procedure amounting to limiting care. Instead, it is providing care with careful and planned management of resources by ensuring rational distribution, taking into account individual requirements and social needs.

David Mechanic (1997) argues that rationing is always a blend rather than a single strategy. According to him, it happens at three levels. First, at the level of healthcare systems, government, health authorities or large health insurance plans, which establish spending levels, the types of services to be covered, the extent of technological development, the location of facilities and the extent of patient cost-sharing. Second, at the intermediate levels, where subunits may determine the number and mix of various providers, the extent of direct access and gatekeeping, waiting times for various services, schedules and the like. Finally, at the clinical level, decisions are made about treatment priorities amidst varying conditions, treatment approaches and types of patients (83).

The fundamental problem we encounter is, as aforementioned, the scarcity of resources. This problem is severe in developing countries where the healthcare system often fails in serving the needs of a vast majority of people. Many countries, when they make decisions about resource allocation, adopt a utilitarian approach. Again, a libertarian spirit may also dominate such scenarios, where the ability to pay may become the sole criterion. Their different approaches ultimately focus on rights. Although the rights-based approach sounds inappropriate on many occasions, we can never dismiss its relevance and importance altogether. The framework of distributive justice may primarily ensure a need-based approach where the needs of patients are individually assessed and balanced against the availability of limited resources.

Technologization and Fragmentation

The introduction of technology into medical care in a major way has stimulated an approach that views the human body as a machine and, more accurately, as a collection of several parts that interact with each other. This conception of the body as a fragmented whole has its advantages as well as disadvantages. Fragmentation manifests at various levels but primarily alters the very nature of the caring process by separating the human body into different functional units and further isolating them for conceiving each part's functional efficiency. Healing and well-being are now viewed distinctly by conceiving each unit as a whole with its integrity and internal efficacy. The human body can thus be viewed as a collection of separate independent units that constitute a whole at an abstract level. This atomistic framework hardly visualizes a holistic conception of well-being and health. This paradigm has some advantages as it helps to resolve issues at a micro-level. However, maladies are not mere deficiencies that affect individual organs in the human body. They are rather deficits that are experienced by the whole body and have psychosomatic and social dimensions. Health and well-being pervade the whole of an individual's being, and the technological approach with its inherent fragmentation may not always be successful in capturing the whole picture.

Many medical traditions in the ancient world have recognized the essential unity of the human body as well as the mind-body unity of individuals. The ways healthcare systems understood the nature of diseases and health depend on this broad philosophy of the human self, and the diagnosis and therapy that follows had their foundations in it. Medicine was earlier an art that treated the body as a single unit. The 2nd-century CE Greek physician Galen, for example, upholds the Aristotelian notion of telos, which affirms that everything has a purpose. Galen more or less accurately describes the human skeleton and muscular system and holds the view that every bone, muscle and organ had a particular function in the body (Forrester 2016). He accepts Hippocrates's theory of the four humours and professes that imbalance in the humours in particular organs results in illness and healing consists in restoring the balance. Underlying these ideas of telos and the equilibrium of the humours is the concept of a human being whose body and mind are integrated into a complex but single unit, where every organ functions towards the well-being of the person concerned. For Aristotle, this idea is captured with the notion of eudaimonia, which is realized in the life of a virtuous person.

This integrative picture has suffered a setback with medicine's adoption of the mechanistic paradigm of modern science. With technological artefacts dominating the practice of medicine, the focus has shifted from the total well-being of the individual to the localized improvements of the human body. The science of medicine now has a lesser number of general physicians, as it has increasingly become a domain of specialists. This scenario has eventually resulted in a fragmented perspective, which becomes the leading viewpoint in medical science. Ever since the turn of the past century, the machine metaphor dominated the scientific understanding of the body that has facilitated and promoted more research on the functions of the different parts of the human body. However, technologization has expedited fragmentation, which eventually resulted in a new paradigm where the human body would appear as an aggregate of discrete parts rather than a synthetic whole that exhibits organic unity. The various sciences and technological enterprises that deal with the different aspects of human reality fail to capture the immense complexity of the human organism. Consequently, they fail to represent the concrete man in his entirety, though their attempts to account for different human problems are reasonably successful.

Dr Alexis Carrel (1959), the Nobel laureate in medicine, in a different context laments that man, as known to the specialists, is far from being the real concrete man, as he is nothing but a schema, consisting of other schemata, built up by the techniques of each science. In the following passage that appears in his book *Man the Unknown*, Carrell reminds us that man is

> at the same time, the corpse dissected by the anatomists, the consciousness observed by the psychologists and the great teachers of the spiritual life, and the personality which introspection shows to everyone as lying in the depth of himself. He is the chemical substances constituting the tissues and humors of the body. He is the amazing community of cells and nutrient fluids whose organic laws are studied by the physiologists. He is the compound of tissues and consciousness that hygienists and educators endeavor to lead to its optimum development while it extends into time. He is the homo-economicus who must ceaselessly consume manufactured products in order that the machines, of which he is made a slave, may be kept at work. But he is also the poet, the hero, and the saint. He is not only the prodigiously complex being analyzed by our scientific techniques but also the tendencies, the conjectures, the aspirations of humanity.
>
> (2)

In its development into a techno-scientific enterprise, medicine lost sight of this extremely complex, multifaceted organism.

Birth, Death and Family Relationships

With new technologies occupying the centre stage, birth and death are no longer mere natural events but are phenomena that can be controlled and manipulated to a large extent. Like birth and death, reproduction also ceases to be a mere natural event. The domain of human reproduction has undergone revolutionary changes with the advent of new technologies as we have now gained better control over the process and can now exercise our choices more effectively in this domain. The possibility of more human intervention in reproduction raises several risks and challenges and presents before us several moral dilemmas as well.

While on the one hand, many of these innovations come as a boon, on the other hand, they raise several confusions and dilemmas. There are several areas where technological innovations can effectively intervene, such as infertility treatment, disability prevention, curing of possible genetic and other disorders, delivery-related issues, problems related to sexual relationship, etc. From the outset, pregnancy and childbirth are monitored by modern medicine with the assistance of new technological appliances and medication. These technologies are growing at such a pace that infertility would very soon be completely expunged. Again, physicians can now effectively intervene in instances of complicated pregnancies, ultimately resulting in substantially reducing the number of delivery-related complications that eventually lead to the death of either the mother or the child or even of both.

However, the potential and actual ways in which physicians can intervene in human reproduction often raise numerous issues. Life and death have always perplexed human beings, and modern science of medicine does not directly respond to such concerns. It also evades ethical questions and tries to focus on the positive benefits that could be attained in an ideal situation. For example, technologization presents these natural phenomena as medical issues where right from sexual relationship to reproduction, medical professionals and institutions now mediate pregnancy and child delivery. Sex and reproduction, which were initially conceived as dynamic natural phenomena, have become events that demand medical intervention in the new medicalized and technological scenario. This technologization is further endorsed by the commodification of health, human body and personality traits.

The technology of in vitro fertilization (IVF) is arguably the most popular among artificial reproductive technologies. IVF enables many couples and even single women to become parent, practically at any stage in their lives, without consideration of age. Traditionally, the child-bearing age of a woman was considered to be much lower than what many women in the world today think it is. Any pregnancy above the age of 40 was treated as unnatural and unsafe. Women today opt for late pregnancy due to several reasons. Many women consider the IVF as a boon as it enables them to be mothers at a relatively later age so that they could build a career and attain financial security in life. This possibility makes women more and more independent and provides them more options when they make decisions about their reproductive choices. On the other hand, many women who have failed to conceive naturally now have started considering IVF that might help them to realize their lifetime dream to become mothers and also to overcome social stigmas associated with infertility in many societies.

In September 2019, 73-year-old Mangayamma Yaramati from Guntur in Andhra Pradesh hit worldwide media headlines, as she gave birth to twin girls using in vitro fertilization (IVF) procedure. Mangayamma conceived using donor eggs and her 82-year-old husband Sitaram Rajarao's sperm. Before Mangayamma, another woman, 72-year-old Daljindar Kaur from

Amritsar in Punjab, realized her dream to be a mother in 2016 by giving birth to a baby, and another woman, Punjiben Patel, who was 60 years old in 2015, gave birth to a baby boy in Mumbai. The stories of these women from the outset convey positive messages of hope and happiness to thousands of couples who remain childless after several years of marriage. Infertility is a global problem that affects nearly 20% of couples, and the new medical technologies offer some practical solutions to overcome this.

However, all these women cited above are post-menopausal women (PMW), and this may generate several medical complications to the mother and even to the child. Besides, such incidents may also generate several psychological and sociological issues. Women above 40 years, who use IVF have elevated rates of preeclampsia, gestational diabetes, preterm and very preterm delivery (Klitzman 2016, 216). The increased risk of complications in older women having IVF includes obstetric haemorrhage, preeclampsia, pregnancy-induced hypertension, gestational diabetes, a higher rate of caesarean-section deliveries and unfavourable perinatal outcomes for the neonate such as preterm delivery, low birth weight and admission to the neonatal intensive care unit (Pokulniewicz et al. 2015, 72). Hence, it is strongly advised to avoid using IVF on older patients. The Royal College of Obstetricians and Gynaecologists (RCOG) in the UK has issued a Clinical National Institute for Health and Care Excellence (NICE) guideline which suggests that only a single embryo transfer should be performed for women aged 39 and under (72). The American Society for Reproductive Medicine (ASRM) goes further and suggests that post-menopausal pregnancy should be discouraged (Klitzman 2016, 217).

There are some other factors that make post-menopausal pregnancy ethically problematic. Daljindar Kaur, who gave birth at the age of 72, later reported to have complained that since her delivery, she has suffered from high blood pressure and weakening joints, and she would be tired very easily. She had consulted several doctors, but with no avail. She now realizes that her body cannot take the efforts and exertion of pregnancy and delivery, which were harder than she thought (Practical Parenting Team 2019). Now her baby is underweight for his age. Such "unusual" pregnancies have attracted criticism from several quarters, to which the parents of the babies turn deaf ears. The Indian Council of Medical Research guidelines recommend that the combined age of the parents should not exceed 110. However, this is not a law but only a guideline, and people have the right to exercise their discretion while making a decision. Dr Anurag Bishnoi of the National Fertility and Test Tube Center at Hisar, from where Daljindar Kaur took IVF treatment, says that since reproduction is a fundamental right, the decision to undergo fertility treatments should be left to the individuals (Dhar 2016).

Merryn Elizabeth Ekberg (2014) critically reviews the arguments for and against making ART available for older women in economically advanced nations that have the resources, expertise and facilities to offer assisted reproductive services. According to Ekberg, ART enhances the reproductive autonomy of women, which consists in the freedom to make independent choices about reproduction, including whether, when and with whom to reproduce, and by removing the age barrier to female reproduction, it facilitates the broader social goal of achieving reproductive equality between men and women (224). Women in their late adulthood become medically infertile due to the natural ageing process, and they become involuntarily childless. ART helps them to overcome this predicament. Moreover, since we have acquired scientific knowledge and have developed the technical capability to apply that knowledge, it is then unethical to deny people the opportunity to use the technology unless it is harmful. It is a fact that people live longer and healthier today, and motherhood may add new meanings and values to the longer lives of women. Finally, the idea that older women lack the required physical and emotional strength to be mothers is a myth of ageing, and to deny them motherhood on this ground is a form of ageism that amounts to a form of discrimination (225).

Ekberg then lists the arguments levelled against assisted reproduction and also their rebuttal. It is commonly argued that ART is against nature and since menopause itself is a natural phenomenon, and menopause-driven infertility is not a disease to be medically addressed. IVF in PMW amounts to altering the course of nature, as nature never intends women to conceive children after menopause. Ekberg points out that the problem with this argument is that, according to this logic, all forms of modern medicine are unnatural. Another argument reminds us that there is a higher probability that an older woman will die or develop a chronic, degenerative illness, and this may have adverse impacts on the future life of the child. However, this may be true for younger women who are employed in risky occupations as well. It is also argued that ARTs challenge the conventional ideas and values around family, marriage and kinship. But family and kinship studies reveal that the traditional model of the nuclear, heterosexual, patrilineal family has already declined (225). The following observations by Fasouliotis and Schenker (2000) summarize the debate on ART on PMW in the following passage:

> older individuals are less capable of coping with the physical and psychological stress of parenting. Having parents of advanced age may cause children to endure a greater generation gap or the lack of grandparents. On the other hand, financial and professional security and a greater motivation for parenthood usually characterize older couples. Taking all this into consideration makes it a reasonable supposition that the interests of the child would be better served by being born to older parents than to never exist at all.
>
> (175)

Fasouliotis and Schenker identify the main issues which raised ethical dilemmas following developments in ART, such as issues related to the moral status of the embryo, the involvement of a third party in the reproductive process by genetic material donation, the practice of surrogacy, human embryo cryopreservation, pre-embryo research, gamete manipulation, etc. Besides, there are several other issues related to maintaining the donor anonymity, for the sake of guarding the privacy of the donor and protecting them from legal liabilities of child maintenance and inheritance rights. But on the other hand, one may emphasize the right of the child to know its biological origin, and this information may become vital in the event of illness, be harmed by not knowing his genetic constitution or family medical history of the donors (172–173).

One important ethical concern related to pre-embryo research is regarding the moral status of the pre-embryo. It could be either viewed as an integral part of the mother's own body, or as an independent entity, whose status as a human being is recognized. The former view denies it any rights, and the mother may decide to abort it or to permit research on it, while according to the latter view, the mother is only a guardian of the pre-embryo, who has rights akin to any other human being. Besides, a third perspective recognizes it as a potential human being, so that it should be handled with dignity, and its rights should be kept as long as they do not harm major social and maternal interests or other interests (172).

The Ethics of Surrogacy

To have children is one of the deepest and strongest human urges, and hence humans adopt practically all methods available to satisfy their parental instincts. Surrogacy is practised as a successful technique (under ideal conditions) available, and like all human endeavours that respond to human needs, surrogacy, too, was employed with commercial and other interests. In the Mahabharata, when King Vichitravirya died at a very young age, leaving his two wives without any progeny, Satyavathi, their mother-in-law, requested her elder son, Vyasa, who was a great scholar and sage, to impregnate his younger brother's wives to continue the lineage. Again, the great Pandavas themselves were Pandu's surrogate sons, as they were born to different persons to his wives. The Bible too has references about instances of surrogacy. There are ample proofs that suggest that surrogacy was a common practice in ancient Egypt, Greece and Roam (Hostiuc et al. 2016, 99).

Surrogacy is performed in different ways, and the technological advances in biotechnology and medicine have revolutionized this domain of assisted reproduction. There are different types of surrogacies such as, genetic surrogacy, total surrogacy and Gestatory surrogacy (Niekerk & Zyl 1995, 345). In "genetic surrogacy" (or partial surrogacy), a woman's egg is fertilized by the sperm of the male partner of the couple desiring a child either through artificial insemination or natural intercourse. Here the surrogate is the genetic mother—and hence it is called genetic surrogacy—and the man's partner is the social and legal mother. In "total surrogacy," the surrogate's egg is fertilized with the sperm of a donor either because the commissioning father is infertile, or in order to prevent the passing of a defective gene. "Gestatory surrogacy" (or full surrogacy) is the process, which employs in vitro fertilization where both the egg and the semen are obtained from the commissioning couple or anonymous donors, and the resultant embryo is implanted into the surrogate or carrying mother (345). In all forms of surrogacy, except where sexual intercourse is employed, technology plays a vital role. The involvement of too many stakeholders may confuse, and it is a highly medicalized reproductive process, where the parents hardly have any firm control after the surrogate woman gets pregnant. However, since it interferes with the reproductive process, where the creation of life is the ultimate result, it raises several complex legal and ethical challenges. In many countries, the process is strictly regulated and is expensive, which is often not covered by insurance plans. Consequently, many intended parents travel to other countries, where the procedure is not very strict and is also relatively inexpensive. However, ethical debates and legal battles are not uncommon surrounding surrogacy in different parts of the world and they are more in countries where regulatory measures are not strong.

Many remarkable incidents took place before surrogacy became a standard practice as it is today. In 1998, the couple William and Elizabeth Stern signed a surrogacy agreement with Mary B. Whitehead, according to which Whitehead would relinquish her parental rights to the Sterns, after delivering the baby. Nevertheless, after the delivery of baby M, Whitehead found it emotionally intolerable to leave the child, and she went away with it and was later caught and arrested by the police. Subsequently, William and Elizabeth Stern approached the court and demanded that they should be recognized as the child's legal parents. The New Jersey Supreme Court decided that Mr Stern was the legal father due to its genetic fatherhood, and Mrs Stern was asked to adopt the baby in order to be recognized as her legal mother. Ms Whitehead received some parental rights, in the form of her visitation right (Margalit 2016, 46).

Baby M's case raised some concerns and issues related to the idea of motherhood concerning surrogacy. Although the court of law resolved many of them, the latter often failed to address the moral issues substantially. Later after, many more instances of surrogacy were reported across the world, more and more complex moral issues surfaced. With more advancements in technology, the process became simplified and ready to hand to humanity, and the only hindrances seem to be factors that are legal and financial. Responding to concerns regarding the rights, health and well-being of the surrogate women and the children to be born, many advanced countries have imposed stringent regulations, which made domestic surrogacy inaccessible to a vast majority of people in such places. They search for legally less cumbersome and economically more viable options in other countries, particularly in the developing countries in Europe and Asia. This scenario made India a favourable destination for intending couples from advanced countries. India had a few other advantages such as the availability of good quality healthcare, English-speaking care providers, easily negotiable legal system and economically feasible care process.

India's Anand, Gujarat, was such a destination, and till recently it was a surrogacy hub. Sat Kaival Hospital and Akanksha Infertility Clinic in Anand headed by Dr Nayana Patel and her husband Hitesh have been facilitating the delivery of over 100 babies a year. Until Minister of Health and Family Welfare, Dr Harsh Vardhan, introduced the Surrogacy (Regulation) Bill in the lower house of Indian Parliament on 15 July 2019, and in the upper house on 5 August 2019, the commercial surrogacy industry in India had a turnover of more than Rs. 13 billion. As mentioned above, a peculiar combination of legal, economic, medical, linguistic and bureaucratic factors made India a favoured destination for intending couples worldwide. The industry was making every stakeholder—the intending couple, surrogate women, donors, care providers, medical tourism companies, the local administration and the government—happy and apparently it looked like a win-win scenario. However, the entire process that usually takes several months and sometimes years may encounter several ethical and legal hiccups that may not be easy to resolve, as it happened in the case of baby Manji.

Manji was born to a surrogate woman, who was commercially commissioned by a Japanese couple Ikufumi and Yuki Yamada in 2007. The embryo was created from Ikufumi Yamada's sperm and the egg donated by an anonymous woman. However, during the pregnancy, the couple got divorced, and when the baby was eventually born, she was disowned by her intended mother. In this scenario, it became difficult to determine the baby's nationality and parentage, as the Japanese embassy in India did not grant Manji a Japanese passport or visa since according to the Japanese Civil Code, the mother is the woman who gives birth to the child, and it does not recognize surrogate children. Again, since the Indian law has no place for commercial surrogacy, Manji's father had to adopt her, which was not possible as there was another Indian law that prohibited single men from adopting children. Nor could Yamada procure an Indian passport for Manji, as she lacked any birth certificate where the names of both mother and father needed to be mentioned. Finally, he managed to get a birth certificate, where only the baby's father's name was mentioned.

Around this time, a Jaipur-based social justice and child welfare organization, Satya, filed a habeas corpus petition with the Rajasthan High Court. Satya accused the clinic of "furthering the illegal trade in infants and selling them to foreigners by taking advantage of the lack of proper surrogacy laws." It further claimed that Manji was a victim of a "child-trafficking racket." However, the Supreme Court of India dismissed Satya's accusations and granted temporary custody of the baby to her grandmother, Emiko Yamada, who was in India on a visiting visa (Points 2009, 6). Later, the Japanese government issued a one-year visa to her on humanitarian grounds, and finally, the baby went to Japan with her grandmother to join her family.

The immediate ethical issues that surface in the context of commercial surrogacy are related to a concern for the surrogate women, who are treated as a commodity and as a mere object by others for gaining their purposes. This happens in the case of commercial surrogacies and not necessary in altruist surrogacies, where the surrogate women undergo the process for the sake of helping the childless couple. In developed countries, the chances of exploitation are less due to very strict regulations. However, in countries like India, where commercial surrogacy is practised, the element of exploitation is almost unavoidable. The poverty of the surrogate forces her to opt for it and hence her volition is not real. The context of commercial surrogacy promotes more and more women "willingly" coming forward to lend their services in the reproductive process. However, this process may facilitate her exploitation and alienation. She may also be under the emotional trauma of forgoing her motherhood due to the legal requirements. The process commercializes and medicalizes her reproductive process and alienates her from the biological function, she is capable of, owing to her gender status.

In 1984, *The Warnock Report* (Warnock 1984) discussed in detail the moral aspects of surrogacy and the factors that made it both acceptable and unacceptable. It brings out some fundamental moral objections to the very idea of surrogacy. Procreation is a process that should be confined to the loving partnership between two people and since surrogacy involves the participation of a third party, it is an attack on the value of the marital relationship, and since the contribution of the carrying mother is greater and more intimate and personal than the contribution of other partners, denying her all rights on the child after its birth challenges basic morality (44–45). Again, the process challenges the concept of human dignity, since in surrogacy the woman uses her uterus for financial profit and treats it as an incubator for someone else's child by entering into an agreement to conceive a child, with the sole purpose of handing the child over to the commissioning couple after birth (45). *The Warnock Report* further says that since in surrogacy, a woman gets pregnant with the intention of giving up the child to whom she gives birth, it distorts the mother and child relationship. It damages the child in many ways. Surrogacy does not permit the child's bond with the carrying mother to continue and the process degrades the child, as for all practical purposes, the child will have been bought for money (45).

Though *The Warnock Report* was compiled in 1984, many points it raised are valid even today. As aforementioned, the two major concerns are regarding the safety of the surrogate women and the child to be born. Pregnancy and childbirth are processes that produce fundamental changes in a woman's psychophysical constitution as it initiates several hormonal changes in her body. The commercial aspects involved in the process of surrogacy reduce her status into a mere object, completely disregarding her individuality and her identity as a mother. The arguments based on autonomy are often raised in support of the commercial surrogacy. However, it is clear that the real issue involved here is not an assertion of individual autonomy, but the denial of it, at a more fundamental level. On most occasions, the social and economic conditions of a surrogate woman do not allow her to realize and assert her autonomy. In a scenario where these conditions do not come her way in asserting her autonomy, she may not be voluntarily willing to take the role of a surrogate for money alone.

Controlling Birth and Designer Babies

As noted above, the primary use of healthcare technology is to have better and stronger control over reproduction and birth. With the new technological know-how, doctors can facilitate parents to have babies with desired traits and features, a procedure that can be termed as "anti-nature." Again, it is assumed that natural bodily functions cease with death. However, medical technologies can actualize this even though they cannot bring the dead person back to life. On 15 August 2019, a woman who was brain dead for 177 days at Brno University Hospital gave birth to a healthy girl child. She was kept alive with the use of medical technologies for 17 weeks in order to facilitate her delivery when after 16-week pregnancy, she became unconscious following an epileptic fit (Cook 2019). Had this happened a few decades ago, the possibility of saving the child's life would not have been imaginable. These biomedical achievements show how advanced medical technologies have become related to human reproduction in the contemporary world.

In the previous section, I have elucidated the triumph of assisted reproduction technologies, and how they facilitate infertile individuals and parents to realize their parenthood ambitions. The potential of IVF ceases to end there. Scientists can now take this technology to the next level, with a combination of other technologies, including the editing of genomes of our cells, and also of children to be born. They can alter the genetic sequences with modern techniques for genetic modification (GM), similar to what is done in the process of genetic selection done in selective breeding of crops, plants and animals.

Technology can now facilitate the analysis of many genetic regions and consequently arrive at a better understanding of the traits that multiple genes govern. This possibility enables scientists to predict the various traits affected by genes such as the IQ of the individual and susceptibility to various diseases like diabetes and cancer. This technology is further growing at a high pace, and soon the screening of embryos for such traits may become a reality. It may reveal a series of other features such as proneness to a wide range of physical and mental diseases, sexual orientation, other dispositions of the individual, etc. Scientists may then be able to effectively intervene in order to "correct" the system with advanced "genome editing" techniques.

In 2012, a team at UC Berkeley developed the "genome editing" technique clustered regularly interspaced short palindromic repeats (CRISPR-Cas9) system approach. Scientists can now modify the CRISPR-Cas9 so that it could target any DNA sequence, and therefore, they can delete, add or modify DNA sequences with precision (Munsie and Gyngel 2018, 7).

Scientists can further extrapolate the use of this gene editing technology for inducing desirable traits in children yet to be born, and therefore, they can virtually "design" future babies. This possibility may disturb many moralists and religious people, as they may find it as an interference with the design of nature or god. The Human Genome Project devote a significant share of funds allocated to the project to studies of the ethical, legal and social issues it raises. Francis Collins, director of the National Institutes of Health (NIH) and who was the director of the Human Genome Project, has stated that concerns over ethical issues were the greatest threat to the success of the project (Buchanan et al. 2009, 27). But if gene editing technologies can be applied in the domain of correcting genetic disorder and other diseases, there should not be any logical opposition to the employment of such technologies in "perfecting" the human race, as any meddling with the human genome is an interference with the natural course of events. The same set of objections applies to the use of cloning as well, though it employs a characteristically different technique and can effectively achieve a very different outcome than the technique of gene editing.

The major sources of moral controversy over genetic research are the social and political concerns raised in connection with its application. There is a possibility that the genetic information collected may be used to deny insurance and employment (27). This possibility makes a large number of people in society vulnerable. The controversial eugenics movement that found enthusiastic advocates in England, Russia and the United States during the late 19th and early 20th centuries may gain new momentum with the new possibilities. Buchanan et al. (2009) observe:

> Nevertheless, the history of eugenics is not a proud one. It is largely remembered for its shoddy science, the blatant race and class biases of many of its leading advocates, and its cruel program of segregation and, later, sterilization of hundreds of thousands of vulnerable people who were judged to have substandard genes. Even worse, eugenics, in the form of "racial hygiene," formed part of the core of Nazi doctrine.
> (28)

They further add that the history of eugenics was marked, in its worst moments, by cruel violations of human rights and hence is instructive for those concerned with the bioethics of the new genetics. It is crucial to identify and counter all those steps that might propel us in this same direction (29–30).

Another important moral problem lies in the question concerning the moral status of an embryo and the zygote, which are to be used for experimentation for furthering knowledge in this domain. The question, "can we interfere with nature/god," is not a pressing issue from the moral perspective, as diseases can also be seen as natural and many therapeutic interferences we make, which have made human life more meaningful and fruitful, try to change the natural course of events. Again, as Smith et al. (2012) point out, a coherent anti-deliberate sequence alteration (DSA) argument would necessitate the rejection of all deliberate forms of alteration, such as selective breeding and GM. But to maintain such an ethical stance against DSA, while accepting natural sequence alterations from evolution, is to subscribe to a form of naturalistic fallacy (492).

However, the major hurdle facing this technology is the difficulty in getting fertilized zygotes for research purposes due to the dubious nature of its moral status. Some may ascribe to the zygote and embryo a human or quasi-human status. Due to this ambiguity, many couples and women would be unwilling to allow research on them. To overcome this, some scholars have proposed the creation of zygotes using donated eggs and sperm for research (Munsie and Gyngel 2018, 8). However, ethical objections have been raised against this, as it involves the creation of an embryo whose sole purpose is to be used as a means for research. It is no doubt a critical challenge for further research in this area as how to source appropriate material to progress germline genome editing (GGM) using human gametes and embryos, and regulating such research poses countless challenges for the field (8).

There are two crucial issues to consider here. First, the abovementioned question concerning the moral status of the embryo, and second, the impacts of the application of such technologies on individual human beings including the elderly and children, human societies and future generations of humankind. According to some moral frameworks, a human embryo is a potential person. As Michael J. Sandal (2005) observes, there are three possible ways of conceiving the moral status of the embryo: as a thing, as a person or as something in between (245). He adds that one way to oppose a degrading, objectifying stance towards nascent human life is to attribute full personhood to the embryo. However, Sandel finds such an "equal moral status" view problematic and argues that it would make embryonic stem cell research morally equivalent to yanking organs from babies, and the former would also be treated as a grisly form of murder, and the scientist who performs it should face life imprisonment or the death penalty (245). It is no doubt trivial to consider the harvesting of stem cells from a six-day-old blastocyst, as morally abhorrent as harvesting organs from a baby. Sandel further states that, although in natural pregnancies, at least half of all embryos either fail to implant or are otherwise lost, we do not regard these events as the moral or religious equivalent of infant mortality. Sandel concludes by arguing in the following line.

The conviction that an embryo is a person derives support not only from certain religious doctrines but also from the Kantian assumption that the moral universe is divided into binary terms: everything is either a person, worthy of respect or a thing, open to use. However, this dualism is overdrawn.

(246)

However, the prospects of genetically modifying the traits of the future generation cause more significant concern, as it implies the idea of designing babies and invokes the fear of eugenics programmes. Many scientists and ethicists are suspicious about the impacts such technologies may have on the children, as they fear that it may harm the latter and their parents by meddling with their relationship. Instead of treating the child as an intrinsically valuable gift, here it is treated as a commodity to be manufactured, which possesses certain desirable traits that can be predetermined by the parents and others. Such children will constitute a group of individuals with designed traits, most of them visibly superior to their natural counterparts and thus exacerbate social inequalities or harm the species by altering our evolutionary trajectory (Munsie and Gyngel 2018, 8).

Human Life and Technological Control

The idea of control has always fascinated humans and has also posed several challenges and threats to individuals and communities. The technology used by physicians can save valuable human life, substantially improve its quality and help humans to overcome many constraints that are imposed by those conditions that make them disabled. On the other hand, as the above discussions reveal, they pose several challenges to our moral assumptions and beliefs. It is noted above how ARTs have already challenged the sanctity of the traditional model of the nuclear, heterosexual, patrilineal family. Again, the idea of parenthood, yet another concept that remained and conceived as sacred for a long time, was also subjected to scrutiny in the changed circumstances. ARTs have transformed the very meaning of parenthood, as now we have genetic, gestational, legal and social parenthood (Morris and Nott 2009, 6–7). However, is there anything precious in such a model of a family and the idea of a parent?

One fundamental aspect of these traditional models of family and conceptions of parenthood is its undeniable patriarchal character. All of them had invariably placed man at the centre of the power configuration, where the role of women was confined to child-bearing and rearing, besides household responsibilities. This traditional structure is often criticized and rejected by many feminist thinkers as patriarchal, which invariably consists of the oppression of women. The new ART possibilities enable us to imagine families with very different patterns, structures and relationships. Women now have more options and control over making decisions about how, when and from whom to get pregnant, and this has substantially strengthened her reproductive autonomy. These possibilities may help her to come out of her "traditionally assigned roles" that predominantly confine her to the private space. Such choices may help her to strengthen her financial status, which may further empower her. Such changes may have ramifications not only within the families but also in society. Hence, this scenario might ultimately lead to the evolution of a different social structure with entirely different equations between the man–woman relationships, the mutual relationships and mutual responsibilities between members of the family and society and between children and their parents.

The actual and potential ways in which technology interferes in our lives today indicate that radical changes are imminent and may happen soon. However, all such changes may not lead to a more fruitful life and may sometime even end up either reinforcing the existing oppressive power structures with more vigour or establish different, but still despotic, structures. Technology not only empowers individuals to have better control over their lives but also to exercise control over the lives of other people. The inherent menaces of the eugenic programme are an example. It creates a minority who are visibly stronger and powerful than the rest.

However, whether we like it or not, novel technological possibilities are bound to redefine human values and make changes in human life. They may keep posing challenges to our moral norms and question our beliefs. Many of the moral issues they raise may not have clear-cut solutions due to the lack of consensus on many fundamental concepts with which they primarily deal. As mentioned above, there are diverse and often contradictory views about the status of the pre-embryo or foetus, and there is no agreement on how far the use of technologies can be regulated in this area. The situation is similar to the ongoing debates about abortion, as some will take up the pro-life position and some others subscribe to the pro-rights perspective. We find different value systems conflicting with each other preventing consensus. This aspect distinguishes our age—which ceases to hold on to one single metaphysical view of religious belief system—from an age where medicine was predominantly an art than a science.

6 Death, Dying and End-of-Life Issues

In 1975, Karen Quinlan, a 21-year-old college student, ingested some drugs and alcohol at a party. She soon started feeling unwell and stopped breathing and eventually lapsed into a coma as her brain was damaged due to a lack of oxygen. She was taken to the hospital where she was kept alive with the help of several devices, like feeding tubes and respirators. It was evident that Karen would be in a persistent vegetative state for the rest of her life without any hope for recovery. The feeding tubes, which began to be used since the late 1960s, prevented Karen from starving to death, and respirators helped her to breathe.

Very soon, her parents lost all hope in their daughter surviving. After consulting their parish priest, they requested her doctors to remove her respirator. However, Karen's primary physician, Dr Robert Morse, refused to end the artificial support. He argued that she was not yet brain dead as there were some activities in one sector of her brain. The matter eventually reached the court where the judge passed a verdict against the wishes of her parents citing that Karen's true wishes on this matter were unknown and the US Constitution was silent about the right to die. The court refused to consider her parents as her legal guardians who could make decisions for her since Karen was over 21 years old.

The legal battle continued, and finally, in January 1976, the New Jersey Supreme Court ruled 7-0 in favour of Karen's parents' position. The court treated them as her legal guardians. Interestingly, the court also provided a new interpretation of the right to privacy by extending it to decisions about refusing medical treatment as well. In cases where it is medically clear that there was no reasonable possibility of a recovery, the state's interests in preserving life are superseded by the individual's right to disconnect her life support systems. In the case of Karen, her parents, as her legal guardians, would exercise her rights to privacy. Even after disconnecting the ventilator in May 1976, Karen continued to be artificially fed. She lived for another nine years in a persistent vegetative state. She finally succumbed to death from respiratory failure on 11 June 1985. The remarkable legal battle her parents fought in various courts initiated a nationwide debate on issues related to the rights of patients to decline

DOI: 10.4324/9781003312697-6

treatment. This right was further linked to the basic bioethical principle of informed consent.[1]

Introduction

Birth and death hardly raise any substantial ethical concerns, as they are natural occurrences, though humans have attempted to manipulate them and control them. However, untimely deaths, due to diseases and accidents, have always caused profound concerns, and the science of medicine is deeply involved in addressing such issues. In many ancient societies, people tried to control these phenomena with religious invocations and therapies. Nevertheless, those practices did not drastically alter natural processes but only made minor amendments. With better understanding of ailments and their cure through medicines, the situation improved. In many societies, early healing practices that used medicines depended largely on plants and herbs. In some civilizations like India and China, these practices advanced further and eventually lead to the development of very detailed pharmacopoeias.

Most ancient societies treated birth and death as natural and only the process of living that figured in between enticed the ethicists. However, there are some isolated exceptions. *Ayurveda*, for example, suggests certain herbal medicines and decoctions for the pregnant women for facilitating the growth of the child in the womb. There are certain medicines given to the ailing, which may result in proper recovery or peaceful death. The latter could be even considered as a method of aiding a speedy death and hence can be treated as a form of euthanasia. Some religious communities, such as Jainism and Buddhism, have the idea of voluntary death, which can also be treated as a form of euthanasia from a modern perspective. But such practices were not very common in the society during ancient times. The developments in biotechnology and the new medicine that emerged during the past few decades of the 20th century have radically redefined the ways we conceive and deal with all these phenomena. Consequently, they have begun to raise moral issues and challenges. I have discussed the ethics surrounding reproduction and birth in the previous chapter, and I shall now discuss the problems surrounding death.

Though it is impossible to avoid death, it is now possible to delay it and prolong life significantly with medicines and medical technologies. Hence, the science of medicine and the physicians come to play an important role here. Since long in many societies, death has become a medical phenomenon, defined in terms of a legal and biomedical paradigm. People hardly die at home, and even if death occurs at home, the hospitals need to certify it officially. Hence, the hospital's role in people's death is fundamental. Most people die in hospitals or reach hospitals in a near-to-death condition, from which they may either recover or succumb to their ultimate fate. Again, if a given society's legal system permits, doctors can facilitate their patients in planning the time of their death and even assist them in the process of dying at a desired time and place. All these possibilities have given medicine the ability to exert significant control over what was otherwise considered as a natural occurrence. For modern man, death is a hospital event.

Two critically vital scenarios that generate the most serious ethical issues concerning the question of death are decision-making regarding end-of-life care and euthanasia. While the latter deals with the termination of life with the direct or indirect assistance of the physician, the former necessarily involves healthcare professionals' support. However, before analyzing them, we need to understand and define death itself as well as the process of dying.

Karen's case, as discussed above, raises a range of issues surrounding the notions of life, death, right to die and euthanasia. It primarily poses an ethical issue before the physicians—whether they can or should allow their patients to die if they can prevent it. Karen's physicians thought that their primary responsibility was to preserve life. According to Dr Morse, no medical precedent allowed him to disconnect his patient's respirator (Pence 2008, 25). The doctors were apprehensive due to several reasons, besides religious beliefs and long-held medical ethics. When these events happened, the American Medical Association treated deaths that occur from withdrawing a respirator as euthanasia and hence murder. They were also reluctant to deviate from the usual standards of medical practice in those days when physicians considered it their duty to continue treatment until the death of their patients (25). It is clear that the doctors were confused and were anxious about several consequences of their actions if they were to oblige the wishes of Karen's parents. The lack of precedence in the medical field was worrisome for the physicians, and the more than 2000-year-old Hippocratic moral tradition also bothered them.

The medico-technological practices physicians employ in their profession have a significant role in creating such moral confusions and anxieties. Such technological practices enable physicians to adopt several life-saving as well as life-sustaining measures for their patients. However, the irony is visible from the outset itself. While these technologies and medicines help to sustain and prolong life, they sometimes fail to assure relief and well-being. They further fail to ensure the quality of life for their patients. An extreme form of dilemma occurs when patients suffer severe pain due to an irremediable illness or when the illness ultimately takes them to an irreversible vegetative state. Death alone may relieve the patient from such a dreadful scenario, which the science of medicine cannot facilitate in the light of its value system. Thousands of patients across the world may wish to die peacefully—with the direct or indirect assistance of physicians—without undergoing the agonies caused by a dreadful disease. Discussions surrounding the notion of euthanasia nevertheless are not new to human societies. However, they find a renewed interest among different societies in the present technological context. They also generate numerous moral confusions. The new scenario exposes certain contradictions in our approach towards healthcare, life and death.

Modern medicine and healthcare technologies are capable of saving significantly more lives and enabling millions of people to enjoy better lives than ever. However, on many occasions, they fail to ensure a better quality of living, and their contributions are largely confined to the prolongation of life. From the perspective of saving and prolonging lives, modern medicine has certainly accomplished substantial gains. However, often these gains come at the expense of another important dimension of well-being; quality of life! However, an altogether techno-pessimistic approach to modern medicine may also not yield any fruits. Hence, while dealing with such scenarios, we may need to adopt a framework that takes into account all aspects of well-being and negotiate with various interests. In Karen's case, the judges made a significant observation in this context. They noted that the quality of life is an essential factor that needs to be taken into account. They further noted that though physicians have a general interest in preserving life, the patients or their surrogates have the right to refuse life-sustaining treatment in the absence of any prospects of returning to a cognitive sapient existence (Fine 2005, 306). Such observations by the judiciary have kindled further ethical and legal debates on such issues, informed by better medical knowledge.

Karen's case has naturally evoked much attention and opened up the possibility of public debates all over the United States and even outside. The believers of the Catholic Church view the case with many suspicions, as they assume that life is inherently valuable and believe that we must preserve it by all means. It raises some fundamental questions about the nature of death and about the criteria to decide whether a person is alive or dead. However, the judiciary eventually contends that it is easy to deal with life than dealing with death. They have, therefore, decided to see issues related to individual privacy and individual choices emerging from such scenarios. Consequently, the use of a technology or taking medicines even to sustain life has become a matter of individual choice.

However, it was essential to arrive at some clarity regarding the question of death as well. Modern medicine and medical technologies have significantly interfered with our traditional approaches to the natural event of death, where it was primarily associated with the absence of heartbeat or breathing. One of the most important contributions of the Karen case is the emergence of the idea and definition of brain death as a criterion for deciding when a person is dead. Doctors knew that she was in a coma. However, the word "coma" was vague and since for her to be declared as "brain dead," the New Jersey law of that time required all of her brain to be dysfunctional, which was not the case (Pence 2008, 24). She was indisputably in an irreversible persistent vegetative state. However, there was some ambiguity about her actual status.

Karen's case further led society to contemplate on the measures to be taken in order to avoid such ethical dilemmas. The judges who heard the proceedings were of the view that, instead of the court adjudicating on such issues, a "prognosis committee" could deal with them. This observation prompted the formation of various clinical ethics committees later (Fine 2005, 306).

The Cases of Nancy Cruzan and Theresa Marie Schiavo

Another important litigation that had attracted substantial public attention was the case of Nancy Cruzan, who met with an accident on the night of 11 January 1983. All attempts to resuscitate her failed. Although she was breathing without the help of ventilators, the doctors eventually diagnosed her to be in a persistent vegetative state. Though her parents wanted her feeding tubes to be removed and allow her to die, her physicians refused to do so. Finally, the matter was placed for judicial scrutiny.

The trial court which heard the case echoed the spirit of the Karen case verdict and observed that it was clear to the court that continuing with nutrition and hydration was not in tune with Cruzan's wishes. The court thus declared that no state interest overweigh Cruzan's "right to liberty." The trial court's decision pointed to a fundamental natural right guaranteed by the Constitution to "refuse or direct the withholding or withdrawal of artificial death prolonging procedures when the person has no more cognitive brain function ... and there is no hope of further recovery" (Gaudin 1991, 1308).

Notwithstanding this, the Missouri Supreme Court reversed the trial court verdict and asserted that no one is entitled to exercise another's right to refuse medical treatment in the absence of the formalities required under Missouri's Living Will statutes or the clear and convincing, inherently reliable evidence (1308). The right to refuse life-saving medical treatment is commonly considered to be based on the idea of the federal right to privacy. However, the court refused to characterize this constitutional right as one based on privacy and instead labelled it a "liberty interest," which can be infringed upon by the state or federal governments if state interests demand. Here the demanding state interest is the preservation of life (3016, 17, 18 and 19). Finally, the US Supreme Court, which ruled on the case in 1990, supported the idea that patients have a fundamental right to refuse life-sustaining treatments. However, the Court added that states might regulate the circumstances under which life-sustaining treatments are withdrawn when the patient cannot speak on his or her behalf (Fine 2005, 306). As mentioned above, Cruzan's case presented several interesting issues, as it is considered as the first case where the judgement explicitly recognized the rights of competent dying patients. It is also worthwhile to note that, even before the final Supreme Court judgement on her case, 20 states in the US had recognized the right of patients to refuse medical life support. Further, all these states had recognized the right of surrogates to make decisions for incompetent patients (Pence 2008, 28).

Terry Schiavo's is another landmark case, which raised similar ethical and legal concerns. Terry was a married woman of 26 years when she suffered a cardiac arrest and subsequently entered a "persistent vegetative state." Her husband, Michael Schiavo, and her parents together took care of her. Till 1994, she underwent several therapies that had no significant impact on her condition. In 1998, Michael Schiavo filed a petition asking the court to allow the removal of her feeding tubes. He argued that Terry would not want to be kept alive in a vegetative state. However, her parents contended this petition. The legal battle continued for several years, and it was clear that she was in a persistent vegetative state, which would be permanent with hardly any chance of recovery. Terry's tube was finally removed on 18 March 2005, and she died on 31 March.

The Ethics of Dying and Technological Interventions

These three cases are milestones in the history of bioethics, where problems related to the notion of death, refusal of treatment, obligation to treat patients who are in permanent vegetative state, ethics of artificial nutrition and hydration, right to take decisions by competent patients and surrogates, prolongation of life vs. quality of life, right to die and euthanasia are extensively discussed.

Though all these cases directly or indirectly raised all these issues, the three central concerns were the right to refuse treatment, the ethics of life support and the conflict between obligations towards preserving life and quality of life. Karen's case was directly confronting the ethics of life-supporting technologies, and the final verdict acknowledged the right to the refusal by the patient/surrogate. In Cruzan's case, though the Missouri Supreme Court explicitly stated that the state's interest in preserving life outweighed the family's concern regarding the quality of life, the US Supreme Court reviewed this decision and upheld the right of competent patients to refuse to undergo medical treatment, even if that may amount to death. This judgement was extremely significant because, for the first time, the Supreme Court underlined the rights of people to decline medical support that they consider was unwanted.

In all these cases, the precondition of discontinuance of medical treatment is the irreversible vegetative state of the patient that amounts to brain death. Hence, it is necessary to understand this central concept in modern bioethics. It is evident that in the absence of modern technologies, we would not have encountered the numerous ethical challenges we face today. For example, had death been conceived today as a simple natural phenomenon, as our ancestors did, it then would not have raised the kind of complex ethical dilemmas it raises today. Earlier, people either entirely or partially recovered from diseases. People who became unconscious would eventually die, as there were no means to supply them with required nourishment.

However, medical technologies now enable physicians to keep them alive for an indefinite time by artificially supplying respiration and nourishment. With the aid of mechanical ventilators and cardiopulmonary resuscitation, modern medicine can keep people alive even in the absence of vital functions in the body. Phenomena that are understood as "brain death" and "persistent vegetative state" (PVS) are such states of the body which are the creations of modern medical technologies. In case of brain death, there is an irreversible loss of the clinical function of the whole brain. In a vegetative state, the upper brain and the midbrain are not integrated into function with the brain stem or the rest of the body, although the brain stem continues to manage the vegetative function (Fine 2005, 303 & 304).

In 1968, an ad hoc committee of the Harvard Medical School was constituted to examine the definition of brain death. It came out with a report (1968) which states two reasons that necessitate such a new definition. One, the burden on patients' relatives, on hospitals and on those in need of hospital beds already occupied by these comatose patients, whose heart continues to beat while their brain is irreversibly damaged. Two, the controversy created by the obsolete criteria of death in obtaining organs for transplantation (337). The report finds the ancient criteria of death, as the stoppage of persistent respiration and heartbeat, as technically valid even today. The cessation of the respiratory function and heartbeat would result in brain death in a few minutes. Though the new resuscitative and supportive measures can revive vital functions, they cannot revive the brain. Earlier people considered the heart to be the central organ in the body and associated death with its stoppage. Now doctors can resuscitate it and enable a person to breathe with the revived heart. The patient appears to "live" with the help of these technologies even after his/her brain is completely damaged (339). With modern scientific knowledge recognizing the centrality of the brain and the central nervous system, it is more appropriate to associate death with the stoppage of brain functions.

The equating of brain death with death has resolved several legal issues that may arise in the context of people dying and harvesting organs from such dead persons for transplantation. It tries to answer the question: Are we ought to treat patients with irreversible and total brain dysfunction as dead or alive? The problem is scientifically resolved with the establishment of the centrality of the brain in defining the life of human beings. Any irreversible dysfunction of the brain is a loss of personhood and hence of life itself. Total damage of the brain, therefore, amounts to death. The question is, however, whether this response is morally satisfactory? Is it acceptable to doctors and other medical professionals? Can the relatives of the patients admit that their loved one is dead while he/she is still breathing?

One important factor that raises serious ethical concerns about brain death is the possibility of organ harvesting from the deceased. Organs need to be harvested at the earliest from the dead person for facilitating transplantation. The recognition of brain death becomes convenient in this context, as it enables surgeons to remove organs before many vital operations of the body cease. Millions of patients benefit from transplantation. Keeping this in mind, many physicians and policymakers have advocated a proactive role in recognizing brain death in order to facilitate the availability of organs for transplantation. However, this is not well received, as most neurosurgeons fear that the general public will view them as organ producers (Ganapathy 2018, 309).

The ambiguity surrounding brain death may lead to the possibility of misappropriation. The concept of brain death is defined differently in different countries, though these differences are not fundamental. India has enacted a law that legalized brain-stem death in 1994, and the Transplantation of Human Organs Act (THOA), 1994, provides its definition. However, this fact has deepened the fear of patients and their relatives that doctors may show undue enthusiasm in declaring more and more people brain dead for the sake of organ harvesting. THOA has relatively rigid criteria for declaring a person brain dead, as it makes the certification of four doctors mandatory that needs to be certified twice, in a gap of six hours. Nevertheless, the notion of brain death has not gained general acceptability either from the medical fraternity or from the general public (Shroff and Navin 2018, 322). The reasons are many, but three of the following are primarily important:

1. Brain death heavily shakes the long-established notion of death, a phenomenon with which humans are familiar since time immemorial. The notion of brain death, as indicated above, is made possible due to the use of life-sustaining medical technologies. Earlier also, people widely used various therapies and techniques in order to preserve life. But the employment of mechanic ventilators and cardiopulmonary resuscitation has revolutionized the scenario. Consequently, it is now possible to preserve several vital functions like breathing and blood circulation for a more extended period. Though those vital functions are indeed sustained with the support of technologies, people generally associate them with the basic criteria to decide whether a person is dead or alive. So long as those signs are visible, whether naturally or through artificial means, it is hard to accept that a person is dead. The lay public finds this idea problematic because of a mix of religious and customary beliefs surrounding death.

2. Modern medicine, which uses sophisticated technologies, operates in a highly specialized domain and, therefore, distances itself from the normal day-to-day activities of human beings. All such developments make the practice of medicine an institutional exercise. The general public then looks for information in the media, which supplies it in a language that they understand. In modern societies, the media plays a crucial role in deciding public opinion about any segment and functional sphere of society. The more the operations of the healthcare sector alienates itself from the general public due to its scientific and technical sophistication,

the more the latter rely on the media for information. The media mostly features stories that highlight the pitfalls of the institution, and this contributes further to an atmosphere of mistrust and suspicion.

3. Due to several factors, there is a growing distrust among the general public about physicians and other healthcare professionals. This factor resulted in the erosion of trust that constituted the backbone of the profession for long. Adding to this general mistrust is the public awareness about the possible misappropriations that can happen concerning organ harvesting. As mentioned above, people now often perceive their physicians as organ producers, and physicians are aware of this.

While recognizing the ethical and legal legitimacy of brain death, it is also essential to recognize the need for discontinuing any form of medical assistance to such patients. Some even argue that death even makes it obligatory to cease treatment and harvesting of organs for transplantation to extend life for others (Gostin 2014, 309). In the United States, all the states have approved the Uniform Determination of Death Act, according to which neurological criteria define brain death. Hence, doctors can withdraw life support once the patient meets this criterion regardless of the patient's or their family's views. However, in New Jersey and New York, it is mandatory to consider the family's religious and moral views before it is unplugged (903). Death is a multidimensional phenomenon, which has religious, cultural and social significances. Hence, in many societies, defining death purely in terms of scientific and neurological terms may not be acceptable to the general public. In India, for instance, many people believe that death is an event that happens as part of a continuous journey of life that does not cease with it. The journey of life continues even after death with the next life, and one's acts and deeds in the present life will have consequences in future life. Whatever criterion is applicable to understand death may have no bearing upon this belief in rebirth. However, the long association of death with respiratory functions cannot be replaced very quickly. A similar situation prevails in most human societies. With more awareness and the growth of rational and scientific temperament, the validity of the neurological criteria becomes increasingly acceptable.

Another critical aspect to note here is the difference between withdrawing life support by discontinuing treatment to a brain-dead patient and withholding support to patients that allows them to die. The latter may be considered as coming into the purview of passive euthanasia and can be legitimized only in the case where there is a "conscious" approval from the patient either directly or through an advance directive. The "Do Not Resuscitate" (DNR) directive in many US states is another example of exercising one's right of refusing to undergo treatment or appointing a surrogate in order to do so, as they are implied by the principle of informed consent, which is one of the fundamental ethical principles of modern bioethics. Since such actions may amount to the death of the patient, they have grave ethical and moral implications. In India, the Supreme Court has made passive euthanasia with advance directive legal with its judgement on 9 March 2018.

In the Karen case, though the final judgement favoured her parents, who wanted her life support to be removed, her feeding tubes continued to be in place even after the ventilator was unplugged. In the case of Cruzan, the feeding tubes were also removed. If the patient is brain dead, then there is hardly any logical difference between ventilators and feeding tubes. One may argue that the latter is associated with nourishment, and we are duty-bound to provide nourishment to a human being who is alive. However, equally important for a human being is respiration. If nourishment could be artificially supplied through feeding tubes, respiration could also be facilitated with the aid of ventilators. This issue is often discussed a little more elaborately by ethicists and hence demands some closer look.

Ethics of Artificial Nutrition and Hydration

The problem of artificial nutrition and hydration (ANH) raises some other ethical issues. ANH is given to patients who are unable to swallow on their own due to several reasons. Hence, to discontinue ANH is equivalent to stopping nourishment to a living human being. The theologians may argue that this goes against the fundamental duty towards life, which is precious and divine in itself. In his Papal allocution of vegetative state and other injuries, Pope John Paul II states that ANH is obligatory even in cases of persistent vegetative states. The Pope reminds that the obligation to provide the "normal care due to the sick in such cases" includes the use of nutrition and hydration. We cannot ethically justify the cessation or interruption of minimal care for the patient, including nutrition and hydration because it leads to death by starvation or dehydration. In this sense, it amounts to be true and proper euthanasia by omission, which by its very nature and intention brings about death. Such an act, even if performed with the purpose of eliminating all pain, is always "a serious violation of the law of God, since it is the deliberate and morally unacceptable killing of a human person" (John Paul II 2004). Life requires nourishment, and all our traditional moral principles support feeding others, especially, those who are deprived of it, as our duty. The patient in a vegetative state is incapable of doing it on her own. Hence, as fellow humans, we need to assist her through all means that are available to us. Before artificial methods were available, such patients had no option but to die of starvation. Modern medicine has technologies that can artificially feed incapacitated patients. The use of other medical technologies, like ventilators, too aid patients to sustain their life.

However, their primary purpose is to aid a particular therapy, and their use is not to be continued indefinitely. Once the patient regains her consciousness and starts breathing naturally, they are removed. They do valuable service in between and aid the therapeutic process fruitfully. For patients who are unable to breathe on their own due to inadequate brain activities, life support technologies may aid sustenance of breathing, and their withdrawal may result in their immediate death. It is clear that their employment in two different contexts has different intents and effects. In the first case, they may assist the therapeutic procedure that facilitates a cure. In the second case, their use helps only to sustain life and hence seems to constitute the core of a therapy that envisages no cure other than indefinitely sustaining breathing and blood circulation. In this sense, their use is not going to benefit anyone. However, due to our conventional association of life with breathing, relatives of the patient and even physicians feel emotionally reluctant to discontinue such aids. The idea of brain death enables them to regulate their employment for the benefit of humanity. By recognizing the legitimacy of the concept of brain death, we can rationalize the use of such life-saving technologies, which are both expensive and often scarce. As stated above, it is now morally obligatory for us to discontinue such facilities to a patient who is brain dead, as the dead does not require medical support.

Implicit in this notion is the view that the life of an individual is associated with her somatic life and not just with a bodily existence. The body, of course, can be preserved for an indefinite period even after the brain functions cease to exist. In other words, the total damage to the brain amounts to the destruction of the person. Afterward, the patient ceases to be a person. Hence, the natural rights we associate with an individual, such as the right to healthcare, no longer remains valid to her.

Nevertheless, the case of a patient who is conscious or may regain consciousness with medical treatment, but has lost his/her natural ability to consume anything for satisfying the basic requirements of nourishment presents a different problem. Since she is not dead, she is entitled to all the fundamental rights of any normal human being. Hence, we are obliged to provide her nourishment through artificial means. With the advances in healthcare and the subsequent rise in the life expectancy of people across different societies, the need for ANH is very high in hospitals and other healthcare centres. Such a scenario raises several other issues than those that are mentioned above. In many such cases, particularly when the patients are old, the decision-makers are members of the family. Their decisions often are influenced by several social, cultural and economic factors, which hardly have any objective bearing on the technical decisions healthcare professionals make. Sometimes, even if the patients are conscious, they are unable to voice their wishes due to several factors. In the typical end-of-life (EOL) situations, this may happen commonly.

ANH becomes ethically problematic due to various other reasons as well. The very status of ANH as a treatment option is questionable. It is not part of any therapy, but only an aid that supports a therapeutic procedure. Hence, it should ideally cease to continue once the medication or surgical procedure ends. ANH is largely used for EOL care, and here it raises several issues. ANH contributes to the prolongation of life. However, it may not contribute to the enhancement of its quality. On the contrary, it may ultimately diminish it. Many patients in the EOL state use it occasionally, and this may, to some extent, help them. But many others use it almost permanently till the end of their life, and this may aid only the prolongation of their sufferings. It may also give false hopes to patients and families about cure or improvement (Heuberger 2010, 354).

Dying Patients and Their Interests

The fundamental ethical approach to the dying patient is to start discussing the dying process and helping the patient to depart peacefully rather than trying to delay the imminent death with the help of therapies, which are often painful and burdensome for both the patient and her family. The introduction of hospitals in our culture has significantly changed the lives of many patients who are in the last stage of their lives. Old age brings several health-related discomforts, and many of them are not terminal. Proper clinical interventions may cure many of them or help patients to manage their diseases in better ways than suffering from them. Many hospitals now have geriatric wards to take care of such issues, and they contribute significantly to alleviating the sufferings of the senior population. However, not all geriatric health issues demand the adoption of a protocol that aims at a complete cure. The usual culture in hospitals focuses on cure and all those procedures that facilitate the same. Often the notion of cure is identified with prolongation of life, and this process may disregard the quality of life a patient rightfully deserves at the end stage of her life. All these have to change, and there should be a shift to a more realistic understanding of patient health. Hospitals are often reluctant to make a diagnosis of dying as they focus on the improvement of the existing state (Ellershaw and Ward 2003, 30).

Often the aged patients admitted to the hospital will be in such a state that they hardly make any decision regarding the treatment and the continuation of the support system. As a combined effect of old age and illness, their ability to make autonomous choices erodes significantly. In many cases, the decisions for them are made by others like close relatives or their children. Their wishes about the same are not known. One primary obligation of the healthcare system to such patients is to help them to make decisions and to know their wishes about their treatment. As far as doctors are concerned, they have to respect life, protect the health of their patients and oblige to make patients' interests their first concern (Kalantri 2003, 260).

EOL is a situation that might require frequent hospitalization and the use of several life support systems. Often the patients become a burden to the family members who assist them. For the doctors, the discussion with the patient and their relatives is a routine process. But for the patient, it is a unique experience and perhaps the first of its kind, she has experienced in her entire life. There are questions and anxieties, sometimes explicitly raised and more often not. The doctor here must be compassionate and responsive to the concerns.

The end stage of a patient demands a more careful and rational approach. What is required is not enthusiasm in preserving life at all costs, but to administer or withdraw medication, ANH and other life support whenever it is appropriate. An ethical approach to ANH and ventilators consists not in withholding them rigorously in all circumstances but sometimes in withdrawing them as well. Doctors may emotionally feel to do the contrary. However, they have to go beyond their emotional leanings and understand the situation where they find their patients. Every patient comes from a social, cultural and family background, and every medical decision will have a different meaning to different patients. Doctors have to negotiate with such situations and try to understand it along with their patient's disease.

Death and Dying: The Changing Perceptions

As observed earlier, phenomena like death and dying, which were considered at some point in history as natural occurrences, have come to be treated very differently later. Earlier people were born and died at home, with many people around. They were public events, and during the dying process, people were rarely alone. As observed by Philippe Aries (1974), the approach of death transformed the room of the dying man into a sort of public place, and the late 18th-century enlightened doctors complained about people crowding into the rooms of the sick people as that may deprive patients of fresh air (539–540). The priest from the church arrived at this point to make the event of dying part of a more significant religious journey of the individual. In Indian villages, relatives and friends used to chant sections from religious scriptures to facilitate the end journey. They stay back with the dying person, till his earthly voyage ends. Making death a social event helps to naturalize it and to make people accept it as a reality that everyone has to encounter. Linking it with religious rituals assures that though one may not be salvaged from one's mortality, the divine salvation will make the tragic event meaningful.

On the contrary, many people die in hospitals today, or even in intensive care units, surrounded by lifeless machines and the beeping voices of medical equipment. They die a lonely death, often with no human being near them. Before this inevitable end, some may spend several days in the hospital with uncertainty about recovery. This possibility alienates death from our day-to-day experience and our social surroundings. It has become a medical event, and the dying person is assisted not by relatives, but by healthcare professionals in unfamiliar circumstances. People today hardly witness the process of dying; instead, they only see the after-death rituals.

More than death, the process of dying has undergone remarkable changes, as the advent of modern medicine made it possible to prolong it indefinitely. It became possible for people to live very long with their diseases, which nevertheless are terminal. For example, during the 1980s and early 1990s, HIV/AIDS was a fatal disease that caused the death of thousands of patients every year. During those days, HIV/AIDS was synonymous with imminent death. With the development of antiretroviral medication, the situation has improved considerably, and today the life expectancy of a patient with HIV infection is not much less from that of an average person (Katz and Maughan-Brown 2017, e325, and Augustyn, Walker and Goss 2012). This has led patients in many places to recognize their infection not as a terminal disease but as any other viral infection, which can be effectively controlled. The management of the disease with medication is a different experience than being in a continuous process of dying with the disease. Many new technologies have improved the experience of living with the disease in significant ways, transforming the miserable plight of a dying patient into the joy of living a life with meaning.

One major problem associated with the general perception of the new technologies is the false hope they have created for dying patients. Regardless of all its achievements, modern medicine can never predict the possibility of a cure with absolute certainty. Many people approach healthcare facilities today with the misapprehension that the new technologies have a magical cure to their diseases. On the contrary, none of the therapeutic procedures adopted by modern medicine, which includes its medication as well as the application of technology, can promise a complete cure. They may sometimes end up receiving ineffective and expensive healthcare assistance.

Perhaps the most significant contribution of modern medicine and medical technologies is the longevity revolution it brought about. In many countries, the average age of the death of people has significantly gone up. We have discussed this aspect in one of the previous chapters. As a consequence, people refuse to accept any death that happens before a person attains that age and consider it as unnatural and unfortunate, which is not always correct. Death is such an evasive phenomenon, as we never know what the right time to die is.

Brain Death and Organ Transplantation

Ever since the idea of brain death was initiated, several controversies surrounding its moral foundations were raised. Subsequently, medical fraternity in different parts of the world began to discuss and debate it. Finally, in 1980, the Uniform Determination of Death Act (UDDA) has made it into law in the United States, and now many countries in the world have adopted this criterion. The new concept has undoubtedly provided a more scientifically accurate definition of death. As discussed above, it drastically changed the long-established beliefs surrounding death, where the heart was treated as the central organ in the body, and its functioning held the key. The new definition never contradicts the traditional view. However, it goes deeper into the phenomenon of death with the assumption that the brain is the central organ in the human body. Metaphors like "breathing one's last" have now become inadequate to describe death.

Since long, the religious and biological ideas of death coexisted. The former focused on the idea of the departing of the "soul," and the latter emphasized the cessation of biological functions like respiration, metabolism, heartbeats, blood circulation, etc. These two accounts hardly contradicted each other, as they dealt with different aspects of the same phenomenon. The idea of brain death adds a deeper dimension to the biological view. Such a definition was made necessary by the advances in medical technologies and some possibilities they offer in providing better care to people who suffer from vital organ failure. Therefore, this new definition of death has resulted in significant advancements in healthcare by facilitating organ transplantation.

Though there is no necessary causal link between brain death and transplantation, the two indeed have some relationship. It is precisely this link with organ transplantation that makes the concept of brain death morally controversial. As stated above, harvesting organs from a brain-dead patient ensures the quality of the organs. This new definition of death may also help physicians to plan better and fruitful EOL management of their patients by discontinuing ineffective medical treatment. The possibility of organ harvesting from the brain dead and the immense benefits that suffering patients gain from it have made organ harvesting popular among the public as well as the medical fraternity. The latter is further anxious about the care of a large number of patients who need transplantation. But critics point out that transplantation may only help the patient who needs it and not the donor. They also point to the possible mistakes physicians may make in diagnosis. Furthermore, the concept of brain death, with its inherent ambiguities, confuses both the patient and her surrogates. Often there arises strong opposition from the families in withdrawing the life-supporting technologies and medication. However, it is also essential to restrict the resources for care. Since the concept of brain death is the chief facilitating factor for organ procurement, there is an intense apprehension that the latter may become the leading cause for the death of the donor. It may also facilitate the wilful and unethical organ trafficking and trading, which are also criminal acts in many countries.

Many scholars argue that decisions regarding brain death should be made for the benefit of the patient, and organ donation should be a consideration of secondary importance. Clarke et al. (2014) argue that although

> facilitating successful transplantation is laudable from a justice perspective, the real utility of the accepted brain death criteria may be in determining hard clinical endpoints where care may be considered

nonrestorative and thus futile, as technological intervention can be viewed as having approached the limits of accepted medical practice.

(45)

In the absence of any organ procurement, there is no reason to affirm the death of a person in terms of any neurologic criterion.

Though many arguments and factors can be arrayed against the legitimacy of such a concept like brain death, the major factor that makes it morally problematic is its failure in being in harmony with our common idea of human death. Moreover, the concept of brain death is the product of modern technology. In order to determine whether a person is brain dead or not, elaborate technological criteria are involved. This reliance on technology makes human death a highly technical phenomenon, which is contrary to our understanding. All such aspects strengthen the view that brain death is an invention of modern technology. It is a product of the technologically reinforced modern industrial civilization, which commodifies everything, including the human body and organs.

However, it is unfair to denounce the idea of brain death as the product of a malicious design that identifies everything, including the human body as a commodity for furthering mere economic interests. From the very outset, its utility in drawing the limit of clinical interventions cannot be ignored. As mentioned above, this new definition of death thus plays a beneficial and essential role in the management of EOL patients. As Michelle J. Clark (Clarke et al. 2016) makes it clear, it is futile to continue to treat a patient who is neurologically dead, and keeping this limit in view is important in preserving the dignity of the person. Clarke further affirms the need to identify the clinical endpoint as death and not just a state where further treatment is simply futile. By simply calling and pronouncing the patient dead, adds Clarke, the patient's true state is respected (2054).

The process of organ transplantation raises another set of ethical problems. Apart from all the complex medical issues it may raise, the very idea of organ procurement fosters several ethical questions. Fredrik Svenaeus (2010) discusses the three metaphors that guide contemporary thinking on organ transplantation. The three metaphors are gift, resource and commodity (164). According to Svenaeus, each of them implies a specific set of values. Svenaeus, adds that although "gift" is the sanctioned metaphor for donating organs, the state authorities and medical organizations perceive the human body and its parts mainly as a resource. We understand the idea of gift by associating it with an act of charity. The person who gifts something to another person does it with full awareness (voluntary) and with no expectation of reciprocity from the latter. The receiver of the gift gets it because the giver wants to give it to the former. Svenaeus further states that a person gifts something she does not want, and in the case of organs, she does not need them after her death. Hence, to refuse to gift them after one's death is irrational. However, when something is perceived as a resource, its utility value is emphasized rather than its charity value. Though in many places an informed consent of the donor or her surrogates is a prerequisite for organ procurement, many countries are now adopting the idea of presumed consent (164). According to this idea, unless the patient explicitly states it otherwise when she was alive, it is legally appropriate to harvest her organs after her death. Again, since there is a huge requirement for organs, they may become a commodity, as anything that is scarce is a commodity in our market-driven economic environment and its value system.

There are very serious moral issues surrounding the perception of organs as resources and commodities, as this is a blow to the dignity of man. The perception as commodities is more problematic as it fits the basic economic equations of capitalism. The value of a product—and in this case the human body and organs—is determined exclusively in terms of demand–supply equations. This particularly raises concerns in the light of the increasing growth in the trafficking of body parts that has global dimensions. Poverty encourages people in many poor countries to sell their organs in order to make money and there are international organ brokers to facilitate such illegal and unethical transfer of body parts (Gunnarson and Svenaeus 2012, 13). This is damaging to all stakeholders involved and to a huge blow to human dignity. Many countries have laws that aim to prevent such immoral trafficking but such exchanges continue to happen primarily due to economic disparities and poverty. The United States has outlawed the buying and selling of organs in 1984 with the introduction of the Anatomical Gift Act and the National Organ Transplant Act. In India, the parliament in 1994 passed the "Transplantation of Human Organ Act (THO)," which specified the provisions under which organ donation and transplantation activities could be legally facilitated. Although various measures governments across the world have adopted, the illegal trafficking of body parts continues in many parts of the world.

From 30 April to 2 May 2008, the Transplantation Society and International Society of Nephrology in Istanbul, Turkey, convened an International Summit on Transplant Tourism and Organ Trafficking, which was attended by more than 150 representatives of scientific and medical bodies from around the world, which included government officials, social scientists and ethicists. The Summit defines organ trafficking as

> the recruitment, transport, transfer, harboring or receipt of living or deceased persons or their organs by means of threat or use of force or other forms of coercion, of abduction, of fraud, of deception, of the abuse of power or of a position of vulnerability, or of the giving to, or the receiving by, a third party of payments or benefits to achieve the transfer of control over the potential donor, for the purpose of exploitation by the removal of organs for transplantation.
>
> (International Summit 2008)

It has been widely observed that the growth of medical tourism for transplant surgery and other advanced procedures have exacerbated the older divisions between the North and South and between the haves and have-nots, as the flow of organs, tissues and body parts follows the modern routes of capital: from South to North, from the Third to the First World, from poor to rich, from black and brown to white, and from female to male bodies (Shroff 2009, 354). The Istanbul Summit (2008), which described transplantation as a symbol of human solidarity, had voiced its anxiety on the reports of trafficking in human beings who are used as sources of organs and of patient-tourists from rich countries who travel abroad to purchase organs from poor people (1227). The Indian scenario is no different. Sunil Shroff compares the organ trade in India with other problems like child labour and prostitution in order to bring out its societal angle. He affirms that here too, there is the exploitation of the poverty-stricken people who look for significant substantial gains in order to meet their requirements. According to him, factors like

> the presence of a growing middle class, the lack of a national health insurance scheme, the growing disparity between the rich and poor, and to some extent the presence of technology in the country makes the process of commodification of organs a simple, quick, and attractive business proposition for some and a solution for others.
>
> (Shroff 2009, 352–353)

There are many other issues involved in illegal organ trading for transplantation. As stated above, since the donors are invariably from the economically underprivileged groups and societies, the medical care they receive after surgery too will be of inferior quality. This may cause additional health problems to them, which may further exacerbate their poverty. Again, since the surgery is performed in such places where the quality and standard of care would be minimal, there is a great danger to both parties.

Organ trading raises some more fundamental moral issues where the question of human dignity comes to focus. The question is: What is fundamentally wrong with selling one's body parts? How does it impair the dignity of a human being? Modern ethical ideas affirm that individual autonomy is one of the central principles to be upheld in modern life. Autonomy assures that an individual is a sole decision-maker regarding her life. She has the right to choose among alternatives she comes across. Furthermore, in healthcare decision-making, she makes final decisions about whether to adopt the suggested course of treatment or refuse any treatment at all. The principle of autonomy further affirms that an individual has rights over her body and she alone can decide what needs to be done with it. In the light of this principle, can we justify prostitution and selling of body parts? It may be true that when body parts are sold for a price, that amounts to the commodification of the individual. It also leads to instrumentalizing the body and organs and this exercise may ultimately harm the poor, who largely sell their body parts for their immediate financial gains (Svenaeus 2010, 125).

As we noted above, selling and buying or organs is illegal in many parts of the world and the reason for the same is the moral ideal that endorses human dignity. These countries—which include most of the world's democratic countries, including India—though recognize the individual's rights over her body, refuse to accept that the individual has the right to sell it partly or completely. However, as Svenaeus observes, the donation of body parts presupposes ownership—an individual is the owner of her organs—and this ownership status may confer to the individual the right to sell or rent her possessions as well. These possessions include her body and its organs. Hence, how can we justify the state imposing restrictions on such activities (164–165)?

This is posed more as a philosophical problem and is an issue, which many societies have to grapple with in the context of the advances they make in transplantation technologies. In Iran, the buying and selling of kidneys are legal, and the government strictly regulates it. The government plays a crucial role in this exercise in Iran and also provides financial assistance to the recipients by making medicines available in subsidized rates (Major 2008, 68). Iran successfully avoids a few dark sides of organ trading with the active involvement of the government in the process. However, the philosophical and ethical questions remain unanswered.

The problem lies in the liberal tradition of the West, which recognizes the property rights of an individual as indisputable. The Lockian tradition has underlined this aspect. John Locke's (2010) concept of property provides some fundamental justifications for legitimizing the idea of private property. With this, he also legitimizes an ethical framework, which bestows upon individuals, certain fundamental rights that enable them to make choices and take decisions and live as independent individuals. Modern bioethics developed in the United States and other advanced Western countries has inherited this spirit of the liberal tradition. Therefore, along with beneficence, nonmaleficence and justice, the principle of autonomy is also projected as foundational. This principle guides the process of decision-making in the practice of medicine. According to this tradition, an individual's ownership over her body is fundamental in order to facilitate gifting or donating of body parts.

However, the body is not an ordinary property like other properties. For example, a pen which I have bought is my property, which I can gift or sell. I am its owner, and I am exercising certain rights I have over my property and even after giving away this property, I remain as an individual with integrity. Such acts of gifting have a moral value, as they are expressions of charity. But the moral value of an act of donating an organ is different from this, as it is more than an act that expresses charity. It is instead a rare act of solidarity, which sometimes involves a sacrifice. It bestows upon the recipient an irreplaceable benefit, which no other person can supply. The donor gives it away for the benefit of her fellow human beings and, in that sense, to universal humanity. Therefore, instead of ending up separating one part of herself for the sake of another, she broadens her selfhood by reaching up to universal humanity.

The material objects I have procured and may sell, or gift are not my natural endowments, like my body and its organs. These objects are owned by me later, as gifts from others or purchased with money. According to the classical definition of property, proposed by Locke, man has a *property* in his own *person* and this nobody has any right to, but himself. The labour of his body and the work of his hands are properly his and he makes his own property mixing his labour with and joined to nature, which commonly belongs to all men (Sec 27). I become the owner of something only after an act of labour. I cease to become its owner after I sell it. In this sense, my ownership over them is contingent. All property we own is like this a contingent commodity. Man can own them and sell them. However, the body is different. It is "with" and "through" the body that man affirms ownership over things. Hence, the body itself is not a thing that we procure as a property. It constitutes man's being. An individual does not own it, but she is constitutive of it and can never cease to own it. Even after transplantation, we describe the recipient as someone who had undergone transplantation. The donor remains the "real" owner of the organ. The procedure, unlike other surgeries, may transform the recipient's identity. The liver or kidney which she carries now hardly becomes hers. She is now described as a recipient.

Organ transplantation is, no doubt, a boon to humanity from modern medicine and technology. It raises multiple ethical and legal issues, and facilitating complex transplantation surgeries by no means is easy. In the present context, this treatment is inaccessible to a vast majority of patients due to several procedural, technological, economic and other reasons. Transplantation surgeries are highly expensive in all parts of the world and this factor alone will make it inaccessible to a large number of patients who require it. The availability of organs causes another major hurdle and governments in different countries are adopting several means to overcome them. Notwithstanding such efforts, the waiting list in many countries is very long. Consequently, many patients may die due to the unavailability of organs. With some changes in the policy and procedures, we may be able to pool the sufficient number of organs required to meet the requirement of patients.

Quality of Life and Moral Dilemmas

As noted above, the modern ethical framework evaluates actions in the light of principles like autonomy, nonmaleficence, beneficence and justice. Such principles need to be considered even in the case of EOL patients. The first one, autonomy, emphasizes the importance of informed consent as well. All therapeutic decisions like the withholding and withdrawing of the ANH and ventilators should be consistent with this principle unless they are taken on purely medical grounds. The expressed or implied wish of the patient is important here. In EOL scenarios, a conflict between longevity and quality is quite common. Doctors may subscribe to different philosophical schools when it comes to the question of choosing between the two. What is important is certainly what the patient desires. However, when the patient moves to comatose state and from there to persistent vegetative state and brain death, the ethical decision to be made by the doctors is to stop all therapeutic interventions, overruling all desires of the relatives.

The question of quality of life is not altogether a technical issue, as what is conceived as a life with quality differs from person to person. It is common to find patients whose legs are amputated finding life meaningless, and they may gradually encounter bouts of depression. On the other hand, some others who are paralyzed below their neck find meaning and happiness in their remaining abilities and lead a life with joy and purpose. Hence, to choose between longevity and quality is not the business of the physician or any other person, but it is the prerogative of the patient herself. However, the physician is not ethically obliged to facilitate all the desires of a patient while the latter continues under his care. Physicians can insist on their patients to satisfy some requirements and follow some protocols as a condition for extending care. The physician is also a moral agent and, therefore, may have to make attempts to convince his patients what he thinks is a morally appropriate and sustainable option. What is important is to avoid any possible coercion as the patient–physician relationship necessarily involves power disparities.

There are certain undeniable circumstances where the physicians can adopt an unequivocal moral stance and inform the relatives of the patients about the futility of continuing therapy. For example, for a patient who is in a persistent vegetative state for a long time and there are no genuine medical reasons to believe in a recovery, the continuation of a treatment or the use of ventilators and even ANH is futile. Such brain-dead patients can be allowed to succumb to the natural process of death and save scarce and expensive resources for another patient who needs them.

It is natural to have moral anxieties and other concerns when patients and their relatives encounter the question of death. Physicians, on the other hand, relate to the death of their patients in a different way. Though emotions may not be completely absent, they often do not dominate in physicians' responses to patients' death. However, in many EOL cases, physicians' views are crucial, particularly in non-Western cultures. Hence, the responsibilities are also high. Many such cultures have huge scarcity issues and also economic problems. The physician may have to consider all such factors while giving her advice to the patients and their relatives. End-of-life state and death are understood very differently in the modern world where various therapies and medical technologies offer multiple options to both physicians and patients. But paradoxically, many such advancements further seem to deepen the moral crisis we face in the healthcare sector.

Dying with Dignity

As stated above, ethically the first step for a physician to adopt in an EOL scenario is to recognize it as a situation where neither cure nor any substantial improvement of the patient's health is a possible outcome. The patient–physician interaction has to begin with the understanding—ideally from both the parties or at least from the part of the physician—of imminent death. The priorities of all the stakeholders in this context are, therefore, significantly different from an ordinary patient–physician relationship where the primary objective is a cure.

However, in the light of the modern technological possibilities, death itself has to be understood very differently. Medical technologies can either assure or deny a patient the possibility to live and die with dignity. These new technologies have significantly reduced the agonies of death by saving millions of lives by effectively interfering on time. In one sense, they have made drastic changes in our ideas about a meaningful life and assumptions about a dignified death. We have seen how effectively they can interfere in sustaining life, particularly in the case of patients who are in the state of temporary coma. Such patients, instead of starving to death, successfully sustain their life with the artificial nourishment and hydration provided to them even without their conscious awareness and once they return to consciousness, may continue to live healthy lives.

With the introduction of more and more new technologies, doctors are now able to arrive at an increasingly better and more accurate diagnosis of their patients' health impediments. These technologies can now predict not only the possibility of diseases but also how and when the patient might die. They enable the doctors to predict how imminent is death, how long their patients are going to live, the feasibility of therapeutic interventions and also other social, cultural and economic aspects of the prognosis of the disease. This enables them to prepare the patient or her relatives to approach death more realistically and well in advance. What is more important in this context is to ensure the dignity of the dying patient and enable them to die with dignity.

The idea of dying with dignity declares that human life has an intrinsic worth and once it loses its worth, it is better to end it. This presumption does not necessarily require any metaphysical basis. However, many religious and metaphysical traditions support this view. Peter Allmark (2002), while discussing this idea of death with dignity, argues that it involves two claims; lives without dignity should be ended and people should be allowed to make the choices necessary to procure a death with dignity (225). However, "dignity" is a term whose meaning is understood by different people in light of their respective values. Hence, how to decide when does life become devoid of dignity is not an easy question to answer. Since the emphasis is on dignity, which is a term derived from the Latin, *dignitas*, meaning worthiness and nobility, the stress is not on death but life. In this sense, the idea implies that it aims to ensure a good life until death and not a good death.

Under normal circumstances, the threat to dignity is not easily noticed in many social contexts. This is partly because of the diversity in the ways in which the concept of human dignity is conceived today. Many conventional and traditional standards that exist in various cultures pose visible threats to the dignity of patients who are old and who are in the last stage of their lives. It is believed that their dignity is not exceedingly threatened in healthcare contexts as they are cared reasonably well in many places by professionals and there are protocols to ensure this. However, this may not be true in the case of many patients, especially those who deserve special attention like older persons and people who are terminally ill. The EOL scenarios involve these groups that are most vulnerable to death. David Sudnow (1967) in his classic study on the sociology of death emphasizes the idea of social death which precedes biological death. This is particularly the case with older patients as they are perceived by the rest of the society in the light of their forthcoming death. According to Sudnow, a person who is socially dead is essentially treated as a corpse, despite the fact that she is still biologically alive (74). This presumption about their imminent death influences all healthcare professionals and shape their attitudes and approaches towards older patients. Moreover, as Jonathan Lieff (1982) points out health providers, and particularly doctors, demonstrate an avoidance towards the dying, elderly and handicapped patients (49), as they believe that talking about death creates a negative self-image (50). Moreover, when dealing with a difficult elderly and dying patient, the doctor may experience a psychological impotence, as they encounter an unfamiliar situation that makes them uneasy. They are "taught to keep people alive at all costs and strive to work with patients in an optimistic and confident manner, in order to instill confidence in patients" (58). The presence of dying patients makes them uneasy and helpless. They thus tend to turn away from such patients than to accept defeat.

This insensitivity and avoidance are widely prevalent in many cultures. For example, in India, where the number of older people is consistently increasing over the past few decades, the instances of elderly abuse also show a constant increase. Though traditionally, Indian culture was respectful to their elders, the changing socio-economic structure and the erosion of the joint family system crippled this approach. In the professional atmosphere in the hospitals, they are widely neglected, and many of them face a sudden decline in health as a consequence of neglected bouts of illnesses by the family. A cross-sectional hospital-based study conducted in the Department of Psychiatry in M.P. Shah Medical College, Jamnagar, India, documents high prevalence of abuse (24%) in elderly patients with depression. The study reports that among depressed elderly, female gender, fewer educational years, widowhood status and living in a joint family are significantly associated with the experience of abuse, with the commonest being psychological (Patel, V.K. et al. 2018, 532).

Similar conditions exist in many other societies. Article 6 of the Inter-American Convention on Protecting the Human Rights of Older Persons stipulates the conditions required to maintain dignity until death. The article states:

> States Parties shall take steps to ensure that public and private institutions offer older persons access without discrimination to comprehensive care, including palliative care; avoid isolation; appropriately manage problems related to the fear of death of the terminally ill and pain; and prevent unnecessary suffering, and futile and useless procedures, in accordance with the right of older persons to express their informed consent.
>
> (Huenchuan 2017, 2)

As mentioned above, the elderly constitutes one of the major sections in society, along with the terminally ill, who are vulnerable to death. This general neglect may add to their agonies during their EOL period. In general, patients in the EOL situations may have to be treated with two basic approaches for safeguarding their dignity. The first, as mentioned above, is to ensure them good life till the end of their life. The other is to provide them the option of a good death, which is also known as euthanasia.

Good Life till Death and Good Death

The idea of a good life till death is a complex mix of medical and emotional comforts that patients in need receive. This is what palliative care aims to provide to patients in the end stage of their life. Palliative care primarily aims at controlling pain and other symptoms and alleviating the social, psychological and spiritual problems of patients. The nature of treatment provided to them are characteristically different from normal, as the goal here is not complete or partial cure, but to ensure good life with fewer pains and sufferings to the patients till the end of their life. In this sense, it is a different paradigm of medical care. On the other hand, palliative care patients do enjoy all the rights of other regular patients. However, their physical and psychological needs are going to be very different from the latter.

There are multiple ethical issues facing EOL and palliative care professionals. Not all patients are at the same stage of their health and hence their individual requirements may significantly vary from each other. Again, another crucial issue that professionals may face while dealing with such patients is in determining their capacity to express their agency. Many of them will be in a declining stage and hence may not possess the ability to determine what they want. Hence, there are difficulties associated with ensuring informed consent and confidentiality. A few of them may still respond to medication, at least partially. Hence, it is essential to continue to treat them. However, how aggressively they are to be subjected to medical treatment is a difficult question. Many therapeutic interventions often generate discomforts to the patients, and hence professionals have to decide how useful is it to continue the treatment that aims at recovery. They may often encounter a problematic situation, where they will have to make a call on whether to continue with or withdraw life-sustaining treatments. The life of the patient may end if they decide to withdraw treatment, and hence many professionals decide to prolong it even if they are convinced of the futility of the treatment. This is ethically wrong in palliative care. What is required is an approach that controls pain and symptoms, ensures psycho-social care and respects the autonomy and other rights of the patients.

On the other hand, the other option of good death mentioned above is a more proactive approach in EOL. Euthanasia is a controversial concept in all societies. Even in those societies where it is made legal, very strict regu-lations, as well as monitoring measures, are in place to oversee the process of its implementation. This is because it deals with ending a life before it comes to a natural end. Life is treated as intrinsically valuable. Hence, the question of ending it is always problematic and societies across the world find it not very easy to legalize it. People may have multiple reasons for ending their own life. Most of these reasons are personal and subjective. A few are due to psychological distress, which may happen due to various reasons. However, the only reason that sounds legitimate is in legally allow-ing people to voluntarily end their life on medical grounds. Such grounds can be easily established with the help of physicians. All other reasons are to be treated as amounting to suicide, which no human society would treat as legally permissible and provides official facilitation. Some societies may not make attempts to commit suicide a criminal offence. But no society would provide help to individuals in order to end their life. Before we get into the details of the concept, we have to understand it from its medical, philosophical and sociological perspectives.

The term "euthanasia" in Greek literally means "good health," as "eu" in Greek means good and "thanatos" means death. It refers to an act of facilitating death for the sake of alleviating pain and suffering due to dis-eases or other health issues. The concept of euthanasia can be seen from various perspectives.

1. Patients go to the physicians or the hospital with the hope of assuaging their pain and suffering caused by diseases. In some cases, medicine fails to provide this intended objective. If the patient suffers from a terminal disease and no improvement is in sight, but suffers excruciat-ing pain, then the doctors feel helpless as they realize their inability to provide her the required medical care. In such situations, death seems to be the only remedy and being professionally bound to help their patients by relieving them from their pain and suffering, the doctor may feel obliged to help his patient die.

2. However, this situation is paradoxical. Typically, doctors are supposed to help their patients to live better lives and not die a good death, as death and dying are not medical issues but natural events. Killing one's

patient is against all values of the medical profession, and it counters one of the fundamental premises of the old Hippocratic tradition of medical ethics.

3. The more improvements we make in medicine, the more we find patients living longer. However, an increase in longevity does not guarantee better health or quality of life. Paradoxically, it may lead to a scenario where the new advancements in medicine make people suffer more by prolonging their life without ensuring a corresponding improvement in health. Hence, it may not be unethical to assist people in ending their lives that are unnecessarily prolonged with medication and technology.

4. The dignity of man is a non-negotiable principle. Hence, it is important to enable a person to live with dignity. When incurable diseases and the sufferings they generate threaten human dignity, in order to restore the latter such patients should be allowed to die with dignity.

5. No one would want to die, and even those who request euthanasia do not actually desire for death, but only freedom from suffering. Killing such patients is not helping them in lessening their pain, as it is not a solution to the problem. Ending the life of a patient cannot be equated with curing his diseases or solving his problem.

6. Legalizing euthanasia may paint the image of physicians in dark colour, as the public may begin to perceive them as agents of death.

7. If euthanasia is ethical and legal, then suicide is also ethical and legal, as the former is not different from the latter. However, ending life is to be disrespectful towards life and also against human dignity.

8. Finally, many philosophical and religious perspectives oppose the idea of euthanasia. Christianity, particularly Catholicism, opposes euthanasia, as it believes in eternal life and affirms that human beings have no right to end the life of oneself or another human being, as all humans are the special creations of God. The strength of these religious perspectives is that they are non-negotiable on certain of their doctrines. The idea of assisting people to die or euthanasia is unacceptable to many such traditions. The prohibition in taking a life applies not only to other human beings but also to oneself.

Euthanasia: Historical and Philosophical Perspectives

We find in the Hippocratic oath a strong disapproval of euthanasia. However, such robust denunciation of euthanasia was not common in the pre-Hippocratic Greek culture. The Spartans never allowed their disabled newborns to live, as they considered such children would be a liability to the society. Among some Greek communities, the magistrates permitted citizens who undergo intense physical or mental sufferings to kill themselves as a final remedy (Ryan, Morgan and Lyons 2011, 44). With the Hippocratic tradition taking prominence, doctors began to refuse partaking in acts that may lead to the death of an individual. Later, with the spread of Christianity, for which the idea of the divinity of life was a central doctrine, euthanasia was both legally and morally condemned.

In most non-Western civilizations, the idea of physicians facilitating the death of their patients was unheard of. In ancient India, it was considered as against the law of *ahimsa*, which most religious traditions treated as sacred. Moreover, it also interfered with the *karma* of a person and hence was treated as a sin. However, there were certain customs prevalent among some religious sects whereby people starve to death, when they decide it is time for them to depart. This custom has no medical significance, as the people who were suffering from incurable diseases were not the one who followed it. Such customs can be viewed as suicides, but not necessarily in the contemporary sense of the term. For many of them who performed it, it was a religious act.

Euthanasia is associated with the idea of mercy killing, where the natural course of a person's life is deliberately put to an end for rescuing her from the agonies and sufferings of a terminal disease. In this sense, euthanasia is classified into several types. There is active or positive euthanasia whereby a physician by means of a lethal injection brings a patient's life to an end. In passive euthanasia, the death of the patient is ensured by not providing her any treatment. Such mercy killings are carried out either with the wish of the patient or without her wish or consent. In the presence of a clear wish of the patient, euthanasia becomes voluntary and otherwise it is involuntary and murder. Sometimes euthanasia is implemented even if there is no clearly expressed wish of the patient, either because the latter is incompetent due to some mental disease or is unconscious and is unable to give such consent. On such occasions, the family members of the patient take the decision. Among these different types of euthanasia, passive euthanasia has wider acceptability and, in some societies, the active or positive euthanasia is also made legal.

The modern views on euthanasia are characteristically different from the ancient contentions. The emergence of medicine as an advanced scientific and technological enterprise has impacted the way human societies conceive death. As discussed above, death has ceased to be a natural event and is now a medical event. Due to technological advancements, the life of people even in permanent vegetative states is extended beyond its natural limits, causing pain and sufferings to both the patients as well as the relatives of the patients. The religious groups who strongly oppose euthanasia, highlighting the intrinsic and sacred value of human life, fail to see this aspect. In circumstances where a terminally ill patient wishes to opt euthanasia in order to end her sufferings, it is clear that no other alternative is less beneficial to the patient than this. But those who argue that life has an internal worth object to this. According to them, this dismisses the internal worthiness of life and makes death beneficial (Keown 2002, 39).

John Keown discusses the three competing views about the value of human life—vitalism, sanctity/inviolability of life and Quality (capital Q) of life (39). Vitalism is the view that affirms the absolute moral value of life and hence argues that it is wrong to either shorten life or fail to lengthen it. No external conditions alter the value of life and it is important to preserve it at any cost. The sanctity/inviolability principle could be traced to the Judaeo-Christian tradition's idea of human life as a creation of God and hence possessing an intrinsic dignity, which entitles it to protection. In non-religious terms, the principle is understood in terms of the radical capacity inherent in human nature, which results in the development of rational abilities such as understanding and choice (40). The term "inviolability" is more appropriate to articulate the principle in this context. Keown points out that this principle holds the idea that human life is not just instrumentally good, but a necessary good, a fundamental basis of human flourishing. However, human life is not the highest good or a good to which all other essential goods must be sacrificed in order to ensure its preservation. Keown, therefore, affirms that the sanctity doctrine is not vitalistic. Hence, the core of this doctrine is a principle that prohibits intentional killing, which does not require the preservation of life at all cost and there is no moral obligation to administer or undergo a treatment that is not worthwhile (41 and 43). Quality is the principle used in assessing the worthwhileness of both the treatment and the patient's life. Diseases, injury and disability are conditions that impair quality of life, says Keown, and hence the worthwhileness of life as well. From the perspective of this principle, some lives are not worth living and hence it is right to end them intentionally. Keown proposes to use Quality of life (with a capital Q) instead of quality of life, to distinguish the worthwhileness of treatment from the worthwhileness of the patient's life (43–44).

The ideas of "good life till death" and "good death" are represented in the conceptions of palliative care and euthanasia. They apparently hold opposing perspectives. Many critics have cautioned about the harmful effects of legalizing euthanasia. The European Association for Palliative Care (EAPC) Ethics Task Force points out that legalizing euthanasia may ultimately harm elderly and disabled people and they propose palliative care as an alternative. They argue that while euthanasia aims at death, palliative care focuses on life. The EAPC Ethics Task Force fears that legalizing euthanasia may have the following undesirable consequences: (i) pressure on vulnerable persons; (ii) the underdevelopment or devaluation of palliative care; (iii) conflict between legal requirements and the personal and professional values of physicians and other healthcare professionals; (iv) widening of the clinical criteria to include other groups in society; (v) an increase in the incidence of nonvoluntary and involuntary medicalized killing; (vi) killing to become accepted within society. However, such fears, though are not completely baseless, seem to propose a comparison between the two different processes. A comparison between euthanasia and palliative care is often misleading. They need to be understood as serving different purposes. The proponents of euthanasia would not argue against patients approaching palliative care, as everyone considers the former, usually as a last resort. Again, the EAPC Ethics Task Force assumes that in euthanasia the intention is to kill the patient. This is not correct. The ultimate objective of euthanasia is to alleviate the suffering of the patient, which is not possible through any other means. In other words, it may become a sensible alternative in the age of advanced medical technologies, when all other means, including palliative care, fail to assuage the pain and sufferings of the patient.

Whether to legalize euthanasia is always a controversial issue in almost all societies. There is a demand from rights groups to legalize it. They argue that it would help some patients to avoid pain and suffering in the last days of their lives and enable them to die with dignity. However, conservatives and other opponents of euthanasia who are concerned about the worthwhileness of human life and also those who raise safety issues, mount strong opposition to this demand. As Ezekiel J. Emanuel (1999) points out, this issue is not about the ethics of having a particular social policy and practice. It is not just about the morality of a specific decision regarding the care of an individual patient (629). Ezekiel reminds that irrespective of the social policy, a society adopts, whether for or against euthanasia or physician-assisted suicide (PAS), there will be both benefits and harms. He continues:

> Legalization would inevitably generate abuses, cases in which people's lives where intentionally ended when they should not have been because they were coerced or because appropriate palliative measures were not provided or because they did not consent. ... Similarly ... if neither euthanasia nor PAS is permitted some patients experiencing unremitting pain will be prevented from entering their lives and will suffer needlessly.
>
> (630)

According to Ezekiel, there are three main benefits to legalization. First, realizing individual autonomy; second, reducing needless pain and suffering; and third, providing psychological reassurance to dying patients (630). On the other hand, according to Ezekiel, the opponents of euthanasia identify six potential harms such as, undermining the integrity of the medical profession, creation of psychological anxiety and distress in patients from the possibility of euthanasia or PAS, coercion of patients to use euthanasia or PAS against their wishes, provision of euthanasia or PAS to patients prior to implementing optimal palliative care interventions, provision of euthanasia or PAS to patients without their full informed consent because of either mental illness or mental incompetence and psychological distress and harm to surviving family members of the patient (635). He adds that for almost all these harms there are few firm data, as they are much harder to empirically evaluate.

While the euthanasia debate is predominantly centred on the question of rights of the individual patients in developed countries, in developing countries, the situation is further complex. The concern for finding a solution for the pain and suffering of the patient is a universal concern. However, pain and sufferings are not always physical. Providing good EOL care involves multiple challenges as it has got emotional, economic and spiritual aspects. Many families may not be able to provide the required care to the patients due to their economic status, as care for many such patients requires the assistance of professionals and such professional assistance is often expensive. Home care is also not very easy due to socio-economic factors. In India, for example, when the joint family system existed, caring for the elderly posed very little challenges. Moreover, many diseases did not have appropriate medication and consequently, the life expectancy was not very high. With the development of better healthcare facilities, people now live longer, but with difficulties and disabilities due to diseases. With the breaking up of the joint family system, there is dearth of manpower to provide adequate care for the elderly at home. Though joint family system ceases to exist, the values enshrined by that system still persist and there is a strong social stigma towards senior living facilities. People who live in such facilities are viewed as unfortunate souls and their relatives as sinners. Moreover, due to such a stigmatized perception, there are very few such senior living facilities functioning in India, which can provide quality professional care to elderly people. The healthcare services extended to them are not very good and there are hardly any government funds for the specific needs of the EOL patients.

These socio-economic factors mentioned above certainly add to the sufferings of millions of elderly people in the country and many of them have agonized EOL days and die a death that lacks dignity. These factors may encourage many elderly patients to consider euthanasia as a possible option, as it provides them a better choice than living and dying without dignity. Moreover, there are possibilities that EOL patients are coerced to opt euthanasia by others, as on most occasions the crucial decisions are taken by relatives who are caretakers of the patients and physicians too often communicate with the caretakers and not the patients directly.

The euthanasia debate in the Indian society has been kindled further by the 2018 Supreme Court judgement. This judgement was the culmination of a process, which began in 2005, with the apex court seeking the central government's response on the appeal that seek the declaration of "right to die with dignity" as a fundamental right under Article 21, which deals with the right to life of the constitution. This was following a public interest litigation filed by an NGO called Common Cause, seeking the Supreme Court's favourable judgement in allowing terminally ill patients to execute a living will for passive euthanasia. Meanwhile, in 2011, the Supreme Court in Aruna Shanbaug's case allowed passive euthanasia for her. Aruna was in a permanent vegetative state since 1973, after a tragic incident in which she was brutally attacked and sexually assaulted by a sweeper in the hospital. Pinki Virani, a social activist, approached the Supreme Court with the plea to euthanize Aruna, to which the nurses at King Edward Memorial (KEM) Hospital in Mumbai, who were caring for Aruna, filed a counter-petition opposing euthanasia. The court rejected Ms Virani's plea, but ruled that if the request for removing life support was from the family of a terminally ill patient, it could be done in the supervision of the doctors and the court. This ruling was later referred to by the Supreme Court, which referred the PIL to the constitution bench. Finally, in March 2018, the Supreme Court recognized "living will" of terminally ill patients for passive euthanasia. It also laid down guidelines for carrying out the procedure.

The apex court has only recognized passive euthanasia and there is a long way to go before India legalizes physician-assisted suicide. If we decide to ignore the moral oppositions to this on grounds such as life's intrinsic value and sacredness, the remaining oppositions are based on procedural issues and safety considerations. Strictly speaking, they are not oppositions on moral grounds. With more patients becoming aware of their right to a death with dignity, the demand for legalizing euthanasia is also becoming stronger and democratic states may find no reasons for denying this right to their citizens.

Note

1 The sources used for preparing this case discussion are the following: Long (2000); Clark (2006); Mukai et al.(1977); Munson (2009).

7 The Social Organization of Medicine and Bioethics

Introduction

So far the focus of these discussions was on the moral anxieties human societies encounter with the practice of medicine. The history of the evolution of modern medicine has several momentous events that significantly shaped the course and destiny of human life on earth. Many of them were milestones in the development of medicine as a science, and many of them empowered physicians and surgeons to alter the course of diseases that harm humans with appropriate technologies. The science of medicine is, as it is repeatedly pointed out, a complex scientific and technological enterprise now with corporate interests dominating its functional dynamics. Different societies grapple with the moral anxieties differently, as the moral values that guide their ethical evaluations and choices are diverse. However, modern medicine by its very nature proposes a unique outlook towards the very nature of human life, body, well-being, social life and human destiny. Some of its technological possibilities testify this. For example, cloning. This new medical possibility redefines the very idea of procreation and questions some very fundamental moral assumptions about family life and relationships.

As is evident from the discussions in the previous chapters, technology plays a key role in the way medicine conducts itself in the present day. Such developments are essential to aid the conceptions of health and well-being projected by medicine as a science that envisages to facilitate human happiness. However, the moral issues related to the practice of medicine are not confined to the use and abuse of technology. There are some other issues related to the broader social, political and economic structures that control the evolution of medicine and biotechnology in our world. Like any other industrial sector, healthcare also requires enormous investments. In a global economy that is controlled by the principle of a free-market system, the healthcare sector relies on investment from the corporate sector. Consequently, medicine is now increasingly getting integrated into a highly complex corporate sector, and the moral expectations of the people do not guide its priorities. Instead, the interests of the shareholders gain importance. These expectations of the people have their roots in the ancient

DOI: 10.4324/9781003312697-7

healing traditions that existed in human societies—such as the Indian, Chinese, Hippocratic and the Arabian traditions of medicine—and all stakeholders are aware of this. Though the old values no longer regulate the patient–physician relationship, they have not become entirely obsolete. The idea of "patient first" and even the concepts like autonomy, consent and confidentiality reflect this value. However, such moral concerns fail to make their voices heard when the social organization of medicine is controlled by corporate interests. Hence, a large section of the stakeholders that constitute today's healthcare sector keeps a deaf ear to such concerns of the general moral community. These include companies that manufacture various healthcare technological devices, dealers and vendors, pharmaceutical firms and insurance companies.

Final solutions to many of the moral problems are not easy to be found. We keep encountering new issues, and we may have to keep looking for solutions. There are problems associated with the reach of healthcare, an issue which I touched upon when I discussed the question of allocation and distributive justice in Chapter 5. Besides other considerations, poverty and affordability are significant elements that affect the proper distribution of healthcare services to a large number of people. The human rights framework is adopted to overcome this problem. Again, in the principlist framework, the proponents give equal weight to all four principles. However, in practice, this may not happen always. Beauchamp and Childress have indicated that the principles can never function like rules and have to be applied to specific situations based on requirements. There has occasionally been a conflict between autonomy and beneficence. This problem is discussed in the fourth chapter. Besides, there is also a conflict between autonomy and justice.

At a very fundamental level, healthcare and healthcare ethics pose specific questions that raise concerns about some social and political aspects that determine health. Besides, they also pose some philosophical questions. This chapter deals with these issues. Ever since medicine began to ally with the emerging natural sciences, both by adopting its principal approaches and methodology and by drawing from their fundamental principles, medicine raised ethical issues of a different category, which essentially differed from those issues raised by traditional medical moralities of different cultures. A shift of focus from physician behaviour to other structural aspects related to the functioning of medicine is an important change that happened in bioethics during the past several decades. However, before we focus on such broader ethical issues, we may have to address a set of ethical challenges certain new medical technologies pose before us. They are important because they propose fundamental changes in the very conception of our identities as humans, or as in a phenomenological sense, embodied beings.

As aforementioned, the development of medicine from discrete healing practices to a well-structured body of scientific knowledge involves several significant events. These include the invention of several therapies, medicines, procedures and technologies based on certain fundamental discoveries about the nature of the human body and its various ways of functioning. Many of them have only historical importance today, as physicians have periodically improved upon them replacing the old with new and better ones. Nevertheless, a few remain valid even today and have developed further with essential improvements. Organ transplantation is such a procedure. Ever since 1954, when Dr Joseph Murray performed the first-ever renal transplantation (for which he received the Nobel Prize in Medicine), the procedure has gone a long way, remarkably improving its success rate. The development of its history has also witnessed the development of different fields of medicine, contributing significantly to its betterment. However, with the ascension of the reputation of this procedure, it began to raise several ethical dilemmas.

If transplantation is an established field of healthcare practice, some other new procedures develop with improvements in technology as well as advanced innovations in the pharmaceutical sector. The development of stem cell therapy, gene-editing techniques and cloning is the most notable among them. These innovative procedures represent the new face of modern medicine. They have the potential to initiate substantial changes in the ways physicians practise medicine. While stem cell therapy can suggest a cure for many diseases and situations that are otherwise incurable and non-treatable, gene editing can even suggest the prevention of fatal diseases. These procedures are yet to develop beyond a state of infancy, and they expect to witness drastic improvements in the near future. Cloning, on the other hand, employs a technology over which we have reasonable mastery. Nevertheless, most countries have prohibited its use it in several fields like reproduction. This aspect, too, gives rise to fascinating ethical debates.

In this chapter, I will discuss the ethical aspects surrounding four important technological procedures: organ transplantation, stem cell therapy, gene therapy and cloning. Except organ transplantation, the other three are not very commonly used by physicians worldwide for therapeutic purposes. Their invention and use began only in the recent past. Transplantation is an old procedure and is already a part of conventional medical treatment. Nevertheless, it has something that makes it drastically different from other conventional procedures. The other three discussed in this chapter can clearly be described as next-generation healthcare procedures, as they adopt a very different approach to healing and curing.

The common element in all the four is the way all of them alter our embodiedness and in that sense our very identity as a being-in-the-world who relates with the world and surroundings in specific ways by means of certain natural endowments. All these four technologies bring about drastic alterations in the patient's body, not just to its outer form but also to its very character. Such fundamental bodily alterations are crucial because a person's body is something that makes all her experiences possible and is her place in the world (Svenaeus 2018, 2). All the processes involve advanced technologies.

This chapter traces the root cause of the ethical crisis in medicine to three fundamental changes humans have made to their approach towards their life. First, the change in a conception of health, where we embrace the idea of artificial health in place of natural health. Second, the growing individualism that redefined our fundamental ideas about well-being, disease, healing and health. Third, the dominance of a market-driven capitalist philosophy governing the entire establishment of modern medicine, which not only makes the benefits of medicine inaccessible to a large number of people but also fosters a disturbing tendency that conceives health as a competitive advantage, which is the consequence of the socio-economic practices that determine our lives.

Many new technologies are introduced which manipulate the functioning of the natural body as well as rectifying it when it malfunctions. As mentioned above, I here identify four important technologies, which actually or potentially suggest fundamental changes to our bodily identity and thereby raise critical moral dilemmas: organ transplantation, stem cell research and therapy, gene therapy and cloning.

Organ Transplantation

Organ transplantation has witnessed remarkable developments in the past 50 years. Successful organ transplantation is the result of both technological and pharmaceutical advancements in medicine. Transplantation began to become significantly successful only after the introduction of efficient immunosuppressants (Watson and Dark 2012, i30). In a similar vein, transplantation surgery involving various organs has evolved and is carried out with great success in many parts of the world today.

The major ethical problem involved in organ transplantation is related to the scarcity of suitable organs, as many organs like a heart will be available for transplantation only after death. Nevertheless, some other organs like kidney, liver, parts of the lung, pancreas and intestine can be donated even while alive. The ethics of organ transplantation deals with several issues ranging from what is known as the organ transplantation scams to various other issues, such as determination of death (discussed in the previous chapter), consent of the individuals, scarcity and allocation. The unethical and criminal involvement of hospitals and doctors where organs are harvested from people without consent raises serious concerns and the wide media publicity such incidents gain results in a significant dip in public trust on medicine as an institution.

The Indian scenario was extremely chaotic before the introduction of the Transplantation of Human Organs and Tissues Act (THOTA). This bill was passed in 1994. Before this, medical practice was largely unregulated in the country, and medical councils hardly interfered in ethical issues (Nagral

1995, 19). THOTA not only helped to enforce regulations but also brought much clarity on some procedures that may lead to confusion. For example, THOTA could mostly curb the sale of organs that was going on without any control. It has clearly distinguished between living organ donation from cadaver donation. It has recognized brain death as the final criterion to determine whether a person is dead or alive so that organs could be harvested from that person before they become useless. It also made regulations more effective by making it mandatory for all institutions conducting transplants to register with the authority appointed by the government (20).

The criterion of brain death is widely accepted in most of the countries today in determining the death of a person and harvesting organs from him/her. However, unlike the traditional conception of death, where the ceasing of the functioning of the heart and the absence of respiration are criteria, the determination of brain death is a technical process. The ambiguity surrounding this concept of death generates a range of issues to doctors, relatives and those who need organs. The relatives of the patient may find it difficult to accept his/her death if respiration is yet to cease. The colourful media coverage about the various organ transplant scams in different parts of the country has already cast suspicions in the minds of the relatives of the brain dead person. In developed countries, there are stringent regulations. In many countries, there is a well-regulated system in place to monitor deceased or cadaver donation and transplantation. However, the situation in most of the developing countries is not very bright. Regulations hardly exist, and most places do not maintain a seniority list. These issues are discussed in detail in the previous chapter.

One way to regulate the process of transplantation is by insisting on consent. There are several kinds of consent, such as "opt-in consent," "opt-out consent" and "mandated choice." Opt-in requires the donor to give explicit consent, or if that is absent, his/her relatives' authorization becomes mandatory. Opt-out consent is consent for retrieving organs after death in the absence of any objection for the same from the relatives. Mandated choice requires all adults to indicate their wishes regarding the use of their organs after death. Another way to regulate it is by introducing a seniority system in every state or district so that transplantation surgeries will happen only based on the available list.

The developments in medical sciences and the introduction of new and more effective immunosuppressants have improved the success rates of transplantation surgeries drastically. Nevertheless, several factors still prevent smooth deceased donation in many parts of the developing world. The gap between demand for and availability of organs is a significant problem across the world. With the increase in life expectancy and the availability of better medicines for many ailments, this gap keeps expanding in many places. However, developing countries pose several other challenges. Lack of proper awareness, religious beliefs, superstitions and emotional reasons prevent deceased donation to a large extent in many developing countries.

Most countries in the world adopt various measures to encourage people to donate their organs. Many countries have already adopted the "opt-out consent" model, so that organs are harvested from every person who dies in the absence of any explicit objection to the same. However, the unethical and illegal practices around organ donation and transplantation are still rampant in many countries. In many developing countries, many factors like poverty, lack of proper education and proper awareness make a large number of people vulnerable and susceptible to exploitation. Many such factors have proliferated transplantation tourism and organ trafficking in such countries in a big way.

Since this discussion happens in the backdrop of an examination that focuses on the transformation from ancient medical morality to modern bioethics, it becomes clear how issues like this define the fundamental characteristic features of contemporary deliberations on bioethics. The anxieties, concerns and dilemmas surrounding our engagements with phenomena like organ transplantation or brain death are alien to the field of ancient medical practice. Here instead of physician behaviour, we deal with the unlawful and criminal activities of underworld rackets that are engaged in organ trafficking, corrupt officials and corporate interests of hospitals and their management. All technologies modern medicine use call for a different approach and they require the employment of tools that are unfamiliar and absent in medical moralities of traditional societies.

Stem Cell Research

Therapies using human embryonic stem cell (HESC) research represent an entirely unconventional and a radically different mode of treatment which goes against all forms of hitherto known therapeutic methods envisaged by the art and science of medicine. It is not a mere technology that aids therapy but a therapeutic measure that is bound to revolutionize the field of medicine. Again, it is not a procedure like surgery, which has existed for long and evolved through constant improvements, but something hitherto unheard of. It is a therapy that is comparable to a fairy tale, and that has evolved out of the imagination of modern understanding of the science of genetics. It is based not just on our understanding of the structure of different organs and knowledge about how they function but on the knowledge of how they have evolved and developed from the embryonic form to the organic complexity that human beings represent.

What makes HESCs so fascinating is their very nature. They are unspecialized cells and have the potential to develop into many different cell types in the body. They can develop from muscle cells to brain cells and, in some cases, can also repair damaged tissues. While normal cells in the body have specific purposes, stem cells do not have a specific role, and they have the potential to become almost any cell in the body. They have the capacity for self-renewal, as they can differentiate into all types of cells of the body. This character of the stem cells makes them clinically potential in the treatment of certain deceases, disabilities and injuries. They are believed to have the ability to replace the defective cells in a patient since they can divide or self-renew indefinitely. Scientists envisage situations where they can be used for generating various cell types from the originating organ by inducing them to become tissue or organ-specific cells with special functions. They can even generate the entire original organ. They expect that the stem cells with their regenerative abilities can be effectively used for the treatment of diabetes and heart disease. As aforementioned, its potentials are yet to be fully tapped, though scientists already use them for research and treatment. They are mainly used to screen new drugs and to develop model systems to study normal growth and identify the causes of birth defects (NIH Stem Cell Information Home Page 2016).

It is clear that these are novel and unconventional methods and is not yet part of the normal therapies we adopt. In other words, this sphere of medicine has incredible potentials, and more research needs to be conducted in order to make it part of the standard treatment protocol of physicians. For conducting further research, stem cells have to be procured, either from the embryos or from adults. These are the two significant kinds of stem cells. The embryonic stem cells are pluripotent, as they can change into any cell in the body, while the adult stem cells are multipotent and can only change into some cells in the body. It is now evident what makes the embryonic stem cells more important in possible therapeutic procedures.

However, procuring stem cells from embryos involves the destruction of the embryos, as they are derived in vitro from the inner cell mass of the 5–7 days old blastocyst, for which the trophoblast has to be removed, and this process virtually stops the growth of the embryo further. In other words, this amounts to the killing of the embryo. It is a human being in a dormant form, and its destruction is a homicide. The moral problem consists precisely in this issue. However, how strong are the ethical issues involved in this scenario? Are they severe enough to prevent further research on embryonic stem cells and using them for potential human benefit?

The question of when human life begins is indeed controversial. The fierce debates surrounding abortion raises this issue in a different way. The issue is with the killing of human beings. We may compare the three situations where an individual is said to be killed. First, the killing of a human being, which is murder, and is regarded by all civilized societies as wrong. Here the human being has full moral status, and killing him/her is considered wrong. Second, in abortion, where the foetus's further development is stopped, and in that course, its life is taken away. Though many may find indiscriminate abortions at an advanced stage of pregnancy as objectionable, hardly anyone would dispute its moral permissibility on occasions where its further growth becomes detrimental to the mother's life. Third, the destruction of embryos, which may happen due to many reasons. Such embryos are created in vitro as part of infertility treatment. However, not all embryos created for reproduction are used, and the remaining are either destroyed or donated for research. If the killing of embryos is morally objectionable, then in vitro fertilization also becomes a morally objectionable procedure. Embryos are sometimes created for research purposes. This may invite more criticism as here a human being is created artificially for researching him/her and in that process gets inevitably killed! However, the fundamental ethical worry here is related to the moral status of a human being. At what point of her existence, an individual comes to be recognized as an autonomous individual? What could be regarded as the beginning of personhood? Does personhood begin with conception or at the state of the emergence of the embryo or foetus? Does it begin only after the actual birth? What if the child is born earlier than the standard gestation period? What criteria can be applied?

There are several ethical issues related to the creation of embryos. Usually, the surplus embryos created as part of infertility treatment are frozen. After the couple that created them are no more in need of them, they are either destroyed or donated, either for research or to other couples who may need them for treating infertility. All these three options involve ethical issues. These various processes will have to honour the rule of consent, which is often violated in many places that lack strict implementation of regulations. Destroying the embryos is a painful alternative for any couples, as they may believe that they are potentially their children. Equally disturbing is the other option of donating them for research, as in that process they eventually get killed.

To donate them to other couples who are childless sounds a better option for many. However, then this introduces a different set of ethical concerns. This makes it possible that your children are born to some other couple, and are brought up by them in ways they consider are right and may not agree with your values. For such reasons, the third alternative, even though it looks more meaningful as it does not involve the destruction of the embryo, appears to be more unacceptable for many. Some studies show that in many developed countries, couples tend more towards donating their frozen embryos for research. Some do not want to give them for infertility treatment as they consider it as psychologically disturbing. This is especially the case in those countries that have abolished donor anonymity and made disclosure possible after a certain period of time (Heng 2006, 381). Many parents are worried about the psychological problems that may affect their children when they come to know about their "donated siblings" at a later stage in their lives. However, such concerns are rooted in our old moral assumptions, which presume an old value system that existed earlier when society had strong patriarchal families with heterosexual composition and well-defined moral orientations. These assumptions are increasingly getting obsolete now.

The debates on the ethics of using embryonic stem cells for research is not very intense in the Indian public sphere, and these are largely confined to the intellectual and practical deliberations carried out by professional bioethicists, physicians, regulatory bodies, policymakers and philosophers. There is no strong public opposition to stem cell procurement or research in India. The Indian Council of Medical Research, Department of Health Research and the Department of Biotechnology have brought out the National Guidelines for Stem Cell Research (2013). The Guidelines summarize its guiding philosophy on such matters as consisting of promoting scientific and ethical stem cell research while preventing premature commercialization and potential exploitation of vulnerable patients. The Guidelines express ethical concerns over using appropriate stem cells for a particular condition and using embryos for creating human embryonic stem cell lines. They caution against the commoditization of human tissues and cells and the exploitation of individuals, particularly those belonging to the underprivileged groups. They further point out the challenges related to the contentious issue of human germline engineering and reproductive cloning (ICMR & DBT 2013, 1). The Guidelines further reiterate the importance of safeguarding human rights, dignity and fundamental freedom of human subjects involved in research and observing the fundamental tenets of beneficence, nonmaleficence, justice and autonomy (3).

Two important aspects of stem cell research demand a particular focus while addressing ethical issues. First, there are concerns regarding the moral status of the embryo, and there is a lack of proper public awareness about this new form of therapy. Second, there are a lot of over expectations about its potentials. Most of the other issues, such as safety considerations, violation of fundamental ethical principles and exploitation, are not specific issues that surface within this domain. Concerns about the moral status of the embryo are not a unique issue in stem cell research. As mentioned earlier, this is the major problem that makes abortion such a huge controversy in the United States and some other countries.

Interestingly, in many developing countries, it does not attract public attention in such a large magnitude. In the United States, it is a factor that even decides public elections in some states. Social factors such as race and religious fundamentalism shape these controversies surrounding abortion in the United States (Nevitte et al. 1993, 19). It is the Christian religious groups who raise the major objections against abortion, as annihilating life is against the fundamental tenets of their beliefs that consider God as the creator. They further believe that God has created man in His image. However, this is not a belief which is shared by many other religious groups in the world. Most of the Indian religions and traditions do not even have a concept of creator God, and hardly any other religion in the world other than those in the Abrahamic traditions believe in human creation in the image of God. The strong anthropocentrism is inherent in the Abrahamic tradition, and the humanistic philosophies of Europe place man at a higher pedestal, and this leads to a belief in the unique moral status of man. It is a fact that the question of abortion is not a very serious moral issue for many non-Abrahamic religious groups in the world and hence in many other societies.

The treatment using this new technology is at a very early stage and is yet to be a popular option among physicians and patients. There are several concerns about the safety of this therapy and research. However, there is a need to promote and encourage more research in this domain, as its potential benefits to humankind look bright. It is necessary to weigh and balance the potential harm and benefit of this technology at every stage of research. Researchers need to adopt several precautions such as

> minimizing the risks of harm, selecting and recruiting appropriate patient-subjects, facilitating informed decision-making through the consent form and process, and avoiding the "therapeutic misconception", whereby unduly high expectations affect all interested parties to a clinical trial, are all significant research ethics considerations.
>
> (King & Perrin 2014, 2)

Gene Therapy

Gene therapy targets to alter what is called the very blueprint of human life, and the very possibility of such manipulations suggests a wide range of possibilities. This new form of therapy was introduced as a new phase of the genetic engineering technology, which became a possibility after the elucidation of the three-dimensional structure of DNA in the 1950s. Typically, the procedure involves the insertion of genes into an individual's cells or tissues to treat diseases or disorders. By this, it is expected to alter the expression of certain specific genes that cause disease. Some of these include highly useful therapies that prevent and cure several diseases. Some other possibilities include altering the reproductive cells by inserting the altered gene into the sperm or egg cells, which are the germ cells. Physicians normally execute this therapy by using viral vectors for the insertion of therapeutic DNA into the defective cells. The human genome sequencing enables scientists to diagnose all related genetic diseases by comparing genes with the help of software, and treat many of them before they progress with the help of gene therapy.

Usually, scientists make a distinction between somatic gene therapy and germline gene therapy. Somatic gene therapy consists of transferring the therapeutic genes into the somatic cells of a patient. According to many bioethicists, somatic gene therapy hardly poses any serious ethical problem, as it is widely viewed as an extension of already-available therapies. On the other hand, reproductive cell therapy or germline gene therapy inserts the gene into the reproductive tissue, sperm or egg cells of the patient, effecting a change not only to the individual patient but also to her future generations. This process effectively corrects the disease causing gene variants that may pass down from generation to generation. This latter form of gene therapy raises various ethical problems, as it impacts future generations as well. However, this distinction is not absolute, and it is not true that somatic gene therapy does not pose ethical issues. Genes are introduced to the body using viruses as vectors, and there is a possibility that they may recombine with other viruses and infect the germ cells. This may lead to the same effect of germline therapy. Therefore, somatic therapy may have an indirect effect on the gene pool (Chadwick 2009, 207).

But what is the problem if it affects future generations? Parents make decisions for their children, and it is also essential to respect the reproductive autonomy of individuals. Of course, the impacts will be on future generations who have not consented to that. However, we usually do not take the consent of our children when we take parental decisions about their health. We do that in light of our values and rear them according to our values. There is no requirement of taking consent for that. If a pregnant woman comes to know that her child has some genetic disease and if there is a means by which this could be eliminated even before delivery, hardly anything would be morally prohibiting her from doing that. Similarly, if we come to know that there is a defective gene in our gene pool that might affect our future generations, there should not be anything that morally stops us from attempting to eliminate such possibilities. Of course, this should be done after taking all necessary safety precautions and also after weighing the benefits with risks. Many issues raised by gene therapy arise from our resistance in accepting it as a form of therapy. It is a different generation therapy, and its acceptance requires us to conceive diseases and therapies in entirely different ways, so that we may be able to arrive at entirely unconventional remedies.

Besides the somatic and germline therapy distinction, we may distinguish a therapy from enhancement in order to have more clarity about the ethics of gene therapy. To the extent to which gene therapy confines to the correction of bona fide disease conditions, many people find it acceptable, at least conditionally. However, what is the definition of therapy, and what are its goals? The definition of health may not entirely confine to the usual meaning given to it as the absence of disease. It has a decisive role to play in human life. In this sense, it contributes to the improvement of the human species so that they can pursue their goals more effectively and efficiently. Conventional medicine, too, has some treatments that aim at such "improvements" and "enhancements." Even traditional medicine has remedies that enhance and optimize specific natural abilities. Gene therapy does it more aggressively with more accuracy and specificity.

On many occasions, the treatment given for common diseases can be used for enhancing natural abilities. For example, the gene therapy designed for Alzheimer's disease patients may help in boosting the memory of ordinary individuals. Again, different gene therapies, which are typically used in certain diseases, can also be used for enhancement purposes, and this may cause serious ethical challenges in the field of sports. Adopting these therapies may give undue advantages to individuals by enhancing their athletic performance, as it results in enhancing a given gene. This practice is known as gene doping, which goes against the norms of the World Anti-Doping

Agency. Gene doping has some advantages over conventional forms of doping, where the doping substances are supplied externally and hence are detected by means of chemical or molecular detection of the doping agent. In gene doping, such detection is difficult, as the introduced gene and the protein expressed from it are almost identical to their endogenous counterparts. Besides, transgene is administrated to the muscle, making the procedure of muscle biopsy a prerequisite in its detection, which is not applied in sports (Baoutina et al. 2010, 1022).

Howsoever narrow the line between therapy and enhancement is, it is believed that it is essential to draw such a line. However, questions such as where do we draw it and what parameters are to be used to draw it deserve satisfactory answers. One way to answer this question concerning sports is emphasizing the importance of human efforts and natural human abilities. However, nature makes us all different from each other and also unequals. If this natural disparity can be levelled with gene therapy, why do we worry about its ethical sanctity? Moreover, is there anything that makes what is natural more ethically valuable than what is cultivated or created? All these questions need satisfactory answers, and in the absence of a single all-encompassing moral framework, we are now bound to witness robust debates on such issues.

There are some other experiments related to germline therapy that involve human embryos, and in this process, the modification is done on early embryos. Here, in addition to the aforementioned ethical issues, there are critical ethical problems related to embryo experimentation, where the inner moral worth of an embryo becomes a question. Since such issues are discussed above, I am not venturing to do that in this context.

Cloning

The procedure and possibilities of cloning raised several ethical controversies when scientists announced that they have created the first mammal, a sheep named Dolly in 1996, cloned from an adult somatic cell. There was a general feeling that with this procedure, scientists have started to meddle with the creation of human beings violating all natural and divine rules. Some of the fears it generated deserve no serious moral examination and are not morally worthy enough for any detailed analysis, as they are obviously over-romanticized issues. The opposition against cloning and also against all forms of artificial reproduction methods that mostly make reproduction asexual is an example. The real issue is whether we consider infertility as something that needs to be medically corrected or not or accept it as fate or the result of past *karmas*. Many couples today are not going to contend with such quietism. They may aggressively pursue all available scientific methods to attain their goals. If conventionally followed ARTs are not yielding results, they may turn to other technologies like cloning. Today many countries have banned reproductive cloning. But such policies lack a strong philosophical basis and are done based on fears about the safety of the procedure. Such oppositions may have to go soon, and with more consensuses favouring cloning as an acceptable technology in ART, many people may turn to it.

However, the opposition to reproductive cloning has some other important dimensions. Though the procedure results in the creation of an infant, it is not a reproductive process in the technical sense of the term. Cloning is different from reproduction as it produces an exact genetic copy as offspring. This aspect distinguishes cloning from other ART and genetic technologies. Hence, it is not truly reproduction, but a mere copying technology, where a genetic copy of a sequence of DNA or the entire genome of an organism is created. The technology involves typically transferring the nucleus of a somatic cell into an oocyte from which the nucleus is removed. With this, scientists can remove most of the DNA. This is stimulated for cell division with an electric current to result in the formation of an embryo that is genetically identical to, and thus a clone of the somatic cell donor (Devolder 2017). Since this procedure cannot be treated as reproduction, one immediate impact of cloning will be on our understanding of family relationships and individual identities.

The parent–child relationship and sibling relations are understood in a certain way by human beings. Our social conventions determine the nature of these relationships. In cloning, as Lee Silver (Making Babies 2019) points out, scientists remove the genetic material from an egg and place into it the genetic material from an adult cell, so that the egg now will have a complete set of genes, with complete genomic material and hence could develop into an embryo. This could grow as a foetus in a uterus. A woman who gives birth to a child using this procedure is, in genetic terms, not the mother of the child, but the genetic sister. Similarly, a person's father's identical brother is not, in genetic terms, her uncle, but her father. But as Silver reminds, we understand such relationships in social terms and categorize them as mother–child and uncle–niece relationships. Contrasting such examples show that such problems related to relationships and identities may arise even in natural pregnancies. Hence, we need not worry too much about such issues only because the procedure adopted is asexual and not natural. The real concern lies in how we are going to use it.

One of the main objections raised against reproductive cloning is the use of embryos in research and discarding the excessively created ones. This, again, is a general criticism against using embryos for any other purposes than reproduction. Michael Sandel (2005) exposes the fundamental weakness of this argument. He says:

> If cloning for stem cell research violates the respect the embryo is due, then so does stem cell research on IVF spares, and so does any version of IVF that creates and discards excess embryos. If morally speaking, these

practices stand or fall together, and it remains to ask whether they stand or fall. And that depends on the moral status of the embryo.

(245)

Since I have already discussed the question of the moral status of embryos in an earlier chapter, I refrain from further discussion of it here. However, there are some other critical concerns.

Several factors make cloning a favoured option in the modern world. This technology aids couples to obtain an offspring who is genetically related to one of them. Besides, it offers parents many procreative options. It also enables them to protect their prospective children from those genetic diseases with which they suffer and also from several diseases that are associated with genetic risk factors. Many parents are enthusiastic about the fact that cloning may allow them to produce enhanced children, though this has created considerable controversy among the general public and policymakers.

Some of these are good reasons to support using this new technology in the area of reproduction. The desire to have children who are genetically related is natural to humans, and they should never be denied an opportunity to satisfy this desire if technology can facilitate it. In addition to this, cloning can also facilitate avoiding the chances of inheriting genetic diseases, which is not possible in sexual reproduction. This is analogous to protecting one's children from several diseases using vaccines. The case of enhancement can be seen as an extension to this, as on many occasions the distinction between enhancement and therapy is not clear.

Nevertheless, the problem of enhancement raises some issues. The arguments favouring genetic enhancement sounds problematic if analyzed from the perspective of the idea of justice, mainly when we see the latter as fairness. Any benefit of science and technology should be available and accessible to a large number of people, if not to all. Or else, it would give the few who have benefitted an undue advantage over those who fail to access it due to factors that are not under their control. As pointed out by Lee Silver, unlike the polio vaccine which is given to all children, the genetic vaccine against AIDS or any other kind of disease (and also genetic enhancement technology) may only be available to those who have money. The poor will be at a disadvantage (Making Babies 2019).

However, this argument cannot be extended too far, as it raises some fundamental questions about social justice. Such disparities exist in all fields. All medical services in the society are not available to all in the same way. The vaccination for polio and similar such treatments are only exceptions and not the norm. In a market-driven economy, where the IPR is to be honoured, the products and services available in the market, including healthcare, are not available to everyone in the same manner. The ability to pay is, unfortunately, the norm in most domains. This may be fundamentally wrong, one may argue, but that is a different-level argument.

The concern about the safety of the people involved, particularly the children who are cloned, is not a real ethical issue, as safety is a prerequisite and should be made legally binding to all researchers and practitioners. The ethical problem is: After all safety issues are addressed, can we proceed with it? Michael Sandel (2005) rightly diagnoses the moral problem involved in cloning as well as in other genetic engineering techniques that meddle with reproduction. He argues that the moral problem with reproductive cloning lies in its assault on the understanding of children as gifts rather than possessions, or projects of our will, or vehicles for our happiness (242). He adds:

> What is most troubling about human cloning and bioengineering is not that they represent a radical departure, but that they carry to full expression troubling tendencies already present in our culture, especially in the way we regard and treat children. ... By contrast, the sense of life as a gift we cannot summon or control is fragile and vulnerable. In the face of the Promethean drive to mastery that animates modern societies, an appreciation of the giftedness of life is in constant need of support.
>
> (243)

Sandel's observation is a reminder. It indicates that the root of many of our ethical problems lies in the ways we have organized our societies. We fail to conceive the value of things independent of their market value. A child with enhanced abilities may fair better in our society, which puts all of us in a competitive environment. We function within it with a basic marketplace mentality that suggests that if you have the money, you can do it (Making Babies 2019). Parents who have money would indeed provide better facilities for their children. We may oppose the underlying inequalities that exist in our society but cannot deny the fact that parents have the right to do so. We have inequalities of all types in our society, many of them are social and a few are genetic. Some people are born with better abilities and some with disabilities, and these are things which we have hardly any control over. Some of the genetic inequalities may contribute significantly to social inequalities. We may have some control over social inequalities, and a just society should strive to bring down those inequalities that have a social origin. In this sense, we should also avoid doing things that widen the social gap by allowing a few to purchase enhanced abilities. This may sound a bit authoritarian and opposing individual autonomy. However, a justice-based moral paradigm is equally vital in bioethics and, sometimes, more important than the autonomy-based paradigm, which emphasizes individual rights more than social justice.

Moral Crisis in Medicine and the Future of Bioethics

While thinking about the future of bioethics, it is essential to look at human health, diseases and medicine from the perspective of other broader aspects.

To understand the moral crisis in medicine and effectively negotiate with it, we need to have a proper idea about the role it plays in human societies in the contemporary world. A broader historical, sociological and philosophical analysis may help in this regard. In many ancient societies, as shown above, medicine was conceived as contributing to the fulfilment of the larger design and teleology of life. Many ancient philosophies of medicine were eudaimonistic. The Greeks thought about flourishing, and the Indians envisaged attaining *purusharthas*, which constituted the fundamental objectives of human life. Even those traditions that went against the Vedic orthodoxy had proposed eudaimonic objectives such as *nirvana* in Buddhism and the hedonistic goal of the materialists, Lokayatas. However, modern societies function on the basis of other norms, which value individual liberty and autonomy. They do not propose up front any fundamental goal for all men; instead, they leave it to the individuals to decide what is good for each of them. In this sense, their objective often becomes defensive and negative. They aim at protecting the individual from the coercion of other people and establishments. Therefore, one essential concern of bioethics today is to protect the individual from the repressive and exploitative powers of the whole social establishment of medicine. Contemporary bioethics, therefore, formulates a set of moral principles that have a wide range of applications. I have discussed these aspects earlier. Despite this preventive goal, the principles of bioethics have a positive target; they all try to contribute to the realization of a larger emancipatory goal, which may progressively contribute to individual and collective human flourishing, as they foster individual autonomy. The principles aim to protect those individuals who are vulnerable due to their predicament of falling ill. They help to safeguard the rights of individuals by highlighting autonomy.

Therefore, medicine at all times seems to be serving two fundamental purposes: social and individual. At the social level, it helps to maintain social order by keeping individuals healthy so that they can participate in the various contractual functions required. At the individual level, it aids individual happiness and flourishing. These two goals are, in one sense, interconnected, as they both presuppose a model of human life and society that people try to give shape to. In the absence of an overarching eudaimonic perspective, most societies try to organize in the light of a contractual arrangement. Society is primarily viewed as constitutive of individuals who are autonomous and equal rights-bearers who enter into different types of covenants and agreements with each other for fulfilling their respective purposes and goals. Hence, in the context of the most primordial professional relationship between the physicians and the patients, they have to be considered as the two parties in a contract with different objectives.

Sociologically, this relationship is very important as it helps to nurture a conducive social life without individual citizens necessarily agreeing upon any fundamental philosophical or religious ideas they have about human life. Diseases and disabilities cause different responses among different individuals, but society in general tries to problematize it in a different manner by seeing how they affect it in the long run. As the sociologist Talcott Parsons (1975) observes, diseases put off individuals from performing their normal functions in society. He refers to Eugene Gallagher's conception of health and illness, which regards the former as a category of the capacity of the human individual and the latter as a state of affairs which would impair, in varying ways and degrees, the capacity of the sick person to function normally (259). The sick here fail to meet their obligatory requirements as well as may become dependent on other people. Society may not only lose their inputs but also will have to spare other individuals for their service. In genuine cases of illness, the individual is not responsible for this scenario. Such incapacitated individuals have to be exempted from their *day-to-day* occupations and such exemptions are given on the basis of the institution-alization of the sick role. The sick role, therefore, is a kind of institutional measure of incapacity (259). However, such exemptions may impact society in various ways, as an illness is a form of social deviance. It is essential to minimize the impacts of this social deviance. When a large number of people become sick and deviate from normal consensual behaviour, it adversely impacts society. Too many people adopting the sick role become a major social concern, and this needs to be regulated. Medicine, as a social institu-tion, therefore, has a very critical role in human life. It has to normalize deviant illness through therapeutic interventions. Modern medicine serves this duty in varying degrees of success. Its various advancements over the past two centuries testify this success. The invention of several vaccines has eradicated a significant number of contagious diseases. Innovative therapies and medications invented in the recent past have proved to be useful for the treatment of a large number of diseases which were terminal earlier. More than the direct impacts on bettering individual lives, they significantly aid in maintaining the socio-economic order in society and alleviating poverty in many countries. Whether this socio-economic order that medicine helps to maintain is morally beneficial is another question that goes beyond the purview of biomedical ethics to answer.

Medical interventions have benefitted individuals more directly, and such benefits have undeniably aided human flourishing, both individual and social. However, as discussed above, modern medicine confronts ethical exi-gency and crisis. There are various aspects of this crisis. Some structural fea-tures of our societies mount hindrances to medicine, aiding the ultimate goal of human flourishing, in the sense of realizing individual liberty, happiness and autonomy in contemporary societies. Most societies in the world are industrialized in different degrees and follow a capitalist economic structure. Though many of them are democracies and, therefore, are explicitly com-mitted to values such as individual liberty and autonomy, certain features of the market-oriented capitalism prevent these values from getting actualized. Max Weber conceives individual autonomy as a central value and believes that individuals can actualize it in modern societies more effortlessly than before. However, Weber holds that capitalism is antithetical to the kind of personality and individuality he values and affirms that although it is the highest economic expression of human rationality, capitalism is dangerous to human value (Kahan 2012, 145).

Medicine is practised in such a context which on the one hand advocates very aggressively a form of socio-economic model that requires its members to follow a certain form of moral order and on the other hand projects an ethical ideal that values individual autonomy and liberty. As a social institution, medicine has to respond to both these requirements. The moral crisis in modern medicine has its roots in the contemporary social organization of medicine and this apparent contradiction between the idea of social order and individual liberty.

The Repressive Nature of Medicine: Medical Gaze, Power and Principles

Foucault demonstrates how contemporary social order hinders the realization of individual autonomy and liberty. As observed by Foucault, criminology has become a standard for professional practices in society. In the same way, it orients itself to surveillance and professional control over the deviant population; it achieves professional power in mental institutions, hospitals and clinics, workplaces and schools with various technologies of surveillance (Waitzkin 1989, 226). Foucault problematizes the institution of medicine in order to know how humans are disciplined and controlled in society. He urges to resist this submission of the self to the power structure dynamics.

One obvious issue with medicine and the patient–physician interaction, which constitutes the basis of all medical encounters, is the power disparity between the two constituents of this relationship. This power disparity may become detrimental to the patients in the modern world, mainly due to the changes in the socio-economic and cultural changes many human societies have undergone with the advent of various historical factors during the past few decades. Many like Foucault argue that the socio-economic structures that determine our lives and institutions are to be found in the discourses of our age, and specific power relations decide them. Foucault demonstrates that the origins of these power structures are in the discourses and codes of knowledge that emerged during the Middle Ages (Kurzweil 1986, 650). Enlightenment had professed human freedom as the central moral value, and our political establishments explicitly assured its preponderance. However, Foucault affirms that power is ubiquitous, and the modern egalitarian social and political establishments are not capable of resisting its repressive character. This repression manifests in several ways in the relationship between patients and their physicians. Patients reveal their experiences about their illness, but the physicians do not receive these patient descriptions passively. They filter out what they consider unnecessary and focus on the presumed necessary facts and sometimes force the patients to narrow down their descriptions to certain specific aspects. This physician gaze captures the patient not as an individual but as an object. Foucault (2003) states:

> Paradoxically, in relation to that which he is suffering from, the patient is only an external fact; the medical reading must take him into account only to place him in parentheses. Of course, the doctor must know "the internal structure of our bodies"; but only in order to subtract it, and to free to the doctor's gaze "the nature and combination of symptoms, crises, and other circumstances that accompany diseases". It is not the pathological that functions, in relation to life, as a counter-nature, but the patient in relation to the disease itself.
>
> (8)

In this essential reductionism inherent in the patient–physician interactions, the two partners speak different languages. From the experiential descriptions of the patient, the physician constructs an account of the disease, which the patient does not understand. After that, the patient's discomforts get baptized into a complex phenomenon and acquire a scientific name, which sounds unfamiliar to the patient. The physician thus defines the disease and prepares a treatment plan for the patient, about which the latter is not familiar. Physicians are the only people who know what the problem is and what the remedies are.

This gaze intensified ever since medicine became a complete science. This was inevitable for its effectiveness and for the society to keep its pace of progress in other domains of life. One immediate impact of such developments is on the patient–physician relationship, as it makes the power disparities further widen. In a scenario where the physicians alone understand the disease and have total control over therapy may lead to physician paternalism that ultimately may reduce the patients to mere objects. Modern societies emphasize values such as personal privacy, autonomy and liberty and consider them to be inevitable for individual flourishing. These aspects are discussed in the previous chapters in detail. Ideally, the modern individual has to be autonomous in the socio-economic and political realms and cannot be otherwise when she takes crucial decisions on her health. Modern bioethics attempts to restrain such paternalistic and coercive propensities with the ethical theories that emphasize individual rights and principles that comprehensively address several issues in healthcare and balance them with individual autonomy and social justice. The four principles aim at liberating individuals from the coercion and exploitation of the physicians, other professionals and other stakeholders.

However, as Foucault points out, they belong to the discourse of our era, reflecting its fundamental concerns and power structures. Therefore, they hardly help in making medicine free from power relations but are pronounced and managed by another set of power relations. The modern professional interactions are seemingly different from the explicitly hierarchical relationships that existed in the Middle Ages. As discussed above, modern societies consider individuals as equal rights-bearers in the socio-economic realm. This was not so earlier when class differences existed in Europe. The equal rights-bearer in modern society is an individual who ideally enjoys her autonomy and privacy and she enters into professional relationships with other rights-bearing individuals like her for conducting her usual socio-economic life. Such relationships are expected to be among equals. However, in actuality, they are hardly so and are mired in other types of power relations. Foucault (1978) analyses the practice of pastoral confessions that began in the Middle Ages. He says, since the Middle Ages, Western societies have established confession as one of the main rituals we rely on for the production of truth and affirms that western man has become a confessing animal (58). Confession, according to him, is a ritual that unfolds within a power relationship, and the production of truth that takes place is permeated with relations of power. One does not confess without the presence of a partner, asserts Foucault. The partner here is the authority who requires the confession, prescribes and appreciates it, and intervenes in order to judge, punish, forgive, console and reconcile (62).

Foucault further notes that confession lost its ritualistic and exclusive localization later with the rise of Protestantism, the Counter-Reformation, 18th-century pedagogy and 19th-century medicine. People began to use it on other occasions and for different purposes in multiple forms in various types of relationships such as children and parents, students and educators, patients and psychiatrists, delinquents and experts (63). While used in other contexts, it changes its nature and objectives, and hence the early power structure becomes obsolete. A new power relation takes over and begins to determine its course.

Foucault presents a comprehensive analysis of the ways power administers over life, and according to him, the power over life evolved in two basic forms. First, it is centred on the idea that the body is a machine. In Foucault's words,

> its disciplining, the optimization of its capabilities, the extortion of its forces, the parallel increase of its usefulness and its docility, its integration into systems of efficient and economic controls, all this was ensured by the procedures of power that characterized the disciplines: an anatomo-politics of the human body.
>
> (139)

The second focuses on

> the species body, the body imbued with the mechanics of life and serving as the basis of the biological processes: propagation, births and mortality, the level of health, life expectancy and longevity, with all the

conditions that can cause these to vary. Their supervision was effected through an entire series of interventions and regulatory controls: a biopolitics of the population.

(139)

The power over life was exerted through the control exercised over the individual and the species bodies. Foucault's observation that criminology has become a standard for professional practices in society has to be understood in light of this fact.

Foucault's analysis reveals how every social institution is engrossed within the whirlpool of different power relationships and how in spite of their overt propagation of an egalitarian polity and the rational organization of the various institutions and establishments, modern societies function quite repressively. Medicine primarily caters to people who are sick, a condition that makes them vulnerable and easily susceptible to repression and exploitation. Therefore, the social organization of medicine inevitably makes it a repressive endeavour. It, therefore, falls short of ensuring patients the autonomy, liberty and privacy that modern bioethics attempts to accomplish. This social organization has already abandoned what Max Weber (2005) terms the "Faustian universality of man" (123), as an individual in our modern society lives a life separated into several individual spheres with no overarching value system.

This social organization robs off medicine its *eudaimonic* goal, and bioethics has already evolved to a state where it has discarded the primeval moral concerns nurtured by ancient philosophers and have adopted a moral paradigm that focused on individual rights and autonomy. This new paradigm helps in resolving many dilemmas practitioners as well as the general public face in their various encounters with different healthcare practices and employment of technologies. However, the essential repressive character that regulates the various professional interactions in medicine further depletes it of its emancipatory potentials. Hence, despite the fact that it helps resolve many dilemmas, many issues and predicaments remain disturbingly unsettled within this new paradigm. All these factors ultimately induce a fundamental moral crisis in contemporary medicine, despite its scintillating contributions. A few of the new medical procedures discussed in this section, including stem cell therapy, gene therapy and cloning, may respond to some of the concerns raised here. However, they eventually make some other issues more intensive.

Artificial Health versus Natural Health

As mentioned above, some important factors that impel this ethical crisis include the crucial changes humans have made to their approach towards their conception of health, well-being and life in its totality. At a fundamental level, it begins with a change in our conception of health, where we embrace the idea of artificial health in place of natural health. Dr Alexis Carrel (1959) refers to two kinds of health: artificial and natural. Artificial health is the creation of modern medicine, and ancient physicians never had any idea about it. Most of the therapies and medicines aim at producing artificial health, as they all try to intervene externally. Almost all therapies, modern medicine recommend and administer, ultimately aim at the creation of artificial health. The idea of artificial health has contributed heavily to making human life drastically better. The whole infrastructure of modern medicine is designed to produce artificial health. The therapies are developed in the light of a deeper understanding of the structural and functional aspects of the human body, its vulnerability to climate, microbial creatures and several other factors in the environment. However, it comes at a high cost. As Carrel says, "man is not content with health that is only lack of malady and depends on special diets, chemicals, endocrine products, vitamins, periodical medical examinations, and the expensive attention of hospitals, doctors and nurses" (289–290). After all, it is artificial and not natural. The idea of natural health searches for health within the body and in its natural environment. Artificial health is health that is externally defined. It can be measured and standardized, and in that sense can be managed in a relatively easy manner. It is a publically defined goal, which a physician understands better than the patient and can guide the latter to reach the goal that she defines for her patient. On the other hand, natural health is an experiential state that enables the individual to harmonize with the world.

As Carrel says, there is a strong desire to discover how to make humans naturally immune to diseases. According to him, the present trend of medicine is towards artificial health, towards a kind of directed physiology and warns that since organic, humoral and mental processes are infinitely more complex than economics and sociological phenomena, while directed economics may ultimately be a success, directed physiology might fail (291). The fundamental failure lies in its incompetency in accomplishing the positive goal of human flourishing. Understood in its philosophical sense, the realization of such a goal is not necessarily the goal of medicine. Nevertheless, considering some form of flourishing as intrinsically valuable is an inspiring goal rather than an externally delineated and directed physiology. It becomes a moral crisis because it presents a dilemma between life with artificial health accomplished at the expense of the quality of living experience.

Besides the problems mentioned above, the concept of artificial health leads to some deeper philosophical worries. Jean Paul Sartre illustrates how a physician experiences her patient's body as in the "midst of the world" (Sartre 1956, 402). A person can emulate such an experience by seeing her own body, its inner organs and their vitality in an ultrasonic screen. For the person concerned, to internalize this "in the midst of the world" experience and understand it, as "one's body" is an unusual experience. Sartre observes that the person who does this externalizing apprehends a wholly constituted object as a "this" among other theses. It is only by a reasoning process that the person refers it back to being hers. Here one refers to it as her property rather than conceiving it as one's being (402). The dichotomy between her person or her being and her body as her property is evident here. In Sartre's terminology, the being that is revealed to her in the typical middle of the world experiences is the "being-for-others." The being-for-others is inauthentic and alienated. It has become apparent that medicine is capable of ensuring only artificial health, and it fails in ensuring human happiness and flourishing. More and more advanced treatment options mostly make modern medicine a highly specialized domain, and this makes it further alienated from human life.

The search for next-generation therapies can be seen as an attempt to remodel modern medicine with appropriate technologies that regenerate the human body at the cellular level. Stem cell and gene therapies endeavour to do this. In transplantation, the machine metaphor of the human body dominates all other narratives. It adopts a view that perceives the different organs as spare parts that are well-assembled for the harmonic functioning of the machine. Here again, the objective is the creation and preservation of artificial health. However, the other three therapies mentioned above are characteristically different. The use of human embryonic stem cells for therapies envisages developing novel therapeutic approaches by the regenerative power of those cells. Here instead of any pharmaceutical product or technology used for curative purposes, the stem cells from the embryo are used in therapy, which will integrate itself with the body. This suggests a new approach to disease and medication. Gene therapy and cloning represent even more radical departures from the conventional approaches to diseases and disabilities as well as methods of treatment. Most of these therapies, except transplantation, are not conventionally adopted methods of treatment, and all three are still at a state of infancy. All of them are not easily accessible to everyone alike. They are all often prohibitively expensive, and only a few in the society can afford them. This raises a fundamental ethical issue: Who benefits from scientific advancements in healthcare?

Medicine, Individualism and Well-Being

The third factor that induces the ethical crisis is related to this important question. One significant feature of the contemporary age is the mounting individualism in many societies across the world. The post-Enlightenment developments in many Western societies have created a world order that pursued a mode of development that had weakened and undermined the metaphysical and religious worldviews that unified all aspects of human life. The resulting emergence of individualism has eventually introduced a strong moral perspective, which emphasized the importance of the rights of individual human beings. The immediate impact of the spirit of this individualism is reflected in principles like patient autonomy, consent, confidentiality and privacy.

Consequently, the idea that "individuals ought to be left to themselves in making decisions about their life" becomes a norm. This idea serves immensely to the cause of the rights of patients and research participants. One of the central concerns of medicine has been the alleviation of human sufferings that result from diseases. Traditionally, physicians were the decision-makers, and patients believed that their physicians knew the best means to attain the goal of overcoming pain and suffering. However, modern physicians and the establishment of medicine can hardly be compared with the largely altruistic individual practitioners that constituted traditional medicine. Modern medicine is a huge corporate network, which employs many state-of-the-art technologies that has the potential to be immensely beneficial to people as well as to be exploitative and coercive. This repressive environment makes moral principles and values like autonomy, consent and rights important.

With the principle of autonomy, acquiring prominence patients gain more control and authority over medical decisions. However, this control has occasionally not served its purpose. On many occasions, patients may find it hard to grapple with the realization about the nature of their prognosis. They may often prefer to leave the decision to those whom they trust. In many societies, especially in non-Western societies, human flourishing is not conceived in purely individualistic terms. In many places, it is not the individual but the family or even the community that constitutes a unit. In such places, all conceptions of well-being are understood in much broader terms.

Such conflicts are not easy to resolve. However, considering the repressive powers of modern medicine, it is important to ensure that the rights of the patient are protected and the recognition of individual autonomy becomes inevitable to facilitate this. However, this is not easy to bring into practice in many non-western societies, in the absence of a culture that fosters individualism. Medical decisions are still made collectively and often by the senior male members, or in smaller families, by the earning member. Patients may not be aware of what is happening to them and what decisions their family members make about the treatment of their ailments. As mentioned above, due to modern medicine's potentially repressive and exploitative character, it is important that patients are aware of their predicament and are properly consulted when any decision is taken while addressing it. On the other hand, in many western societies, the fundamental individualism that prevails in the society may hamper patient well-being, as it fails to ensure the patient the much-required emotional support, which invariably comes from a family environment. The context of medical practice in the contemporary world may have to grapple with such contrasting scenarios. It is futile to search for a universal moral framework, which is constitutive of a set of rigid principles. Instead, we may need to formulate a set of essential principles, which nevertheless need to be interpretatively applied to actual contexts in different parts of the world. This, however, is not an easy task and demands physicians and other medical practitioners to be more than experts in their respective technical domains. Regaining the lost unity is not a feasible undertaking for the professional world of medicine.

A related issue is a clash between some of the important ethical principles of bioethics when they are implemented in different contexts. The principlist approach has certain advantages, as they are not rigid theoretical positions but are only broad principles, which can be applied to any context as and when required. The four of them emphasize different aspects and may not agree with each other in spirit. Yet, since each of them emphasizes one or other vital moral aspect, they together form a comprehensive framework, which can be applied in a specific cultural context. Nevertheless, as pointed out above, the four principles approach is more conducive to a western society rather than Asian and African contexts. In societies, which still make collective medical decisions, deeply patriarchal, hierarchical and financially backward, each of these principles will have different meaning and some of them like autonomy may hardly find a relevant place at all. Even the principles of beneficence, nonmaleficence and justice have very different meanings. Often a clash between the autonomy-based paradigm of moral assumptions and the justice-based paradigm of moral contemplations surface in many non-western countries. Such societies may find the overt individualism reflected in the principle of autonomy as problematic. As mentioned earlier, health is still conceptualized as a collective flourishing in such societies rather than an individual accomplishment, as it appears to people living in many western countries.

The individualistic paradigm may often lead to other stalemates, as it may also lead to the conflict between different moral values held by different stakeholders. Sometimes terminally ill patients may find themselves in immense pain and suffering, and they may wish to end their sufferings by employing euthanasia instead of prolonging their life with the help of medication and technologies. A few medical technologies may enable physicians to prolong the life of their patients. Here the desire of the patient to end her life may be in conflict with the personal morality of the physician and her professional morality that insists on nonmaleficence and beneficence. Such a scenario, in the contemporary world, witnesses a clash between multiple moral claims. On the one hand, there is an autonomous choice made by the patient. The physician, in turn, may believe that it is against her moral values to assist the patient to end her life. There is the belief that life is eternal, and man has no right to end it. If a person suffers, she is only reaping the fruits of her *karmas*, and any interference by the physician would be morally unwarranted. Such a scenario may expose the limitations of the principles-based ethical approach. The clash is not only between different value systems but also with the quality of life and its intrinsic worth.

One way to resolve such issues is to translate them into the legal framework and find a solution. This is particularly the case in societies where the moral and social values are in conflict with the individualistic rights-based frameworks that have legal authority. The collective decision-making that prevails in many such societies may go against the interests of the individual patients, and proper legislation on important matters may help to protect human rights. The Supreme Court of India, in a landmark judgement in *Common Cause v. Union of India & Anr.* delivered on 9 March 2018, held that the right to die with dignity is an intrinsic aspect of the right to life under Article 21 of the Constitution of India. Hence, terminally ill patients have the right to decide whether or not to accept medical intervention. The judgement reiterated that the right to live with dignity gives individuals the right to choose not to undergo pain and suffering. However, this is not a solution to the ethical problem. It only affirms the rights of the individual to refuse to undergo any treatment. The Supreme Court also has emphasized the value of individual autonomy. In order to avoid any clash between the patient's autonomous choice and physicians' commitment to nonmaleficence, it makes the individual the sole authority of her life. The physician's decisive role is to provide the patient with the right kind of recommendations and help her to arrive at the right decisions considering her views about the dignity of life. The Supreme Court, in its verdict, does not pronounce provisions on active euthanasia. Nonetheless, it observes the physician's role in the process as an advisor and facilitator.

Medicine and Market: Genuine Medical Needs versus Market Demand and Health as a Competitive Advantage

Another factor that induces the modern moral crisis in medicine is the dominance of a market-driven capitalist philosophy governing the entire establishment of modern medicine. This has impacted society in many ways. It has severely impaired the accessibility of the benefits of modern medicine to a large section of the population who cannot afford it. The affordability of quality healthcare is a significant concern for most societies. In the third world, the vast income disparities and other social inequalities make the situation even grave. Poverty makes people sick, and this necessitates them to go to hospitals and spend on healthcare. This will intensify their poverty. Many poor people are thrown into the streets after they recover from an illness. The cost of quality healthcare products and services, therefore, widens the gap between haves and have-nots in society. Such issues may become severe with the introduction of new technologies. The idea of genetic vaccines for various ailments is mentioned above. If successfully developed, this technology with gene-editing procedure may prevent several diseases from the embryonic state itself. However, this is going to remain for a long time an expensive therapy and hence will not be affordable/accessible for a large number of people in the society. The children of those who can afford it may constitute a separate class. The prospects of cloning, as aforementioned, may induce the fear of eugenics, which again will result in further stratification of the society. Medicine may unintentionally become a tool for widening social inequalities and proliferating unjust social stratification.

Historically, many medical discoveries have significantly improved the conditions of human life and made it more meaningful and satisfying. These contributions are cherished, not because they have made a few human lives better, but because they have benefitted the entire humanity and have aided in alleviating its sufferings. However, one major flaw of the medicine of this age is its inability to benefit humanity in large. Many of its specialized therapies and procedures are not affordable to a large number of people or are not accessible to rural people. Technological innovations should ideally make it more accessible and affordable, as in many other sectors. But paradoxically, in medicine, the more advanced a therapeutic intervention is, the more limited and confined is its reach. This is ironic, and it exposes an essential dimension of the moral crisis that the healthcare sector faces in the contemporary world.

Medicine is often unable to respond to the genuine health requirements of a large number of people due to their inability to pay for the required services, despite availability. Michael A. Santoro (2005), in his introduction to the edited volume *Ethics and the Pharmaceutical Industry*, discusses in detail the core issues in need of resolution. The first is the imperfect alignment of private profit-maximizing objectives with public health needs. Quite often, private enterprise drives restrict access and distort medical priorities. Despite being invented, the patients in the third world find many life-saving drugs inaccessible, as they are unaffordable to them. On the other hand, for heart ailments and hypertension that are common in developing economies, there are multiple treatment options available (5). The distinction is here between genuine medical needs and market for medicines, requirement and affordability, and also between necessity and profitability. This disconnect is more intense and grave in the developing countries. It is a known fact that effective medication is available for many diseases that consume precious human lives in the third world. The pricing policies of pharmaceutical firms, the greed of management, and the various marketing techniques they adopt are responsible for the calamity.

Santoro cites an example that testifies how strong and detrimental is the influence of the market and the capitalist ideology for human well-being. He highlights the gulf between commerce and medicine by contrasting the needs of a poor child suffering from malaria in sub-Saharan Africa with a middle-aged American man suffering from hair loss. On purely medical grounds, the child should have priority. However, argues Santoro, the balding American man is a valued customer through the prism of capitalism, where the African child barely exists. He points to the fact that, while malaria research attracts 20 cents in research dollars for each infection, ailments prevalent in developed countries attract hundreds of dollars per case. The most pressing medical needs require, asserts Santoro, nonmarket solutions (10).

Similar tendencies and disconnects are ubiquitous in the present-day healthcare sector. There are fundamentally two challenges. First, the discovery, development, manufacturing, registration and distribution of a new drug will cost pharmaceutical companies colossal expenditure. Recovering this investment requires the company to generate sales that would result in a reasonable profit correspondingly. Hence, as Jurgen Drews (2005) points out, in order to ensure good returns from investment and the risks taken, pharmaceutical companies tend to focus on the needs of people in economically developed countries and may incline to neglect the genuine medical needs of people in those countries who have limited purchasing power (28). The other issue is what Drews terms as the apparent conflict between the goals of medical or Hippocratic ethics and corporate interests. The former requires the following of the scientific opportunity in addressing various medical indications, while the latter calls for maximizing profits (29).

This essential disconnect points to a more fundamental tendency that exists in our society. It has to do with deeper issues regarding the social and cultural lives we give shape to and the ways we organize our society in accordance with the rules of the market. These rules make every human endeavour and activity legitimate in the light of such rules. Subsequently, disease and health are also determined by market rules. Health becomes a possession that is ultimately viewed as a competitive advantage. It becomes a commodity that facilitates us a life with better success and happiness. This tendency, however, is not confined to healthcare alone. It is a more significant propensity to evaluate all human endeavours and achievements in the light of an idea of success in the marketplace. In this sense, it is the consequence of the capitalist moral system that gives shape to our day-to-day life.

This moral framework has impacted social and individual lives in diverse ways. While discussing the ethics of human cloning and bioengineering, Michael Sandel argues that they simply carry to full expression the troubling tendencies that are already present in our culture, especially in the way we regard and treat children (Sandel 2005, 243). He complains that we consider children as vehicles for our ambitions or fulfilment (243). There exists a blind drive for success, and this affects children more than any other section in the society. Some reports validate the number of children with attention deficit hyperactivity disorder (ADHD) is on the rise every year. One reason for this is the concern of parents over their wards' prospective academic and professional success. ADHD is a common chronic neurobehavioral disorder of childhood, and it affects school-age children impacting their academic performance. Over the past two decades, the number of children with ADHD has gone up from 6% to 10% in the United States (Gordon 2018). Studies conducted in India show a higher rate of 11.5% (Venkata and Panicker 2013). There is little evidence in proving this increase in number is due to overdiagnosis. However, there exists a tendency to medicalize every phenomenon that fails to meet our expectations.

The fact that children's academic performance is associated with success in life makes education the most problematic sphere in our society. The current trend defies all those ideals proposed by the Greek thinkers such as "care for the self," providing a true science and art of politics, developing moral character and living a good life. Education becomes a tool for competing better. About one million students appear for the Joint Entrance Examinations (JEE) in India every year and they compete to get admission to the 23 IITs and 31 NITs and a few other premium engineering institutes in the country. Similarly, approximately 1.3 million candidates compete to get admissions to the 529 medical colleges in the country. There are specialized coaching institutes in several parts of the country that train students for these examinations since their early teens. These students spent a significant amount of time in such centres preparing for the one exam which their parents and society consider as the most important event in their lives. Such efforts keep them aloof from all other regular activities children of their age would be engaging. For millions of parents in India, success has only one meaning; admission to these premium institutes. They attach hardly any intrinsic value to education. People share a general outlook that treats only those who emerge victorious in the competition as being successful in life. Things gain value in so far as they facilitate this success. Therefore, all that gives one a competitive advantage becomes valuable and will be sought after. Health becomes a competitive advantage, as healthy people can compete better.

Again, this competition has several dimensions. Parents thus desire to have children with better intelligence, better mathematical abilities, above-average height, bright complexion, resistance to several diseases and several other physical as well as psychical features that make them competitively superior to their peers. All these will function as competitive advantages in a world that determines success in terms of market rules. However, there is something fundamentally wrong in this approach of seeing health as a competitive advantage. Health is indeed a competitive advantage, as good health enables us to excel in what we are engaged. However, to excel is not to be equated with winning a competition. Vaghbhata affirms that medicine aims to aid humanity in their pursuit of the three virtues of *dharma*, *artha* and *sukha* (Thirumulpad 2006, 7). In other words, good health enables one to be in the path of righteous actions, relish money, fame and other material gains of life and finally pursue physical pleasure or spiritual emancipation. Hence, the purposes good health serves are multidimensional. It ultimately has a eudaimonic goal to accomplish.

The Social Organization of Medicine and Bioethics

It is evident that most of the factors that induce the crisis emanates from the way we situate medicine and its establishment in our society and value it in accordance with our broad objectives and goals. Since most societies today have discarded eudaimonic objectives, it is hard to regain what Weber terms as the "Faustian universality," which would have resolved many issues, as it hardly raises the problems related to fragmented spheres and their individual well-being that may often contradict with each other. We need to find out how medicine can be properly regulated in the modern fragmented social environment which witnesses the constant conflict between several important aspects that constitute social life; corporate interests versus human values, individual rights versus rights of corporate organizations and institutions, and individual liberty versus social well-being.

It is evident that the social context which gives rise to the wide range of bioethical issues today is larger and wider than what a set of principles and theories can effectively address. It needs proper social organization in the light of better planning and arrangement of the various segments that constitute our social life. We need a better economy, a better planning of living habitats, better governance and the development of better communication channels and solidarity among human beings, groups and communities. But it also demands much more than that as it is important to understand the co-evolution of human beings as biological and social entities in the community (Whitehouse 2003, W29). We need to adopt a comprehensive approach towards understanding and evaluation of ethical problems and issues. In other words, it demands to broaden the scope of bioethics, perhaps by recapturing the original meanings Van Rensselaer Potter (1971), the American oncologist who initially tried to establish a strong relationship between ethics and biological sciences in his attempts to adopt an integrated approach in ethics. The opening statement of his book *Bioethics: Bridge to the Future* states that mankind is urgently in need of new wisdom that will provide the "knowledge of how to use knowledge" (1). It is in this what the ancient philosophers considered wisdom consisting in, which is the "knowledge of how to use knowledge" for the social good, which according to him is the prerequisite to improvement in the quality of life. Ethics for him is broader and comprehensive than we usually understand it in the academic world, as along with medical and environmental ethics it also includes social and religious ethics (1). Potter says:

> I take the position that the science of survival must be built on the science of biology and enlarged beyond the traditional boundaries to include the essential elements of the social sciences and the humanities with an emphasis on philosophy in the strict sense, meaning "love of wisdom." A science of survival must be more than science alone, and I therefore propose the term *Bioethics* in order to emphasize the two most important ingredients in achieving the new wisdom that is so desperately needed: biological knowledge and human values.
>
> (1–2)

With Potter's work, bioethics begins as a new initiative that envisages linking diverse aspects of life on earth to ensure survival. Potter's vision encompasses a philosophy of life, which is much akin to the old philosophical wisdom and he understood the term "ethics" as standing for general human values (Jonsen 2003, 27). Around the same time, theologians and philosophers of the Catholic university at Georgetown used the word "bioethics" to name an institute the university was planning to open with funds from the Kennedy Foundation. They primarily regarded bioethics as a branch of applied ethics (Cooter 2004, 1749). As Albert R. Jonsen (2003) notes, bioethics had been translated from a neologism in a scholarly article into the title of an institution and was on its way towards becoming the name of a new discipline and the meaning of the word "bioethics" narrowed from what Potter had in mind as an endeavour that seeks to ensure global future to more specific problems of biomedicine (27).

Many developments in the field of medicine as well as in the history of humankind in the past few decades during the post-war period have significantly contributed to the further development of bioethics as an academic discipline and practical venture. Hrvoje Jurić (2017) observes that there are different conceptions or self-conceptions of bioethics. The prominent Anglo-American view takes it as a discipline dealing with issues pertaining to clinical practice, healthcare systems, biological, biomedical and pharmaceutical research and research result applications, and other issues concerning human life and health in general. According to Jurić, they narrow the concept of "bioethics" down to medical or "biomedical ethics" and often use these terms as synonymous. They hardly deal with questions that are not directly related to human health or those directly related to other living beings and nature as a whole. Hence, the first group of authors often uses the terms "bioethics" and "biomedical ethics" as synonymous. Jurić adds that the bioethical discourse has become increasingly aware of the fact that bioethics is simply not synonymous with new medical or biomedical ethics, and that it embraces a much wider array of issues, ranging from clinical-medical to global-ecological (128). Jurić tries to give a more synthetic definition to bioethics reflecting the essential interlacement of relationships within the living world, and the interlacement of the problems that humanity is facing in this techno-scientific era on the one hand, and that also concern other living beings and nature as a whole on the other. He states:

> Bioethics is an open field of encounters and dialogue between different sciences and professions, and diverse approaches and worldviews, which gather to articulate, discuss and solve ethical questions concerning life, life as a whole and each of its parts, life in all its forms, shapes, degrees, stages and manifestations.
>
> (132)

The discussions in the previous chapters, particularly those dealing with traditional bioethics, display that such an essential interlacing was present in many ancient societies. Even today, many eastern cultures possess this intimate connection between the different aspects of life, such as human life, nature, religion, ethics and science. The *Ying Yang* symbol, for example, points to the dynamic relationship between nature and nurture and suggests that within each force alone, one finds the other (Whitehouse 2003, W29). The Indian philosophical and religious traditions categorically affirm the unity of nature and consciousness with ideas like *prakriti* and *purusha*, and *siva* and *sakthi* and further reiterates the fundamental non-differentiation of the individual with the cosmic reality. However, as Peter J. Whitehouse observes, the American bioethics and culture tend to focus on individual autonomy as a dominant value (W27). In a prominent manner, this derives its nourishment from the western anthropocentric philosophical tradition and the Abrahamic religious traditions, where nature and the other living creatures are pushed to a lesser status of existence below man. Whitehouse, while discussing Potter's contributions to bioethics, argues that extending bioethics to consider not only human communitarian values but also to include communities of other living creatures is needed (W27). This is evident from Potter's repeated insistence on evolutionary biology and ecology while discussing the biological framework for medicine, instead of mere molecular biology and genetics (Whitehouse 2001, 47). But this is about the science of biology and medicine. The ethics part requires more careful attention and planning. Potter (1998) adds:

> Cultural evolution has failed to reflect on the lessons of biological evolution and to develop a civilization that can delay its own extinction. The course of cultural evolution must be radically changed. Deep and global bioethics that is a well-researched, comprehensive, and worldwide morality must evolve in the first few decades of the 21st century. After that it may be too late.

Potter's alternative is, therefore, not just a scheme for healthcare ethics, as he believes that medicine has to look beyond molecular biology and genetics. Human health can never be isolated from the dynamics of life in its totality, with all its possible dimensions. Many traditions of indigenous medicine had been integrated with a much broader framework of values that reflect the diverse concerns of life. *Ayurveda*, for instance, is often understood as offering a comprehensive programme for a healthy life with peaceful coexistence with fellow human beings as well as the other living creatures and the inanimate nature. This is true for many other ancient healing traditions in varying degrees of accuracy and details. However, to revive and relive those values in the contemporary world is not a viable option before us.

Potter proposes a reasonably comprehensive framework, which of course needs further expansion and development. However, the historical course of the development of bioethics in the west has eventually taken a different route. One reason for this is due to its predominant Anglo-American origin. Bioethics in the modern world as a discipline has originated in the United States during the last quarter of the 20th century. Physicians, philosophers and others who took initiatives in developing the discipline had to deal with a moral crisis created by several inhuman experiments conducted by the medical world. Following such disruptions, the American courts had witnessed several litigations filed by individuals and groups of individuals, questioning the abuses involved in terms of violations to individual rights to life and privacy. Unethical and illegal medical experiments such as the Nazi experiments on Jews and others, the Tuskegee syphilis study and the Willowbrook experiments discussed in the previous chapters have played a significant role in the course of development of contemporary bioethics. Moreover, the extensive media coverage such violations attracted has also stimulated ethical debates to orient in a specific direction in the United States.

These various controversies and debates have given contemporary American bioethics a visible individual-centric character. The principlist framework reflects this spirit. The principles of autonomy, beneficence, nonmaleficence and justice, when applied to specific situations, have certain advantages over other theories such as utilitarianism or virtue ethics. Since they are broad principles, they can be applied to any context. However, the emphasis is visibly on individual rights and entitlements. Although all the four principles have equal importance, autonomy acquires predominance as the primary objective is to protect the individual from the coercion of others. On the other hand, in most non-western civilizations, the primary unit in the society is not the individual, but the family or the community and decisions are often taken jointly, keeping in mind the well-being of the collective group. More importantly, this focus on the individual blurs the value of other aspects such as the environment and the society to which the individual is intimately related.

This overt focus on the individual manifests in the methodological approach of modern medicine, as it focuses mainly on the genetic constitution of the individual patient in order to define her disease besides focusing on other external microbial causes that are observable. Medicine thus limits the location of the disease to the individual and further to one or two organs in the patient's body. This is to disregard the value of other social and environmental factors that facilitate the origination and spread of any disease. In the medical professional's enthusiasm to heal, she has to narrow down her focus to the extent of bracketing the individuality of her patient.

Potter's deep bioethics aspires to encompass such aspects and also introduces a spiritual dimension at the core of bioethics, as it bases some of the moral beliefs on their spiritual connection to nature (Whitehouse 2003, W27). Bioethics, Potter believed, has a more profound role to perform rather than merely serving the individual patients by protecting them from the coercion of their physicians and the exploitation of the corporate medical establishment. Of course, they are important objectives of bioethics. But as ethics of life, it should go beyond that and pursue to make essential contributions to the future of life on this planet, a goal it can attain only by making changes in our attitudes towards health, particularly environmental, public and community (Whitehouse 2001, 48).

Concluding Remarks

With the improvements it made in terms of developing effective medications and advanced medical technologies, modern medicine makes laudable critical contributions to the development of human health. However, its failure in augmenting such developments with the overall development of human civilization indicates a moral failure. I do not propose a deep bioethics alternative as a solution to this failure, as no solution for a moral crisis of this nature and magnitude can be simplistic and one-dimensional. Modern medicine is practised all over the world and the fundamental reasons for the crisis are to be sought in different places. As mentioned above, the very nature of medicine as science, which develops in a certain manner with an overt focus on the immediate causes of human diseases, is one such problem. Another factor is the capitalist economic philosophy, which treats medicine as one of its corporate arms. The third aspect points to the fragmentation of healthcare from other larger aspects of human life that address the challenges posed to human well-being and survival.

The post-Enlightenment developments in science facilitated the emergence and growth of medicine into a complete scientific and rational enterprise. Ironically, the same post-Enlightenment sociocultural scenario was responsible for its fragmentation from the rest of life projects. This fragmentation ultimately separated the domain of values from other important domains that define human life. When bioethics was developed in the aftermath of the World Wars in response to various violations of individual rights in the United States, it overtly emphasized protecting the individual. The individualistic culture in Western societies, too, found bioethics which protects the individuals from coercion as valuable.

But it is an equally important ethical imperative to salvage the individual from loneliness and the terrible solitude of human existence. For this, the individual needs to be reunited with the groups and communities. Many non-western cultures still nurture group identities and make decisions collectively. The human communities have to be further reunited with nature from where they have been separated from social and economic developments. Hence, the solution to the moral crisis calls for a comprehensive reorganization of individual and social life in the light of new values that foster human solidarity. As Potter reminds us, such a worldwide morality must evolve very soon, before it is too late.

Bibliography

Afzal, Hina, Khadija Zahid, Qurban Ali, Kubra Sarwar, Sana Shakoor, Ujala Nasir, and Idrees Ahmad Nasir. 2016. "Role of Biotechnology in Improving Human Health." *Journal of Molecular Biomarkers and Diagnosis* 8 (1). Accessed 23 February 2019. https://doi.org/10.4172/2155-9929.1000309.

Agence France-Presse. 2019. "Second Woman Carrying Gene-Edited Baby, Chinese Authorities Confirm." *The Guardian*, 22 January 2019 01.10 GMT. Accessed 13 December 2019. https://www.theguardian.com/science/2019/jan/22/second -woman-carrying-gene-edited-baby-chinese-authorities-confirm.

Akhmad, Syaefudin Ali and Linda Rosita. 2012. "Islamic Bioethics: The Art of Decision Making." *Indonesian Journal of Legal and Forensic Sciences* 2 (1): 8–12. Accessed 12 July 2019. https://ojs.unud.ac.id/index.php/ijlfs/article/view /3251.

Akker, Olga B.A. van den. 2010. "Surrogate Motherhood: A Critical Perspective." *Expert Review of Obstetrics & Gynecology* 5 (1): 5–7. Accessed 11 September 2019. https://doi.org/10.1586/eog.09.69.

Alexander, Shana. 1962. "They Decide Who Lives, Who Dies." *Life*, 9 November. Accessed 16 September 2019. https://books.google.co.in/books ?id=qUoEAAAAMBAJ&lpg=PA1&dq=life+magazine+nov+1962&pg=PA101 &redir_esc=y&hl=en#v=onepage&q&f=false.

Allmark, Peter. 2002. "Death with Dignity." *Journal of Medical Ethics* 28 (4): 255–257. Accessed 24 November 2019. https://doi.org/10.1136/jme.28.4.255.

al-Almany, Mika'il, ed. 2009. *Sahih Bukhari*. Translated by M. Muhsin Khan. Accessed 15 January 2020. https://d1.islamhouse.com/data/en/ih_books/single/ en_Sahih_Al-Bukhari.pdf.

Anderlik, Mary R. 2001. *The Ethics of Managed Care: A Pragmatic Approach*. Bloomington,: Indiana University Press.

Anilkumar, Kappillil and K.I. Anitha. 2015. "Clinical Research—History of Regulations on Experiments: A Global Perspective." In *Clinical Aspects of Functional Foods and Nutraceuticals*, edited by Dilip Ghosh, Debasis Bagchi, and Tetsuya Konishi. 257–276. Florida: CRC Press.

Aries, Philippe. 1974. "The Reversal of Death: Changes in Attitudes Toward Death in Western Societies." *American Quarterly* 26 (5): 536–560. Accessed 19 January 2020. https://doi.org/10.2307/2711889.

Aristotle. 1893. *The Nicomachean Ethics of Aristotle* (5th Edn). Translated by F.H. Peters. London: Kegal Paul, Trench, Trubner & Co., Ltd.

Aronson, J.K. 2009. "Medication Errors: What They Are, How They Happen, and How to Avoid Them." *Quarterly Journal of Medicine* 102 (8): 513–521. Accessed 22 October 2019. https://doi.org/10.1093/qjmed/hcp052.

Augustyn, Catherine, Brigham Walker, and Thomas F. Goss. 2012. "Recognizing the Value of Innovation in HIV/AIDS Therapy." Boston Healthcare Associates, Inc., Boston, MA and Washington, DC, White Paper. Accessed 19 January 2020. http://phrma-docs.phrma.org/sites/default/files/flash/phrma_innovation_value.pdf.

Ayer, A.J. 1971. *Language, Truth and Logic*. London: Penguin Books.

Azeem, Majeed. 2005. "How Islam Changed Medicine." *British Medical Journal* 331 (7531): 1486–1487. Accessed 8 June 2019. https://doi.org/10.1136/bmj.331.7531.1486.

Babu, Ramesh, D.C. Katoch, and M.M. Padhi. 2012. *Ayurveda: The Science of Life*. New Delhi: Department of AYUSH Ministry of Health & Family Welfare Government of India New Delhi. Accessed 4 February 2020. http://www.ccras.nic.in/sites/default/files/viewpdf/Publication/AYURVEDA_The_Science_of_Life(Dossier).pdf.

Banerjee, Anirban D., Haim Ezer, and Anil Namda. 2011. "Susruta and Ancient Indian Neurosurgery." *World Neurosurgery* 75 (2): 320–323. Accessed 25 December 2019. https://doi.org/10.1016/j.wneu.2010.09.007.

Baoutina, A., T. Coldham, G.S. Bains, and K.R. Emslie. 2010. "Gene Doping Detection: Evaluation of Approach for Direct Detection of Gene Transfer Using Erythropoietin as a Model System." *Gene Therapy* 17 (8): 1022–1032. Accessed 21 January 2020. https://doi.org/10.1038/gt.2010.49.

Barrett, Cyril, ed. 1966. *Wittgenstein: Lectures and Conversations on Aesthetics, Psychology and Religious Belief*. Oxford: Blackwell.

Beauchamp, Tom L. 1995. "Principlism and its Alleged Competitors." *Kennedy Institute of Ethics Journal* 5 (3): 181–198. Accessed 27 October 2019. https://doi.org/10.1353/ken.0.0111.

Beauchamp, Tom L. and James F. Childress. 1994. *Principles of Biomedical Ethics* (4th Edn). New York and Oxford: Oxford University Press.

Beecher, Henry K. 1966. "Ethics and Clinical Research." *The New England Journal of Medicine* 274 (24): 367–372. Accessed 5 November 2019. https://doi.org/10.1056/NEJM196606162742405.

Bentham, Jeremy. 2000. *An Introduction to the Principles of Morals and Legislation*. Kitchener: Batoche Books.

Berman, Daniel and Suerie Moon, eds. 2001. *Fatal Imbalance: The Crisis in Research and Development for Drugs for Neglected Diseases*. Geneva: Médecins Sans Frontières Access to Essential Medicines Campaign and the Drugs for Neglected Diseases Working Group. I September 2001. Accessed 20 November 2019. Available: https://dndi.org/wp-content/uploads/2009/03/fatal_imbalance_2001.pdf.

Bhatnagar, Mukti and Abhishek Gupta. 2013. "Hippocratic Oath: Revisiting in the Present Medical Scenario." *Medicine Update 2013* 23: 667–668. Mumbai: The Association of Physicians of India. Accessed 7 June 2019. http://www.apiindia.org/medicine_update_2013/chap149.pdf.

Blackledge, Paul. 2012. *Marxism and Ethics; Freedom, Desire and Revolution*. Albany: State University of New York Press.

Buchanan, Allen, Dan W. Brock, Norman Daniels, and Daniel Wilker. 2009. *From Chance to Choice: Genetics and Justice*. Cambridge: Cambridge University Press.

Carrel, Alexis. 1959. *Man the Unknown*. Bombay: Wico Publishing House.

Cernadas, José María Ceriani. 2017. "Medical Practice in the Technological Age." *Archivos Argentinos de Pediatria* 115 (2): 106–107. Accessed 20 December 2019. https://doi.org/10.5546/aap.2017.eng.106.

Chadwick, Ruth. 2009. "Gene Therapy." In *A Companion to Bioethics*, 2nd Edn, edited by Helga Kuhse and Peter Singer. 207–215. Oxford. Wiley-Blackwell.

Chakravarty, Abhijit and Pawan Kapoor. 2012. "Concepts and Debates in End-of-Life Care." *Indian Journal of Meical Ethics* 9 (3): 202–206. Accessed 22 October 2019. https://doi.org/10.20529/IJME.2012.066.

Clark, Annette E. 2006. "The Right to Die: The Broken Road from Quinlan to Schiavo." *Loyola University Chicago Law Journal* 37 (2): 385–405. Accessed 18 July 2020. https://lawecommons.luc.edu/luclj/vol37/iss2/5.

Clarke, Michelle J., Megan S. Remtema, and Keith M. Swetz. 2014. "Beyond Transplantation: Considering Brain Death as a Hard Clinical Endpoint." *American Journal of Bioethics* 14 (8): 43–45. Accessed 19 January 2020. https://doi.org/10.1080/15265161.2014.925166.

Clarke, Michelle J., Kathleen N. Fenton, and Robert M. Sade. 2016. "Does Declaration of Brain Death Serve the Best Interest of Organ Donors Rather Than Merely Facilitating Organ Transplantation?" *Annals of Thoracic Surgery* 101 (6): 2053–2058. Accessed 6 July 2019. https://doi.org/10.1016/j.athoracsur.2016.01.100.

Clemens, Maria. 2017. "Technology and Rising Health Care Costs." *Technology Council*, 26 October. Accessed 3 February 2019. https://www.forbes.com/sites/forbestechcouncil/2017/10/26/technology-and-rising-health-care-costs/#45c82a3e766b.

Coleman, Carl H., Marie-Charlotte Bouësseaub, and Andreas Reis. 2008. "The Contribution of Ethics to Public Health." *Bulletin of the World Health Organization* 86 (8): 578–579. Accessed 18 March 2019. https://doi.org/10.2471/BLT.08.055954.

Conrad, Peter. 2007. *The Medicalization of Society*. Baltimore: The Johns Hopkins University Press.

Cook, Michael. 2019. "Brain-Dead Czech Woman Gives Birth After 117 Days." *BioEdge*, 11 September. Accessed 11 October 2019. https://www.bioedge.org/bioethics/brain-dead-czech-woman-gives-birth-after-117-days/13205.

Cooter, Roger. 2004. "Historical Keywords: Bioethics." *The Lancet* 364 (13): 1749. Accessed 25 January 2020. https://doi.org/10.1016/S0140-6736(04)17381-9.

Daar, Abdallah S. and Peter A. Singer. 2009. "Bioethics and Biotechnology." In *Global Perspectives in Health*, Vol. II, edited by Boutros Pierre Mansourian, 70–205. Oxford: Eolss Publishers.

Daniels, Norman. 2003. "Is There a Right to Health Care and, if so, What Does it Encompass?" In *Contemporary Issues in Bioethics*, 6th Edn, edited by Tom L. Beauchamp and LeRoy Walters, 316–325. Wadsworth: Belmont.

Devolder, Katrien. 2017. "Cloning." In *The Stanford Encyclopedia of Philosophy*, edited by Edward N. Zalta. Fall 2017 Edition. Accessed 20 December 2019. https://plato.stanford.edu/archives/fall2017/entries/cloning/.

Dhar, Shobita. 2016. "The Doctor Who Got 72-Year-Old Daljinder Kaur Pregnant Says the Decision to Undergo IVF Should be Left to the Patient." *The Times of India*, 15 May. Accessed 20 November. https://timesofindia.indiatimes.com/india/The-doctor-who-got-72-year-old-Daljinder-Kaur-pregnant-says-the

-decision-to-undergo-IVF-should-be-left-to-the-patient/articleshow/52279761
.cms.

Dobken, Jeffrey Hall. 2018. "The 'New' Medical Morality: Hippocrates or Bioethics?" *Journal of American Physicians and Surgeons* 23 (2): 46–51. Accessed 18 January 2020. https://www.jpands.org/vol23no2/dobken.pdf.

Drews, Jurgen. 2005. "Dug Research." In *Ethics and the Pharmaceutical Industry*, edited by Michael A. Santoro and Thomas M. Gorrie. 21–36. Cambridge: Cambridge University Press.

Ead, Hamed. 2016. "Medical Knowledge Pre Islamic Times." In *Islamic Alchamy in the Context of Islamic Science*, edited by Hamed Ead. Accessed 12 November 2019. https://www.alchemywebsite.com/islam.html.

Ekberg, Merryn Elizabeth. 2014. "Assisted Reproduction for Postmenopausal Women." *Human Fertility* 17 (3): 223–230. Accessed 18 September 2019. https://doi.org/10.3109/14647273.2014.948080.

Ellershaw, John and Chris Ward. 2003. "Care of the Dying Patient: The Last Hours or Days of Life." *British Medical Journal* 326 (7379): 30–34. Accessed 1 July 2019. https://doi.org/10.1136/bmj.326.7379.30.

Emanuel, Ezekiel J. 1999. "What is the Great Benefit of Legalizing Euthanasia or Physician-Assisted Suicide?" *Ethics* 109 (3): 629–642. Accessed 20 July 2019. https://doi.org/10.1086/233925.

Emanuel, Ezekiel J. 2013. "The art of Medicine Reconsidering the Declaration of Helsinki." *The Lancet* 381 (9877): 1532–1533. Accessed 22 October 2019. https://doi.org/10.1016/S0140-6736(13)60970-8.

Fasouliotis, Sozos J. and Schenker G. Joseph. 2000. "Ethics and Assisted Reproduction." *European Journal of Obstetrics & Gynecology and Reproductive Biology* 90 (2): 171–180. Accessed 11 March 2019. https://doi.org/10.1016/S0301-2115(00)00271-2.

Ferngren, Gary B. 2014. *Medicine and Religion: A Historical Introduction.* Baltimore: John Hopkins University Press.

Fine, Robert L. 2005. "From Quinlan to Schiavo: Medical, Ethical, and Legal Issues in Severe Brain Injury." *Baylor University Medical Center Proceedings* 18 (4): 303–310. Accessed 9 July 2019. https://doi.org/10.1080/08998280.2005.11928086.

Forrester, Rochelle. 2016, November 7. "The History of Medicine." In *How Change Happens: A Theory of Philosophy of History, Social Change and Cultural Evolution*, edited by Rochelle Forrester. Best Publications Limited (2009). Accessed 11 October 2019. https://doi.org/10.2139/ssrn.2867148.

Foucault, Michel. 1978. *The History of Sexuality.* Translated by Robert Hurley. New York: Pantheon Books.

Foucault, Michel. 2003. *The Birth of the Clinic: An Archaeology of Medical Perception.* Translated by A.M. Sheridan. London: Routledge.

Friesen, Phoebe, Lisa Kearns, Barbara Redman, and Arthur L. Caplan. 2017. "Rethinking the Belmont Report?" *The American Journal of Bioethics* 17 (7): 15–21. Accessed 7 October 2019. https://doi.org/10.1080/15265161.2017.1329482.

Galarneau, Charlene A. 1998. "The Ethics of Access to Health Care." *The Annual of the Society of Christian Ethics* 18: 305–314. Accessed 17 September 2019. https://doi.org/10.5840/asce19981824.

Ganapathy, K. 2018. "Brain Death Revisited." *Neurology India* 66 (2): 308–315. Accessed 29 June 2019. https://doi.org/10.4103/0028-3886.227287.

Gaudin, Anne Marie. 1991. "Cruzan v. Director, Missouri Department of Health: To Die or Not to Die: That is the Question - But Who Decides?" *Louisiana Law Review* 51 (6): 1308–1345. Accessed 22 July 2019. https://digitalcommons.law .lsu.edu/lalrev/vol51/iss6/7.

George, Sobin. 2015. "Caste and Care: Is Indian Healthcare Delivery System Favourable for Dalits?", Working Paper. The Institute for Social and Economic Change, Bangalore. Accessed 20 January 2020. http://www.isec.ac.in/WP%20 350%20-%20Sobin%20George.pdf.

Ghooi, Ravindra B. 2011. "The Nuremberg Code–A Critique." *Perspectives in Clinical Research* 2 (2): 72–76. Accessed 20 June 2019. https://doi.org/10.4103 /2229-3485.80371.

Gillon, Raanan. 2015. "Defending the Four Principles Approach as a Good Basis for Good Medical Practice and therefore for Good Medical Ethics." *Journal of Medical Ethics* 41 (1): 111–116. Accessed 27 October 2019. https://doi.org/10 .1136/medethics-2014-102282.

Gordon, Serena. 2018. "Youngest Kids in Class may be Over-Diagnosed with ADHD." *CBS News*, 28 November. Accessed 7 November 2019. https://www .cbsnews.com/news/adhd-youngest-kids-in-class-may-be-over-diagnosed-with -attention-deficit-hyperactivity-disorder/.

Gostin, Lawrence O. 2014. "Legal and Ethical Responsibilities Following Brain Death: The McMath and Munoz Cases." *The Journal of the American Medical Association* 311: 903–904. Accessed 12 July 2019. https://doi.org/10.1001/ama.2014.660.

Gunnarson, Martin and Svenaeus Fredrik, ed. 2012. *The Body as Gift, Resource, and Commodity Exchanging Organs, Tissues, and Cells in the 21st Century.* Stockholm: Södertörns högskola.

Haidt, Jonathan and Craig Joseph. 2007. "The Moral Mind: How Five Sets of Innate Intuitions Guide the Development of Many Culture-Specific Virtues, and Perhaps Even Modules." In *The Innate Mind: Volume 3: Foundations and the Future*, edited by Peter Carruthers, Stephen Laurence, and Stephen Stich, 367–391. Oxford: Oxford University Press.

Hall, Mark A., Elizabeth Dugan, Beiyano Zheng, and Aneil K. Mishra. 2001. "Trust in Physicians and Medical Institutions: What is it, Can it be Measured, and Does it Matter?" *Millbank Quarterly* 79 (4): 613–639. Accessed 15 October 2019. https://doi.org/10.1111/1468-0009.00223.

Häyry, Matti. 2005. "A Defense of Ethical Relativism." *Cambridge Quarterly of Healthcare Ethics* 14 (1): 7–12. Accessed 28 September 2019. https://doi.org/10 .1017/s0963180105050024.

Hazard, Geoffrey C. Jr. 1995. "Law, Morals, and Ethics." *Southern Illinois University Law Journal* 19 (3): 447–458. Accessed 20 December 2018. https:// digitalcommons.law.yale.edu/cgi/viewcontent.cgi?article=3322&context=fss _papers.

Heng, Boon Chin. 2006. "Donation of Surplus Frozen Embryos for Stem Cell Research or Fertility Treatment—Should Medical Professionals and Healthcare Institutions be Allowed to Exercise Undue Influence on the Informed Decision of Their Former Patients?" *Journal of Assist Reproduction and Genetics* 23: 381–382. Accessed 7 October 2019. https://doi.org/10.1007/s10815-006-9070-0.

Heuberger, Roschelle A. 2010. "Artificial Nutrition and Hydration at the End of Life." *Journal of Nutrition For the Elderly* 29 (4): 347–385. Accessed 1 July 2019. https://doi.org/10.1080/01639366.2010.521020.

Holder, Angela R. 1988. "Constraints on Experimentation: Protecting Children to Death." *Yale Law & Policy Review* 6 (1): 137–156. Accessed 21 June 2019. http://digitalcommons.law.yale.edu/ylpr/vol6/iss1/8.

Hostiuc, Sorin, Iancu Cristian Bogdan, Irina Rentea, Edward Drima, Maria Aluas, Tony L Hangan, Diana Badiu, Dan Navolan, Simona Vladareanu, and Nastasel Valentina. 2016. "Ethical Controversies in Maternal Surrogacy." *Gineco.eu* 12: 99–102. Accessed 21 September 2019. https://doi.org/10.18643/gieu.2016 .99.

Huenchuan, Sandra. 2017. "The Right to End-of-Life Palliative Care and a Dignified Death." Contribution from Un-Eclac for the Expert Group Meeting on "Care and Older Persons: Links to Decent Work, Migration and Gender" 5–7 December 2017. New York. Accessed 24 July 2019. https://www.un.org/development/desa/ageing/wp-content/uploads/sites/24/2017/11/ECLAC-contribution.pdf.

Huntoon, Lawrence R. 2005. "Editorial: Modern Bioethics." *Journal of American Physicians and Surgeons* 10 (4): 101–102. Accessed 9 June 2019. https://www .jpands.org/vol10no4/huntoon.pdf.

Irvin, Terence. 2007. *The Development of Ethics: A Historical and Critical Study. Volume I: From Socrates to the Reformation.* Oxford: Oxford University Press.

Jackson, Robert. 1949. *Report of Robert H. Jackson United States Representative to the International Conference on Military Trials.* Washington: Department of State. Accessed 18 June 2019. https://www.loc.gov/rr/frd/Military_Law/pdf/jackson-rpt-military-trials.pdf.

Jackson, Robert. 2005. "Nuremberg Trials: Opening Address for the United States." Florida Center for Instructional Technology, College of Education, University of South Florida. Accessed 18 June 2019. https://fcit.usf.edu/holocaust/resource/document/DocJac01.htm.

Jahr, Fritz. 2010. "Bio-Ethics Reviewing the Ethical Relations of Humans Towards Animals and Plants." *JAHR—European Journal of Bioethics* 1 (2): 227–223. Accessed 12 September 2019. https://www.jahr-bioethics-journal.com/index.php /JAHR/article/view/208.

John Paul, I.I. 2004. "Address of John Paul II to the Participants in the International Congress on 'Life-Sustaining Treatments and Vegetative State: Scientific Advances and Ethical Dilemmas'." 20 March 2004. Accessed 12 August 2019. http://www .vatican.va/content/john-paul-ii/en/speeches/2004/march/documents/hf_jp-ii_spe _20040320_congress-fiamc.html.

Jonsen, Albert R. 1990. *The New Medicine and the Old Ethics.* Cambridge: Harvard University Press.

Jonsen, Albert R. 2003. *The Birth of Bioethics.* Oxford: Oxford University Press.

Jurić, Hrvoje. 2017. "The Footholds of an Integrative Bioethics in the Work of Van Rensselaer Potter." *Facta Universitatis* (Law and Politics Series) 15 (2): 127–144. Accessed 15 October 2019. https://doi.org/10.22190/FULP1702127J.

Kahan, Alan S. 2012. "Max Weber and Warren Buffett: Looking for the Lost Charisma of Capitalism." *Society* 49: 144–150. Accessed 22 January 2020. https://doi.org/10.1007/s12115-011-9518-4.

Kalantri, S.P. 2003. "Dying with Dignity." *Indian Journal of Anaesthesia* 47 (4): 260–262. Accessed 19 January 2020. http://medind.nic.in/iad/t03/i4/iadt03i4p260.pdf.

Kangle, R.P., ed. 2010. *Kautilya Arthasastra, Part 1.* New Delhi: Motilal Banarsidass Publishers Pvt. Ltd.

Kant, Immanuel. 1997. *Groundwork of the Metaphysics of Morals.* Translate and Edited by Mary Gregor. Cambridge: Cambridge University Press.

Kant, Immanuel. 2018. *Fundamental Principles of Metaphysics of Morals.* Global Grey ebooks. Accessed 22 September 2019. https://www.globalgreyebooks.com/fundamental-principles-of-the-metaphysic-of-morals-ebook.html.

Kateb, George. 2011. *Human Dignity.* Cambridge: Harvard University Press.

Katz, Ingrid T. and Brendan Maughan-Brown. 2017. "Improved Life Expectancy of People Living with HIV: Who is Left Behind?" 4 (8): 324–326. Accessed 19 January 2020. https://doi.org/10.1016/S2352-3018(17)30086-3.

Keane, Michael and Ramna Thakur. 2018. "Health Care Spending and Hidden Poverty in India." *Research in Economics* 72 (4): 435–451. Accessed 5 March 2019. https://doi.org/10.1016/j.rie.2018.08.002.

Keown, John. 2002. *Euthanasia, Ethics and Public Policy.* Cambridge: Cambridge University Press.

King Jr, Henry T. 2003. "Robert H. Jackson and the Triumph of Justice at Nuremberg." *Case Western Reserve Journal of International Law* 35 (2): 253–272. Accessed 19 June 2019. https://scholarlycommons.law.case.edu/jil/vol35/iss2/7.

King, Nancy M.P. and Jacob Perrin. 2014. "Ethical Issues in Stem Cell Research and Therapy." *Stem Cell Research and Therapy* 5 (85): 1–6. Accessed 30 October 2019. https://doi.org/10.1186/scrt474.

Klitzman, Robert L. 2016. "How Old is too Old? Challenges Faced by Clinicians Concerning Age Cutoffs for Patients Undergoing in Vitro Fertilization." *Fertility and Sterility* 106 (1): 216–224. Accessed 18 September 2019. https://doi.org/10.1016/j.fertnstert.2016.03.030.

Koenig, Harold G. 2000. "Religion and Medicine I: Historical Background and Reasons for Separation." *International Journal of Psychiatry in Medicine* 30 (4): 385–398. Accessed 29 January 2020. https://doi.org/10.2190/2RWB-3AE1-M1E5-TVHK.

Kohli, Arunima Sarvdeep. 2012. "Medicalization: A Growing Menace." *Delhi Psychiatry Journal* 15 (2): 255–259. Accessed 17 February 2019. http://medind.nic.in/daa/t12/i2/daat12i2p255.pdf.

Komrad, Mark S. 1983. "A Defence of Medical Paternalism: Maximising Patients 'Autonomy'." *Journal of Medical Ethics* 9 (1): 38–44. Accessed 25 October 2019. https://doi.org/10.1136/jme.9.1.38.

Krugman, Saul. 1986. "The Willowbrook Hepatitis Studies Revisited: Ethical Aspects." *Reviews of Infectious Diseases* 8 (1): 157–162. Accessed 20 June 2019. https://doi.org/10.1093/clinids/8.1.157.

Kumar, R. Krishna. 2011. "Technology and Healthcare Costs." *Annals of Pediatric Cardiology* 4 (1): 84–86. Accessed 18 January 2020. https://doi.org/10.4103/0974-2069.79634.

Kurzweil, Edith. 1986. "Michel Foucault's History of Sexuality as Interpreted by Feminists and Marxists." *Social Research* 53 (4): 647–663. Accessed 7 November 2019. https://www.jstor.org/stable/pdf/40970437.pdf?refreqid=excelsior%3Ae b5a75d1c78de66402ae7dff11f5b0e3.

Lawrence, Dana J. 2007. "The Four Principles of Biomedical Ethics: A Foundation for Current Bioethical Debate." *Journal of Chiropractic Humanities* 14: 34–40. Accessed 27 October 2019. https://doi.org/10.1016/S1556-3499(13)60161-8.

Lieff, Jonathan. 1982. "Eight Reasons Why Doctors Fear the Elderly, Chronic Disease, and Death." *Journal of Transpersonal Psychology* 14 (1): 47–60.

Accessed 14 November 2019. https://pdfs.semanticscholar.org/4a6d/8226a5a8eab0bfaf25efec102bca071e1a23.pdf.

Lillie, William. 1957. *An Introduction to Ethics* (3rd Edn). London: Methuen & Co Ltd.

Lima, Natacha Salomé and Predrag Cicovacki. 2014. "Bio-Ethics: Past, Present, and Future." *JAHR—European Journal of Bioethics* 5 (2): 263–274. Accessed 14 October 2019. https://hrcak.srce.hr/ojs/index.php/jahr/article/view/15559/8130.

Locke, John. 2010. *Second Treatise of Government*. London: The Project Gutenberg Ebook. Accessed 24 February 2020. https://www.gutenberg.org/files/7370/7370-h/7370-h.htm#CHAPTER_VII.

Long, Tony. 2000. "June 11, 1985: Karen Quinlan Dies, But the Issue Lives On." https://www.wired.com/2008/06/dayintech-0611-2/.

MacIntyre, Alasdair C. 1998. *A History of Moral Philosophy*. London: Routledge.

Magner, Lois N. and Oliver J. Kim. 2018. *A History of Medicine* (3rd Edn). Boca Raton: CRC Press.

Majeed, Azeem. 2011. "Arabic Roots of Modern Medicine." *The Lancet* 378 (9803): e4–e5. Accessed 18 December 2018. https://doi.org/10.1016/S0140-6736(11)61701-7.

Major, A. Edward. 2012. "Law and Ethics in Command Decision Making." *Military Review* XCII (3): 61–74. Accessed 20 December 2018. https://www.law.upenn.edu/institutes/cerl/conferences/cyberwar/papers/reading/Major.pdf.

Major, Rupert W.L. 2008. "Paying Kidney Donors: Time to Follow Iran?" *Mcgill Journal of Medicine* 11 (1): 67–69. Accessed 11 February 2020. https://www.ncbi.nlm.nih.gov/pmc/articles/PMC2322914/pdf/mjm11_1p67.pdf.

Margalit, Yehezkel. 2016. "From Baby M to Baby M(anji): Regulating International Surrogacy Agreements." *Journal of Law and Policy* 24 (1): 41–92. Accessed 19 September 2019. https://brooklynworks.brooklaw.edu/jlp/vol24/iss1/2.

Materstvedt, Lars Johan, David Clark, John Ellershaw, Reidun Førde, Anne-Marie Boeck Gravgaard, H. Christof Müller-Busch, Josep Porta Sales, and Charles-Henri Rapin. 2003. "Euthanasia and Physician-Assisted Suicide: A View from an EAPC Ethics Task Force." *Palliative Medicine* 17 (2): 97–101. Accessed 10 July 2019. https://doi.org/10.1055/s-2004-834590.

Mechanic, David. 1997. "Muddling Through Elegantly: Finding the Proper Balance in Rationing." *Health Affairs* 16 (5): 83–92. Accessed 12 October 2019. https://doi.org/10.1377/hlthaff.16.5.83.

Miles, Steven H. 2005. *The Hippocratic Oath and the Ethics of Medicine*. Oxford: Oxford University Press.

Mill, John Stuart. 1864. *On Liberty* (3rd Edn). London: Longman, Green, Longman, Roberts & Green.

Mitscherlich, Atexander and Fred Mielke. 1949. *Doctors of Infamy: The Story of the Nazi Medical Crimes*. New York: Schuman.

Moazam, Farhat. 2007. *Bioethics and Organ Transplantation in a Muslim Society: A Study in Culture, Ethnography and Religion*. Bloomington and Indianapolis: Indiana University Press.

Moazam, Farhat. 2012. "'Doing Bioethics' in Pakistan." *The Hastings Center*. Bioethics Forum Essay. Accessed 4 February 2020. https://www.thehastingscenter.org/doing-bioethics-in-pakistan/.

Morris, Anne and Sue Nott. 2009. "Rights and Responsibilities: Contested Parenthood." *Journal of Social & Family Law* 31 (1): 3–16. Accessed 16 February 2019. https://doi.org/10.1080/09649060902761594.

Mukai, Christine, Hilary K. Josephs, and Linda Luli Nakasone, eds. 1977. "Towards a Definition of Death." State of Hawaii Legislative Reference Bureau, January 1977. https://lrb.hawaii.gov/wp-content/uploads/1977_TowardsADefinitionOfDeath.pdf.

Muller, Denis. 2008. "The Role and Influence of Religions in Bioethics." In *Global Bioethics: Issues of Conscience for the 21st Century*, edited by Ronald M. Green, Aine Donovan, and Steven A. Jauss. 279–294. Oxford: Oxford University Press.

Munsie, Megan and Christopher Gyngel. 2018. "Ethical Issues in Genetic Modification and Why Application Matters." *Current Opinion in Genetics & Development* 52: 7–12. Accessed 24 September 2019. https://doi.org/10.1016/j.gde.2018.05.002.

Munson, Ronald. 2008. *Intervention and Reflection Basic Issues in Medical Ethics* (8th Edn). Belmont: Thomson Hiher Learning.

Munson, Ronald. 2009. "Deciding to Die: The Case of Karen Quinlan." *OUPblog*, June 22 2009. https://blog.oup.com/2009/06/karen_quinlan/

Nagral, Sanjay. 1995. "Ethics of Organ Transplantation." *Indian Journal of Medical Ethics* 3 (2): 19–22. Accessed 21 October 2019. https://ijme.in/articles/ethics-of-organ-transplantation/?galley=pdf.

Ndebele, Paul. 2013. "The Declaration of Helsinki, 50 Years Later." *Journal of the American Medical Association* 310 (20): 2145–2146. Accessed 13 October 2019. https://doi.org/10.1001/jama.2013.281316.

Nellickappilly, Sreekumar. 2010. "Science, Religion and Ethics: The Religious-Ethical Basis of Indian Science of Medicine." *Acta Bioethica* 16 (1): 31–39. Accessed 22 May 2014. https://doi.org/10.4067/S1726-569X2010000100005.

Nevitte, Neil, William P. Brandon, and Lori Davi. 1993. "The American Abortion Controversy: Lessons from Cross-National Evidence." *Politics and the Life Sciences* 12 (1): 19–30. https://doi.org/10.1017/S0730938400011217.

Niekerk, Anton van and Liezl van Zyl. 1995. "The Ethics of Surrogacy: Women's Reproductive Labour." *Journal of Medical Ethics* 21 (6): 345–349. Accessed 18 September 2019. https://doi.org/10.1136/jme.21.6.345.

Nietzsche, Friedrich. 2006. *Thus Spoke Zarathustra*. Edited by Adrian Del Caro and Robert B. Pippin. Translated by Adrian Del Caro. Cambridge: Cambridge University Press.

Padela, Aasim I. 2007. "Islamic Medical Ethics: A Primer." *Bioethics* 21 (3): 169–178. Accessed 20 December 2018. https://doi.org/10.1111/j.1467-8519.2007.00540.x.

Pai-Dhungat, J.V. 2015. "Hippocrates - Father of Medicine." *Journal of the Association of Physicians of India* 63 (3): 18. Accessed 13 November 2019. https://www.japi.org/r2f484/hippocrates-father-of-medicine.

Parsons, Talcott. 1975. "The Sick Role and the Role of the Physician Reconsidered." *The Milbank Memorial Fund Quarterly Health and Society* 53 (3): 257–278. Accessed 20 January 2020. https://doi.org/10.2307/3349493.

Patel, V.K., D.S. Tiwari, V.R. Shahl, M.G. Patel, H.H. Raja, and D.S. Patel. 2018. "Prevalence and Predictors of Abuse in Elderly Patients with Depression at a Tertiary Care Centre in Saurashtra, India." *Indian Journal of Psychological*

Medicine 40 (6): 528–533. Accessed 20 January 2020. https://doi.org/10.4103 /IJPSYM.IJPSYM_18_18.

Pellegrino, Edmund D. and David C. Thomasma. 1987. "The Conflict between Autonomy and Beneficence in Medical Ethics: Proposal for a Resolution." *Journal of Contemporary Health Law and Policy* 3 (1): 23–46. Accessed 7 February 2010. https://scholarship.law.edu/jchlp/vol3/iss1/7/.

Pence, Gregory. 2008. *Classic Cases in Medical Ethics: Accounts of the Cases and Issues that Define Medical Ethics* (5th Edn). New York: McGraw-Hill Higher Education.

Plato. 2018. *Apology*. Translated by Benjamin Jowett. Global Grey ebooks. Accessed 11 January 2019. https://www.globalgreyebooks.com/apology-ebook.html.

Plomp, H.N. and N. Ballast. 2010. "Trust and Vulnerability in Doctor-Patient Relations in Occupational Health." *Occupational Medicine* 60 (4): 261–269. Accessed 10 September 2019. https://doi.org/10.1093/occmed/kqq067.

Points, Kari. 2009. "Commercial Surrogacy and Fertility Tourism in India: The Case of Baby Manji." *The Case Studies in Ethics*. The Kenan Institute of Ethics at Duke University. Accessed 6 June 2021. https://kenan.ethics.duke.edu/wp -content/uploads/2018/01/BabyManji_Case2015.pdf.

Poitras, Geoffrey and Lindsay Meredith. 2009. "Ethical Transparency and Economic Medicalization." *Journal of Business Ethics* 86 (3): 313–325. Accessed 17 February 2020. https://doi.org/10.1007/s10551-008-9849-2.

Pokulniewicz, M., T. Issat, and A. Jakimiuk. 2015. "In Vitro Fertilization and Age: When Old is Too Old?" *Przegląd Menopauzalny* 14 (1): 71–73. Accessed 18 September 2019. https://doi.org/10.5114/pm.2015.49531.

Potter, Van Rensselaer. 1971. *Bioethics: Bridge to the Future*. New Jersey: Prentice-Hall, Inc.

Potter, Van Rensselaer. 1998. "Deep and Global Bioethics for a Livable Third Millennium." *The Scientist*, 4 January. Accessed 19 February 2020. https:// www.the-scientist.com/opinion-old/deep-and-global-bioethics-for-a-livable-third -millennium-57186.

Practical Parenting Team. 2019. "Woman Who Gave Birth at 72 Says She Struggles to Cope With Her Son." *Practical Parenting*, 3 April. Accessed 25 November 2019. https://www.practicalparenting.com.au/indian-woman-daljinder-kaur -who-gave-birth-at-72-says-she-struggles-to-cope-with-baby.

Pratley, Peter. 1997. *The Essence of Business Ethics*. New Delhi: Prentice-Hal of India.

Rachels, James. 1975. "Why Privacy is Important." *Philosophy & Public Affairs* 4 (4): 323–333. Accessed 16 January 2020. https://www.jstor.org/stable/2265077.

Rachels, James and Stuart Rachels. 2012. *Elements of Moral Philosophy* (5–7th Edns). New York: McGraw-Hill.

Rajput, Vijay and Carolyn E. Bekes. 2001. "Ethical Issues in Hospital Medicine." *Medical Clinics of North America* 86 (4): 869–886. Accessed 12 September 2019. https://doi.org/10.1016/s0025-7125(02)00013-5.

Rand, Ayn. 1964. *The Virtue of Selfishness: A New Concept of Egoism*. New York: Penguine.

Rao, Desiraju Hanumanta. 2004. *Valmiki Ramayana: Book III: Aranya Kanda - The Forest Trek*. Chapter [Sarga] 37. Accessed 11 January 2020. https:// sanskritdocuments.org/sites/valmikiramayan/aranya/sarga37/aranya_37_frame .htm.

Rao, K. Srinivasa. 2015. "Private Hospitals Adopting Unethical Practices: Study." *The Hindu*, 23 February and updated: 28 September, 2016. Accessed 12 October 2029. https://www.thehindu.com/news/cities/Vijayawada/Private-hospitals -adopting-unethical-practices-Study/article10693014.ece.

Ray, Priyaranjan and Hirendra Nath Gupta. 1965. *Caraka Samhita: A Scientific Synopsis*. New Delhi: Indian National Science Academy.

Risse, Guenter. 1992. "Medicine in the Age of Enlightenment." In *Historical Essays*, edited by Andrew Wear, 149–195. Cambridge: Cambridge University Press.

Robinson, Walter M. and Brandon T. Unruh. 2008. "The Hepatitis Experiments at the Willowbrook State School." In *The Oxford Textbook of Clinical Research Ethics*, edited by Ezekiel J. Emanuel, Christine Grady, Robert A. Crouch, Reidar K. Lie, Franklin G. Miller, and David Wendler. 80–85. Oxford and New York: Oxford University Press.

Roelcke, Volker. 2004. "Nazi Medicine and Research on Human Beings, Medicine, Crime, and Punishment." *The Lancet* 364: 6–7. Accessed 10 November 2019. https://doi.org/10.1016/S0140-6736(04)17619-8.

Rothman, David J. 1991. *Strangers at the Bedside: A History of How Law and Bioethics Transformed Medical Decision Making*. New York: Basic Books.

Ryan, Ann, Mandy Morgan, and Antonia Lyons. 2011. "The Problem with Death: The Genealogy of Euthanasia." In *Refereed Proceedings of Doing Psychology: Manawatu Doctoral Research Symposium 2011*. 43–48. Accessed 5 January 2010. http://hdl.handle.net/10179/3387.

Sandel, Michael J. 2005. "The Ethical Implications of Human Cloning." *Perspectives in Biology and Medicine* 48 (2): 241–247. Accessed 12 September 2019. https://doi.org/10.1353/pbm.2005.0063.

Santoro, Michael A. 2005. "Introduction: Charting a Sustainable Path for the Twenty First Century Pharmaceutical Industry." In *Ethics and the Pharmaceutical Industry*, edited by Michael A. Santoro and Thomas M. Gorrie. 1–5. Cambridge: Cambridge University Press.

Sartre, Jean-Paul. 1956. *Being And Nothingness*. Translated by Hazel E. Barnes. New York: Pocket Books.

Schee, E.V.D., P.P. Groenewegen, and R.D. Friele. 2006. "Public Trust in Health Care: A Performance Indicator?" *Journal of Health Organization and Management* 20 (5): 468–476. Accessed 15 September 2019. https://doi.org/10.1108/14777260610701821.

Shafer-Landau, Russ, ed. 2013. *Ethical Theory an Anthology*. Chichester: Wiley-Blackwell.

Sharples, R.W. 2003. *Stoics, Epicureans and Sceptics: An Introduction to Hellenistic Philosophy*. London and New York: Routledge.

Sherwin, Susan. 2010. "Gender, Race, and Class in the Delivery of Health Care." In *Bioethics: An Introduction to the History, Methods and Practice*, 2nd Edn, edited by, Nancy S. Jecker, Albert R. Johnson, and Robert A. Pearlman. 392–404. New Delhi: Jones and Bartlett India Pvt. Ltd.

Shroff, Sunil. 2009. "Legal and Ethical Aspects of Organ Donation and Transplantation." *Indian Journal of Urology* 25 (3): 348–355. Accessed 19 January 2020. https://doi.org/10.4103/0970-1591.56203.

Shroff, Sunil and Sumana Navin. 2018. "'Brain Death' and 'Circulatory Death': Need for a Uniform Definition of Death in India." *Indian Journal of Medical Ethics* 3 (4): 321–323. Accessed 15 November 2019. https://doi.org/10.20529/IJME.2018.070.

Shuster, Evelyne. 1997. "Fifty Years Later: The Significance of the Nuremberg Code." *The New England Journal of Medicine* 337 (20): 1436–1440. Accessed 25 June 2019. https://doi.org/10.1056/NEJM199711133372006.

Skutch, Alexander F. 2007. *Moral Foundations: An Introduction to Ethics.* Mount Jackson: Axios Press.

Smith, George P. 2002. "Distributive Justice and Health Care." *The Journal of Contemporary Health Law & Policy* 18: 421–430. Accessed 23 September 2019. https://scholarship.law.edu/jchlp/vol18/iss2/3.

Smith, Kevin R., Sarah Chan, and John Harri. 2012. "Human Germline Genetic Modification: Scientific and Bioethical Perspectives." *Archives of Medical Research* 43 (7): 491–513. Accessed 18 September 2019. https://doi.org/10.1016/j.arcmed.2012.09.003.

Sudnow, D. 1967. *Passing On: The Social Organization of Dying.* New Jersey: Prentice Hall.

Svenaeus, Fredrik. 2010. "The Body as Gift, Resource or Commodity? Heidegger and the Ethics of Organ Transplantation." *Bioethical Inquiry* 7 (2): 163–172. Accessed 19 November 2019. https://doi.org/10.1007/s11673-010-9222-x.

Svenaeus, Fredrik. 2018. *Phenomenological Bioethics.* Oxon: Routledge.

Taher, Mohammad Abu, Abdul Mannan, and Shahinoor Rahman Dulal. 2018. "Contribution of Greek Mythology and Civilization on Medical Science – A Brief Analysis." *International Journal of Advanced Research* 6 (11): 1095–1102. Accessed 20 January 2020. https://doi.org/10.21474/IJAR01/8098.

Tan, L.T.H. and Ong, K.L. 2002. "The Impact of Medical Technology on Healthcare Today." *Hong Kong Journal of Emergency Medicine* 9 (4): 231–236. Accessed 16 January 2020. https://doi.org/10.1177/102490790200900410.

Thirumulpad, K. Raghavan. 2006. *Ashtangasangraha (Prakasika Vyakhya): Swasthavritham.* Chalakudi: Prakashika.

Thompson, Dennis F. 2005. *Restoring Responsibility: Ethics in Government, Business, and Healthcare.* Cambridge: Cambiridge University Press.

Tsai, Daniel Fu-Chang. 1999. "Ancient Chinese Medical Ethics and the Four Principles of Biomedical Ethics." *Journal of Medical Ethics* 25 (3): 315–321. Accessed 6 June 2020. https://doi.org/10.1136/jme.25.4.315.

Venkata, Jyothsna Akam and Anuja A. Panicker. 2013. "Prevalence of Attention Deficit Hyperactivity Disorder in Primary School Children." *Indian Journal of Psychiatry* 55 (4): 338–342. Accessed 22 September 2019. https://doi.org/10.4103/0019-5545.120544.

Vidyanath, R. 2013. *Illustrated Astanga Hrdaya of Vagbhata: Sutra-sthana.* Varanasi: Chaukhamba Surbharati Prakashan.

Waitzkin, Howard. 1989. "A Critical Theory of Medical Discourse: Ideology, Social Control, and the Processing of Social Context in Medical Encounters." *Journal of Health and Social Behavior* 30 (2): 220–239. Accessed 27 November 2019. https://doi.org/10.2307/2137015.

Wang, Chen, Xiaomei Zhai, Xinqing Zhang, Limin Li, Jianwei Wang, and De-pei Liu. 2019. "Gene-Edited Babies: Chinese Academy of Medical Sciences' Response and Action." *Lancet* 393 (10166): 25–26. Accessed 10 January 2020. https://doi.org/10.1016/S0140-6736(18)33080-0.

Warmington, Eric H. and Philip G. Rouse, eds. 1984. *Great Dialogues of Plato.* Transated by W.H.D. Rouse. New York: Mentor Book.

Warnock, Dame Mary. 1984. *Report of the Committee of Inquiry into Human Fertilisation and Embryology.* London: Her Majesty's Stationery Office. Accessed 22 September 2019. https://www.bioeticacs.org/iceb/documentos/ Warnock_Report_of_the_Committee_of_Inquiry_into_Human_Fertilisation _and_Embryology_1984.pdf.

Watson, C.J.E. and J.H. Dark. 2012. "Organ Transplantation: Historical Perspective and Current Practice." *British Journal of Anaesthesia* 108 (S_): i29–i42. Accessed 21 January 2019. https://doi.org/10.1093/bja/aer384.

Wear, Stephen. 1998. *Informed Consent: Patient Autonomy and Clinician Beneficence within Health Care.* Washington: Georgetown University Press.

Weber, Max. 2005. *The Protestant Ethic and the Spirit of Capitalism.* Translated by Talcott Parsons. London: Routledge.

Whitehouse, Peter J. 2001. "In Memoriam. Van Rensselaer Potter: The Original Bioethicist." *Global Bioethics* 14 (4): 47–48. Accessed 19 February 2020. https:// doi.org/10.1080/11287462.2001.10800814.

Whitehouse, Peter J. 2003. "The Rebirth of Bioethics: Extending the Original Formulations of Van Rensselaer Potter." *The American Journal of Bioethics* 3 (4): W26–W31. Accessed 17 February 2020. https://doi.org/10.1162 /152651603322614751.

Yadavar, Swagata. 2018. "Budget 2018: India's Healthcare Crisis is Holding back National Potential." *IndiaSpend.* Accessed 13 November 2019. https://www .indiaspend.com/budget-2018-indias-healthcare-crisis-is-holding-back-national -potential-29517/.

Yu, Jiyuan. 2005. "The Beginning of Ethics: Confucius and Socrates." *Asian Philosophy* 15 (2): 173–189. Accessed 20 May 2020. https://doi.org/10.1080 /09552360500165304.

Zhang, Boli, Zuoning Chen, Jian Yi, Haiying Tang, and Chen Wamg. 2019. "Chinese Academy of Engineering Calls for Actions on the Birth of Gene-Edited Infants." *Lancet* 393 (10166): 25. Accessed 30 January 2019. https://doi.org/10 .1016/S0140-6736(18)33081-2.

Zhang, Linqi, Ping Zhong, Xiaomei Zhai, Yiming Shao, and Shan Lu. 2019. "Open Letter from Chinese HIV Professionals on Human Genome Editing." *Lancet* 393 (10166): 26–27. Accessed 30 January 2019. https://doi.org/10.1016/S0140 -6736(18)33082-4.

Zhao, Zhongzhen, Ping Guo, and Eric Brand. 2018. "A Concise Classifcation of Bencao (Materia Medica)." *Chinese Medicine* 13 (18). Accessed 12 May 2021. https://doi.org/10.1186/s13020-018-0176-y.

Other Web Resources

A definition of Irreversible Coma. Report of the Ad Hoc Committee of the Harvard Medical School to Examine the Definition of Brain Death. 1968. *Journal of the American Medical Association* 205 (6): 337–340. Accessed 15 November 2019. https://doi.org/10.1001/jama.1968.03140320031009.

Akanni S. 2013. "An exposition of Islamic Medication in the Light of the Quran and Hadith." 1st Annual International Interdisciplinary Conference, AIIC 2013, 24–26 April, Azores, Portugal – Proceedings: 176–182. Accessed 23 March 2019. https://core.ac.uk/download/pdf/236412819.pdf.

Alexander, Larry and Michael Moore. 2016. "Deontological Ethics." In *The Stanford Encyclopedia of Philosophy*, edited by Edward N. Zalta. Accessed 12 January 2020. https://plato.stanford.edu/archives/win2016/entries/ethics-deontological/>.

Asian Development Bank (ADB). 2011. *Understanding Poverty in India*. Asian Development Bank. Accessed 29 October 2019. https://www.adb.org/sites/default/files/publication/28930/understanding-poverty-india.pdf.

Augustyn, Adam et al. 2019. "Hippocratic Oath: Ethical Code." Accessed 7 June 2019. http://www.britannica.com/EBchecked/topic/266652/Hippocratic-Oath.

"Ayushman Bharat." 2019. Accessed 10 September 2019. https://www.india.gov.in /spotlight/rashtriya-swasthya-bima-yojana.

Brown, DeNeen. 2017. "'You've Got Bad Blood': The Horror of the Tuskegee Syphilis Experiment." *The Washington Post*. Accessed 19 May 2019. https://www.washingtonpost.com/news/retropolis/wp/2017/05/16/youve-got-bad-blood -the-horror-of-the-tuskegee-syphilis-experiment/.

Centers for Disease Control and Prevention (CDC). "The U.S. Public Health Service Syphilis Study at Tuskegee: The Tuskegee Timeline." Accessed 19 May 2021. https://www.cdc.gov/tuskegee/timeline.htm.

"Center for Medicare and Mdicaid Services" (CMS). Accessed 28 December 2019. https://www.cms.gov/Research-Statistics-Data-and-Systems/Statistics-Trends -and-Reports/NationalHealthExpendData/NationalHealthAccountsHistorical .html.

Economic and Social Commission for Western Asia (ESCWA). 2013. "Social Justice and Participation: Policy Brief." 26 December 2013. Accessed 16 October 2019. https://www.unescwa.org/publications/social-justice-participation-policy-brief.

Gender Reassignment Surgery (GRS). 2020. Aetna. - Medical Clinical Policy Bulletins. No. 0615. Accessed 21 January 2020. http://www.aetna.com/cpb/ medical/data/600_699/0615.html.

India Today Web Desk. 2019. "Death Toll From Acute Encephalitis Syndrome Rises to 142." 21 June, 2019. Accessed 10 January 2020. https://www.indiatoday.in /india/story/bihar-acute-encephalitis-syndrome-death-toll-rises-1553477-2019 -06-21.

Indian Council of Medical Researchand and Department of Biotechnology. (ICMR & DBT). 2013. *National Guidelines for Stem Cell Research*. New Delhi: Indian Council of Medical Research. Accessed 21 January 2020. https://www.ncbs.res .in/sites/default/files/policies/NGSCR%202013.pdf.

MacDougall, Heather and G. Ross Langley. 2019. "Medical Ethics: Past, Present and Future." Executive Summary, Royal College Physicians and Surgeons of Canada. Accessed 26 November 2019. https://www.royalcollege.ca/rcsite/documents/ bioethics/medical-ethics-summary-e.pdf.

"Making Babies. Human Cloning: How Close is it?" 2019. Interview with Lee Silver. *Frontline*. Accessed 3 November 2019. https://www.pbs.org/wgbh/pages/ frontline/shows/fertility/interviews/silver.html.

Mathur, Roli, compiled and ed. 2017. *National Ethical Guidelines for Biomedical and Health Research Involving Human Participants*. New Delhi: Indian Council of Medical Research. Accessed 18 October 2019. https://www.icmr.nic.in/sites/ default/files/guidelines/ICMR_Ethical_Guidelines_2017.pdf.

National Health Mission. 2019. "National Health Rural Mission." Ministry of Health and Family Welfare, Government of India. Accessed 13 November 2019. https://nhm.gov.in/index1.php?lang=1&level=1&sublinkid=969&lid=49.

NIH Stem Cell Information Home Page. 2016. "Stem Cell Information." National Institute of Health. U.S. Department of Health and Human Services. Accessed 21 January 2020. https://stemcells.nih.gov/info/basics/1.htm.

Participants in the International Summit on Transplant Tourism and Organ Trafficking Convened by The Transplantation Society and International Society of Nephrology in Istanbul, Turkey, April 30 through May 2, 2008. 2008. "The Declaration of Istanbul on Organ Trafficking and Transplant Tourism." *Clinical Journal of the American Society of Nephrology* 3 (5): 1227–1231. Accessed 19 January 2020. https://doi.org/10.2215/CJN.03320708.

Pitts, David. 2001. "Backgrounder: Nuremberg War Crimes Legacy - Part One ('Crimes Against Humanity')." *Washington File*, 9 March. Accessed 26 August 2019. https://wfile.ait.org.tw/wf-archive/2001/010309/epf508.htm.

Public Health Foundation of India (PHFI). 2018. "Annual Report 2017–18." Public Health Foundation of India. Accessed 10 November 2019. https://phfi.org/wp -content/uploads/2018/11/Annual_Report_2017-18.pdf.

"Rashtriya Swasthya Bima Yojana." Accessed 10 September 2019. https://www .india.gov.in/spotlight/rashtriya-swasthya-bima-yojana.

Regional Committee for the Eastern Mediterranean of the World Health Organization (EM/RC52/7). 2005. "Islamic Code of Medical and Health Ethics." Fifty-second Session, Agenda item 8. Accessed 15 January 2020. http://applications.emro.who .int/docs/EM_RC52_7_en.pdf.

Sachs, Joe. 2019. "Aristotle: Ethics." *Internet Encyclopedia of Philosophy*. Accessed 10 August 2019. https://www.iep.utm.edu/aris-eth/.

Science Daily. 2015. "'Unethical' Targets in India's Private Hospitals." *ScienceDaily*, 3 September. Accessed 16 January 2019. https://www.sciencedaily.com/releases /2015/09/150903223247.htm.

The Case of Nancy Cruzan: U.S.-Supreme Court vs. Director, Missouri Department of Health, 1990, 407 U.S. 261, 110 S. Ct. 2841, 111 L. Ed. 2nd 224. Accessed 11 July 2019. https://www.practicalbioethics.org/wp-content/uploads/2021/10/ Case-Study-The-Case-of-Nancy-Cruzan.pdf.

"The Nuremberg Code." Accessed 12 October 2019. https://history.nih.gov/research /downloads/nuremberg.pdf.

United Nations Population Fund (UAPA). 2002. "Statement at the Launch of HelpAge International's State of the World's Older People." 8 April. Accessed 18 January 2020. https://www.unfpa.org/press/statement-launch-helpage -internationals-state-worlds-older-people.

Williams, John Reynold. 2005. "Medical Ethics Manuel." The World Medical Association. Accessed 12 January 2020. http://www.wrcaonline.org/uploads/ publications/em_en.pdf.

World Health Organization (WHO). 2018. *Integrating Palliative Care and Symptom Relief into Primary Health Care: A WHO Guide for Planners, Implementers and Managers*. Geneva: World Health Organization. Accessed 20 November 2019. https://apps.who.int/iris/bitstream/handle/10665/274559/9789241514477-eng .pdf?sequence=1&isAllowed=y.

World Medical Association (WMA). 2013. "World Medical Association Declaration of Helsinki: Ethical Principles for Medical Research Involving Human Subjects." *Journal of the American Medical Association* 310 (20): 2191–2194. Accessed 17 January 2020. https://www.wma.net/wp-content/uploads/2016/11/DoH -Oct2013-JAMA.pdf.

Index

For Product Safety Concerns and Information please contact our EU
representative GPSR@taylorandfrancis.com
Taylor & Francis Verlag GmbH, Kaufingerstraße 24, 80331 München, Germany

www.ingramcontent.com/pod-product-compliance
Lightning Source LLC
Chambersburg PA
CBHW060250220326
41598CB00027B/4047

9 7 8 1 0 3 2 3 2 0 6 2 5